Perspectives in Animal Ecology and Reproduction

Perspectives in Animal Ecology and Reproduction

— *Volume 8* —

Editor-in-Chief
Dr. V.K. Gupta

Editors
Dr. Anil K. Verma
Dr. G.D. Singh

2011
DAYA PUBLISHING HOUSE®
Delhi - 110 002

ISBN 978-81-7035-747-6

Published by : **Daya Publishing House®**
4760-61/23, Ansari Road, Darya Ganj,
New Delhi - 110 002
Phone: 23245578, 23244987
Fax: (011) 23260116
e-mail : dayabooks@vsnl.com
website : www.dayabooks.com

Laser Typesetting : **Classic Computer Services**
Delhi - 110 035

Printed at : **Chawla Offset Printers**
Delhi - 110 052

PRINTED IN INDIA

Editorial Board

– Members –

Prof. Clement A. Tisdell
Professor Emeritus,
School of Economics,
The University of Queensland, Brisbane,
Australia
E-mail: c.tisdell@economics.uq.edu.au

Prof. Tej Kumar Sherstha
Head,
Central Department of Zoology,
Tribhuvan University,
Kathmandu, Nepal
E-mail: drtks@ccsl.com.np

Dr. Justin Gerlach
Chief Scientist,
The Nature Protection of Seychelles,
133 Cherry Hinton Road,
Cambridge CBI 7BX,UK
E-mail: justgerlach@aol.com

Prof. Vanitha Kumari
Head,
Department of Zoology,
Bharathiar University,
Coimbatore, India
E-mail: regr@bharathiaruni.org

Dr. Sunil Kumar
Deputy Director (Sr. Grade),
Division of Reproductive Toxicology & Histochemistry,
National Institute of Occupational Health,
Meghani Nagar, Ahmedabad – 380 016, India
E-mail: sunilnioh@yahoo.com

Centre of Excellence in Biocontrol of Insect Pests
Department of Zoology
University of Lucknow
Lucknow-226007 (INDIA)

Dr. Omkar
MNASc, FZSI, FESI, FAEB, FAB, FBRS, FAS (AW)
Professor & Coordinator, Centre of Excellence
Member, UP Biodiversity Board
*Executive Editor, **Journal of Applied Bioscience***

March 5, 2011

Foreword

It gives me great pleasure to write the *Foreword* to the book series "*Perspectives in Animal Ecology and Reproduction Vol. 8*". The very fact that this is the foreword to the eighth volume speaks multitudes about the success of this book series. This series has for years brought together critical papers and reviews on animal ecology and reproduction and the current volume is no exception.

Dr. V K Gupta has made herculean efforts to bring out this comprehensive book series which have contained chapters on different topics by experts of different fields from different geographical areas dealing with various aspects of animal–environment interactions and adaptations by different life forms in different habitats. Taxa-wise it has covered the entire range from Protozoa to Mammalia and subject wise has taken up areas ranging from behaviour, ecology, adaptations, interactions, thermoregulation, reproduction, haematology, immunology, physiology, biochemistry and effects of different xenobiotics on various behavioural, histopathological, physiological and biochemical aspects and their secondary effects, *viz.* mutagenicity, teratogenicity and carcinogenicity. To bring out such a comprehensive book series in *eight volumes*, as of now, covering such diverse chapters from the experts and senior persons of different fields is not an easy task.

The present volume has been arranged in *TWO* sections; first on *Animal Ecology* containing sixteen chapters and the second on *Animal Reproduction* having eight chapters. While some of the chapters are research work, others are overviews or reviews. The animal ecology section of the current series concentrates primarily on chemicals and natural products and their positive or negative influences on various behavioural, physiological and biochemical parameters of animals ranging from insects to human beings. It also deals with fisheries and aquaculture in India, predation and life style of copepods, age related changes in the activity of some enzymes and osmoregulatory adaptations in fishes, behavioural displays of axis deer, anuran integument, body size variation in African snail, useful plants, and prospects and limitations of biopesticides.

Section Two deals with chapters on improving reproductive output in fishes and reducing it effectively in human beings; both scenarios being highly pertinent. More specifically issues like, sexual selection and mating systems across the animal world, mating behaviour of Portunid crab, Leydig cell differentiation in adult amphibian, effects of different hormones on induced spawning of *Clarias*, fluoride on reproductive potential of fish, carbamate on biochemical changes in ovary and uterus of mice, herbal drugs enhancing male fertility and *Trypterygium wilfordii* as a new hope for male contraception are included. All these are very important and pertinent contributions from different experts and senior researchers in respective fields.

The volume covers vast topics and up-to-date information with unlimited usefulness not only to the researchers in the field but also to the policy planners, teachers as well as students, especially the PG students of Animal Science, Zoology, Environmental Biology and Toxicology, and those from the disciplines of Reproductive Biology, Endocrinology, etc.

I congratulate the editors for publishing an excellent scientific compendium by bringing together expertise from different disciplines and geographical areas.

Omkar

Preface

The earth contains countless places to live, and therefore a great diversity of life is observed all over. There are more than two million different kinds of living things on this earth. When we look around, we notice that the world abound with diverse living things which exhibit a marvelous spectrum of colours, shapes and forms. Life occurs almost everywhere on earth, from the highest mountain peaks to the deepest ocean trenches and the organisms display a great diversity in their rich ecology and reproductive strategies.

All living things reproduce members of their own kind. Since living things eventually die, reproduction ensures survival of the group. Reproduction is simple in some of the smaller forms of life, but the great majority of animals and plants possess sexually reproducing capability. The living things also respond to stimuli in their environment and their ability to adjust to their environment is one of their most striking characteristics.

In current century, enormous information has to be gathered from the field of biology. Biologists, in modern days are in much demand and will continue to be so in future. The science of biology affect our daily lives and our future too and a battery of researchers are engaged in researches on animal ecology and their breeding patterns.

It was in light of this the current book series was planned. The text in the book has been organized into two units containing 24 chapters. The unit one of the present volume contains 16 chapters which deals with the animal ecological studies. Unit two contains 8 chapters on reproductive strategies adopted by the animals. The highlights of the present volume are the topics *viz.* Sodium fluoride induced toxicity in the eggs and larvae of *Drosophila melanogaster;* Body metric variation in populations of the giant African snail, *Achatina fulica* from two different environ; Ionic variability of aquatic environment and osmoregulatory adaptations in teleost fishes: an ecological perspective; Behavioural alterations of freshwater air breathing teleost, *Channa punctatus* in response to heavy metal exposure; A critical review on certain aspects of anuran integument; Time budget activity pattern of behavioural displays of captive axis deer (*Axis axis*); Study of age related changes in the activity of some metabolic enzymes in *Cyprinus carpio* as biomarkers; Biopesticides- its prospects and limitations: an overview; *Trypterygium wilfordii*: a new hope for male contraception; Mating behaviour of commercially important portunid crab *Portunus pelagicus;* Biochemical changes in ovary and uterus of mice after exposure to indoxacarb; reproductive potential of fresh water fish in fluoride contaminated water; and a review on the sexual selection and mating systems across the animal world.

With the enormous volume of researches in the fields of animal ecology and reproduction each year, it becomes rather difficult to sort out the meaningful and to present it in a comprehensive manner. It needs constant examination of the data in the light of recent knowledge. It is a matter of great pleasure and satisfaction that the book "*Perspective in Animal Ecology and Reproduction*" has been warmly accepted by the learned scholars, scientists and teachers of the colleges, universities and research institutes of the country and abroad. We are, therefore, pleased to place before our readers the next volume *i.e.*, Volume 8 of the series which shall prove more useful to them.

We are grateful to the readers and contributors for their unflinching support and confidence and we shall be thankful to receive constructive suggestions for further improvement of the book series. We would also like to put on record our sincere appreciation for the publisher for co-operation in bringing out the present volume within the stipulated period inspite of our demand for high quality.

Jammu

Dr. V.K. Gupta
Dr. Anil K. Verma
Dr. G.D. Singh

Contents

Section II: Animal Reproduction

Section I
Animal Ecology

Chapter 1

Sodium Fluoride Induced Toxicity in the Eggs and Larvae of *Drosophila melanogaster*

H.P. Gurushankara[1]*, *M. Shanthala*[2] *and V. Vasudev*[1]

[1]*Department of P.G. Studies and Research in Bioscience, University of Mysore, PG Center, Hemagangothri, Hassan – 573 220, Karnataka, India*

[2]*Center for Applied Genetics, Bangalore University, Jnanabharathi Campus, Bengaluru – 560 056, Karnataka, India*

ABSTRACT

The effect of sodium fluoride was studied on eggs and larvae of *Drosophila melanogaster*. Rate of development, viability and sex ratio were the parameters employed to assess the toxicity of the chemical. The eclosion of flies in control and lower concentrations commenced on 9th day and at higher concentrations, it was prolonged in both stage treatments. There was a significant increase in mean developmental time in higher concentrations ($p< 0.05$). The viability has been reduced from control to 1mM concentration; the highest lethality was noticed in the highest concentration employed. Thus, there was a gradual increase in the percentage of lethality from the lowest to the highest concentrations of sodium fluoride. The reduction was significant compared to control ($p< 0.0001$). The LD_{50} was

* Corresponding author: E-mail: hpgurushiva@yahoo.com

estimated to be 12.80 mM and 13.5 mM sodium fluoride for 3rd instar larvae and egg stages of *D. melanogaster*. Sex ratio distortion has been observed at higher concentrations of sodium fluoride treatment. The results obtained are compared with toxicity of sodium fluoride to both eggs and larval stages of *D. melanogaster*. From this, we opined that development and viability of any non-target organism could be interrupted by fluoride like pollutants. Furthermore, this would witness the decline of beneficial non-target organisms like *Drosophila* in particular and faunal diversity in general in fluoride endemic areas.

Keywords: *Drosophila melanogaster, Sodium fluoride, Developmental toxicity, Fluorosis.*

Introduction

Fluoride compounds cause drastic damage to biological systems (Pillai and Stanley, 2002). Fluorosis is a serious health problem in many parts of the world caused by excessive toxic levels of fluoride in many foods and drinking water supplies, especially in fluoride endemic areas (Meenakshi and Maheshwari, 2006). Fluorides are synthetic chemicals that are being extensively used in agricultural pesticides, fertilizers and for fluorinating drinking water, as they are major source of fluoride pollution (Meenakshi *et al.*, 2004). Fluoride in the form of sodium fluoride is one such chemical compound, which has to be tested for its genotypic and phenotypic effects, using different test systems. There are reports to demonstrate the detrimental effects of sodium fluoride to terrestrial and aquatic ecosystem. Of the battery of test systems available *Drosophila* is being used to study the mutagenic and/or genotoxic effects of different chemicals including environmental agents, due to its many advantages (Luning, 1966; Vogel and Sobels, 1976; Vasudev and Krishnamurthy, 1991). The data on differential sensitivity of *D. melanogaster* eggs and larvae to sodium fluoride are wanting, and hence the present investigations were undertaken.

Materials and Methods

The standard Oregon K (OK) strain of *D. melanogaster* formed the experimental material. Sodium fluoride was obtained from the S.D. fine chemicals Bangalore (Product no- 40139, Batch no –

701819411). The flies were reared in standard wheat cream agar food medium seeded with yeast

Toxicity Analysis

Different concentrations of sodium fluoride ranging from 1 to 50 mM were used. These were separately put into 100ml wheat cream agar medium; which was completely mixed after preparation to facilitate uniform spreading of the chemical in the medium and dispersed in equal quantities into 3x1 vials. The untreated medium was used as control. Eggs of the same age (± 4 hours) collected by Delcour procedure (Delcour, 1969) was placed in the vials containing normal or chemical supplemented medium at equal density of 50 eggs/vial. Eight replicates of each concentration total 400 eggs were allocated. Similarly, 3rd instar larva was allocated to test the toxic effects on larval stage of *D. melanogaster*.

The flies were counted and sex was recorded every day from the first day of eclosion to the last day of emergence. From this data, the pattern of emergence as well the mean developmental time of whole group and of the two sexes and percentage of viability of the whole group in each of the concentrations and control was calculated. The sex ratio in different concentrations was also calculated. All the experiments were conducted at the uniform temperature of 24 ± 1ºC.

Statistical Analysis

In the present study, all the data were recorded on data sheet and then transferred to Microsoft Excel. Later the data were processed using SPSS 10.00 for windows. Mean developmental time was calculated by using the formula $\overline{X} = \Sigma fx/N$ for which standard deviation and standard error were calculated. The test of significance between the two means was made using simple t-test. Analysis of variance was used to calculate the statistical significance between the control and treated series for viability. Simple chi square test was used to calculate the difference between the two sexes. Probit analysis was used to analyze the dose effect relationship of sodium fluoride.

Results

The results on the effects of the sodium fluoride on rate of development, viability and sex ratio of *D. melanogaster* treated at eggs and larval stages are presented in Tables 1.1–1.3 and depicted in Figures 1.1–1. 3.

Rate of Development

The present results revealed that there was variation in the development time at different concentrations compared to control (Figure 1.1) treated at egg stage. The eclosion of flies in the control and 1mM to 20mM concentrations eclosion commenced on 9th day; but the emergence of flies were reduced in treated groups compare to control in the order of 60, 57.5, 67.5, 87.5 and 77.5 per cent in 1, 5, 10, 15 and 20mM sodium fluoride treated groups respectively. While in 25, 30 and 40 mM concentrations, the eclosion commenced on 10th,

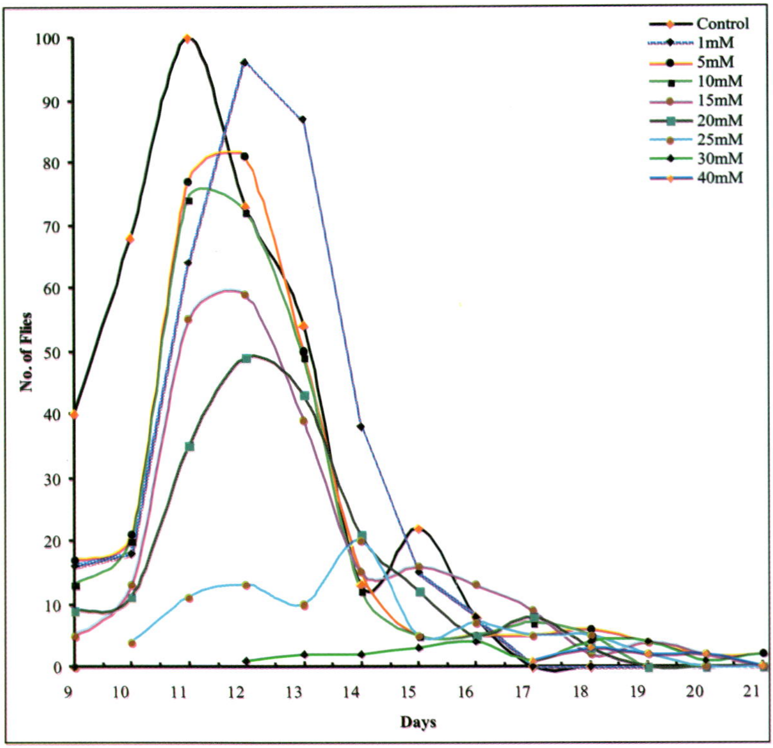

Figure 1.1: Pattern of Emergence of *D. melanogaster* Flies in Different Concentrations of Sodium Fluoride and Control Treated at Egg Stage

12th and 17th day. In control, the eclosion ended on the 16th day. On the other hand, the emergence was terminated on 21st and 20th day in concentrations of 30 and 40mM sodium fluoride treated groups respectively. No eclosion was noticed in concentrations at 50mM treated group.

The graphical representation of variation in the pattern of emergence of flies at different concentrations of sodium fluoride compared to control is presented in Figure 1.2 treated at larval stage. The eclosion of flies in the control and 1 to 15mM concentrations commenced on 9th day; but the emergences of flies were reduced in treated batches compared to control in the order of 68.29, 90.24, 95.12 and 92.68 per cent in 1, 5, 10 and 15mM sodium fluoride

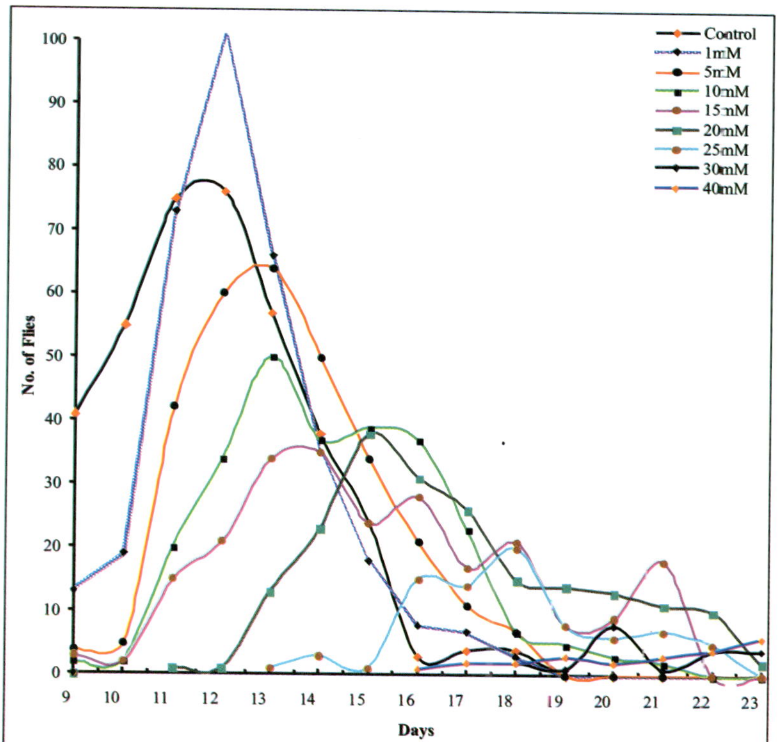

Figure 1.2: Pattern of Emergence of *D. melanogaster* Flies in Different Concentrations of Sodium Fluoride and Control Treated at 3rd Instar Larval Stage

treated concentrations respectively. While in 20, 25, 30 and 40 mM concentrations, the eclosion was commenced on 11th, 13th, 18th and 16th day. In control, the highest peak of emergence was observed at 12th day with a gradual decline and the eclosion was ended on the 18th day. Interesting to note that at 1mM treated group the highest peak of emergence was noticed at 11th day itself and the eclosion was terminated on the 18th day. On the other hand, the emergence was terminated on 23rd day in highest concentrations of 30 and 40mM sodium fluoride treated groups. No eclosion was noticed in concentrations above 50mM treated group.

Table 1.1: Mean Developmental Time (days ± SE) of *D. melanogaster* Group in Control and Different Concentrations of Sodium Fluoride Treated at Egg and 3rd Instar Larval Stage

Concentrations of Sodium Fluoride (in mM)	*Mean Developmental Time of Group (in days)*	
	Treated Eggs	*Treated 3rd Instar larva*
Control	11.53 ± 0.051	11.88 ± 0.107
1	12.27 ± 0.079†	12.36 ± 0.072
5	12.24 ± 0.194*	13.27 ± 0.219*
10	12.48 ± 0.093†	14.27 ± 0.440†
15	13.14 ± 0.127†	15.48 ± 0.375†
20	13.55 ± 0.225†	16.92 ± 0.565†
25	14.34 ± 0.262†	18.43 ± 0.192†
30	16.69 ± 0.701†	20.99 ± 0.285†
40	18.95 ± 0.310†	21.70 ± 0.302†

Significant compared to control at *$p < 0.05$; †$p < 0.01$.

No sign: Not-significant.

The mean developmental time for the group as well for different sexes (days ± SE) of *D. melanogaster* in control and different concentrations of sodium fluoride treated at egg stage are presented in Table 1.1. The mean developmental time has been extended from 11.53 ± 0.051 days in control to 12.27 ± 0.079 in the lowest concentration (1mM) employed. The highest developmental delay was noticed at the highest concentrations (Table 1.1). The mean developmental time of different concentrations was found to be significant ($p< 0.05$) compared to control. There was a dose effect prolongation of the rate of development from the lowest to the highest concentration. Contrary to group, in case of males and females developmental rate has been extended from 11.39 ± 0.069 and 11.66 ± 0.052 for control to 12.19 ± 0.075 and 12.34 ± 0.102 in the lowest concentration treated (1mM). The significant mean difference was observed in male's developmental time ($p < 0.05$) at 1mM sodium fluoride treated concentration; but this was insignificant ($p > 0.05$) in females at same low concentration. Similar to group in case of males and females also shown there was a significant dose effect prolongation of development from the lowest to the highest concentration.

The mean developmental rate for the group as well for different sexes (days ± SE) of *D. melanogaster* in control and different concentrations of sodium fluoride treated at 3rd instar larval stage presented in Table 1.2. The mean developmental time has been extended from 11.88 ± 0.107 days in control to 12.36 ± 0.072 in the lowest concentration (1mM) employed. This extended difference (1mM) low concentration was statistically insignificant ($p > 0.05$) when compared to control. The highest developmental delay was noticed at the highest concentrations (Table 1.2). The mean developmental time of different concentrations was found to be significant ($p < 0.05$) compared to control. Contrary to group, in case of males and females developmental rate has been extended from 11.89 ± 0.136 and 11.75 ± 0.015 for control to 12.58 ± 0. 152 and 12.12 ± 0.074 in the lowest concentration treated (1mM). Comparison between egg and larval stage, larval stage treated group have shown the significant mean difference observed in females developmental time ($p < 0.01$) at 1mM sodium fluoride treated concentration; but this was insignificant ($p > 0.05$) in males at same low concentration. The present results revealed that the mean developmental time is significantly prolonged even in the lowest concentrations. The significant highest delay was noticed in the highest concentrations tested ($p < 0.05$).

Viability

Percentage of lethality as a measure of sodium fluoride toxicity treated at egg stage is shown in the Figure 1.3. In the present experiments, viability has been reduced at different concentrations of the sodium fluoride. The reduction is due to chemical environment because other factors were not variables. Perusal of Table 1.3 reveals that the viability has been reduced from 94.50 per cent in control to 85.50 per cent in 1mM concentration. The highest lethality was produced in the highest concentration tested (40mM). The extent of lethality is directly proportional to the concentration. By applying ANOVA it has been shown that sodium fluoride induced significant effect on male ($F = 85.04$; $p = 0.0001$), female ($F = 125.93$; $p = 0.0001$) and total ($F = 4264.52$; $p = 0.0001$) viability even in the lowest concentrations analyzed.

Table 1.2: Mean Developmental Time (days ± SE) of *D. melanogaster* Males and Females in Control and Different Concentrations of Sodium Fluoride Treated at Egg and 3rd Instar Larval Stage

Conc. of Sodium Fluoride (in mM)	*Mean Developmental Time (in days)*			
	Treated Eggs		*Treated 3rd Instar larva*	
	Males	*Females*	*Males*	*Females*
Control	11.39 ± 0.069	11.66 ± 0.052	11.86 ± 0.136	11.75 ± 0.015
1	12.19 ± 0.075†	12.34 ± 0.102	12.58 ± 0.152	12.12 ± 0.074*
5	12.28 ± 0.123†	12.20 ± 0.299†	13.16 ± 0.196*	13.33 ± 0.304*
10	12.85 ± 0.089†	12.52 ± 0.119†	14.34 ± 0.535*	14.17 ± 0.297†
15	13.25 ± 0.048†	13.48 ± 0.103†	15.84 ± 0.529†	15.49 ± 0.428†
20	14.07 ± 0.296†	13.82 ± 0.253†	17.29 ± 0.594†	16.97 ± 0.597†
25	14.42 ± 0.064†	15.39 ± 0.392†	18.81 ± 0.216†	18.78 ± 0.189†
30	16.79 ± 0.771†	16.63 ± 0.703†	20.96 ± 0.336†	20.73 ± 0.178†
40	18.31 ± 0.373†	18.73 ± 0.328†	21.76 ± 0.472†	21.91 ± 0.164†

Significant compared to control at *$p < 0.05$; †$p < 0.01$.

No sign: Not-significant.

Similar to egg stage, the treatment even in larval form also shows that the viability has been reduced at different concentrations of the sodium fluoride (Figure 1.3). The viability has been reduced from 94.25 per cent in control to 85.75 per cent in 1mM concentration. The highest lethality (5.75 per cent) was produced in the highest concentration tested (40mM). The extent of lethality is directly proportional to the increasing concentration. By applying ANOVA it has been shown that sodium fluoride induced significant effect on male ($F = 293.20$; $p = 0.0001$), female ($F = 176.04$; $p = 0.0001$) and total

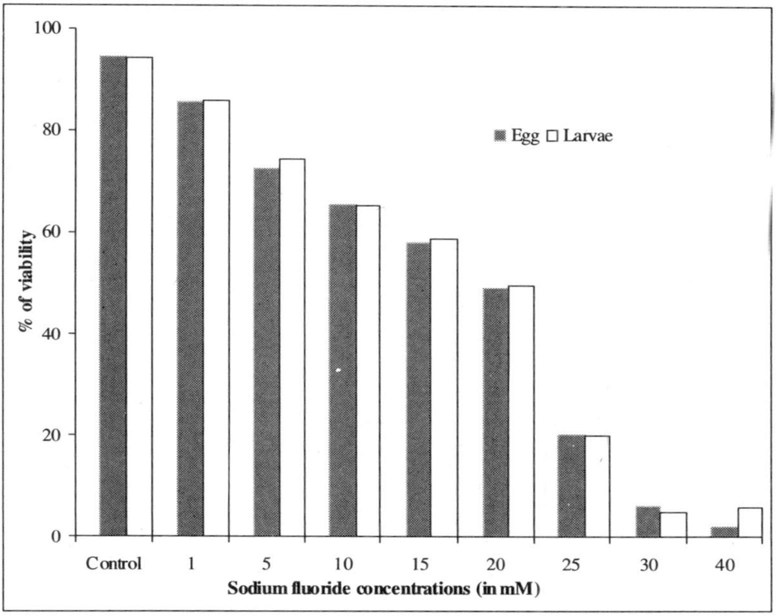

Figure 1.3: Percentage Viability of *D. melanogaster* in Different Concentrations of Sodium Fluoride and Control Treated at 3rd Instar Larval and Egg Stage

($F = 444.83$ $p = 0.0001$) viability even in the lowest concentration studied.

There was a gradual increase in the percentage of lethality from the lowest to the highest concentration of sodium fluoride (Table 1.3). The LD_{50} for 3rd Instar larva and egg stage was 12.80 mM and 13.5 mM respectively.

Sex-Ratio

The effect of sodium fluoride on sex ratio in *D. melanogaster* treated at egg stage represented in Table 1.3. It is clear from the table that control and none of the low concentrations had any discernible effect on the development of either sex ($p > 0.05$). The discernible effect was observed at higher concentrations. By applying chi-square homogeneity test it has been shown that sodium fluoride induced significant sex–ratio distortion at higher concentrations of sodium fluoride treatment ($p < 0.05$). The data on the males and females flies emerged out from 400 larvae. No sex- ratio distortion was observed at control and low concentration (1mM) sodium fluoride treatment ($p > 0.05$). Similar to egg stage treated group, here also sex – ratio distortion was noticed at higher concentrations above 5mM ($p < 0.05$). The significant sex- ratio distortion in *D. melanogaster* is good indication of effect of sodium fluoride during sex determination.

Table 1.3: Effect of Sodium Fluoride on Sex Ratio in *D. melanogaster* Treated at Egg and 3rd Instar Larval Stage

Conc. of Sodium Fluoride (in mM)	No. of Males and Females Emerged Out of 400 Eggs							
	Treated Eggs				Treated 3rd instar larva			
	Males	Females	x^2	p-value	Males	Females	x^2	p-value
Control	179	199	1.058	0.30	188	189	0.002	0.95
1	167	175	0.1916	0.70	165	178	0.4186	0.50
5	156	134	1.669	0.20	132	166	3.879	0.05*
10	117	145	2.992	0.10	158	103	11.590	0.001‡
15	97	135	6.224	0.01†	96	139	7.868	0.01†
20	83	113	4.592	0.05*	75	123	11.636	0.001‡
25	60	22	17.609	0.001‡	60	20	20.00	0.001‡
30	6	17	5.260	0.05*	5	15	5.00	0.05*
40	7	1	4.000	0.05*	7	16	3.5217	0.05*

Significant sex distortion observed at *$p < 0.05$; †$p < 0.01$; ‡$p < 0.001$.

No sign: Not significant.

Discussion

Utility of *Drosophila*, as a test system in screening programmes is based on many important advantages. One of them is the presence of microsomal enzyme systems in this animal, which is similar to that of mammalian liver (Vogel and Sobels, 1976). It also offers the facility to test the effect of different germ cell stages. This is important because one of the characteristic features of chemicals is their specificity of action. Short generation time, less expensive laboratory maintenance, potential to breed in large numbers, presence of well established genetic markers are other important requisites that qualify *Drosophila* as a good organism of choice for quick screening of the effects of environmental agents. Hence, this animal has been used to test the toxic effects of fluoride.

Rate of development and survival value (viability) are the best characters to observe the somatic effects, which in turn reveals the extent of toxicity of the chemical (Luning, 1966). The present results reveal that the mean developmental time is significantly prolonged even in all the concentrations tested with a dose effect relationship (Figure 1.1 and Table 1.1, $p < 0.05$). These results support the view of Luning (1966) wherein the lengthening of developmental time is a good indication of somatic effects caused by the chemical. Vasudev and Krishnamurthy (1982-83; 1979a and b) using Dithane M-45, a carbamate pesticide, cadmium chloride and a lead compound, Sorsa and Pfeifer (1973) using organomerculials, Laamanen *et al.* (1976) using amitrole and Basheer *et al.* (1999) using Dunet have shown similar effects in *D. melanogaster* and came to the same conclusions. Apart from chemicals, other environmental factors such as crowding and temperature have been demonstrated to have effect on rate of development for example relative developmental time was prolonged in crowded condition in *D. malarkotliana, D. bipectinata* and *D. n. nasuta* (Krishnamurthy *et al.*, 1993). Budnik *et al.* (1971) based on their investigations in *D. pavani* have demonstrated that development at 16°C varies significantly between the males and females while at 25°C the difference in the rate of development is insignificant. Thus, it can be said that any variability in the environment is having profound influence on the rate of development. In the present investigations, it is concluded that chemical environment is responsible for increased developmental time in the treated groups.

Viability is one of the adaptive traits of any population and determines the rate of increase or decrease of population in an environment. Environmental factors such as temperature, food, space, etc. are also known to affect the viability. In the present experiment, viability has been reduced at different concentrations of sodium fluoride. The reduction is due to the chemical environment because other factors were not variable. The extent of lethality is directly proportional to the concentration. Earlier workers using different chemicals made similar observations (Budnik, 1971; Sorsa M Pfeifer, 1973; Laamanen *et al.*, 1976; Rajasekarashetty, 1978; Vasudev and Krishnamurthy, 1991, 1982-83, 1979a; Krishnamurthy *et al.*, 1993; Basheer *et al.*, 1999).

Probit analysis, which is the method to determine the dose – effect relationship between the doses of the chemical gives us the indication of dose effect relationship. Thus, the estimated LD_{50} of sodium fluoride to *D. melanogaster* is 12.80 mM for larvae. Similarly, Vasudev and Krishnamurthy (1991; 1982-83) have demonstrated that the LD_{50} of two pesticides namely Dithane M-45 and Baygon was 175 and 12.5 ppm respectively. The LD_{50} of Dunet to *D. melanogaster* was 0.177µl/100ml (Basheer *et al.*, 1999). It is clear from LD_{50} values that pesticides are more toxic than sodium fluoride. It is but natural that pesticides are more toxic to insects but, toxicity of fluorides cannot be ignored because of continuous use of fluorinated drinking water, fluoride containing pesticides and fertilizers. The LD_{50} of this chemical to male mouse is 54.4 mg/kg body weight (Pillai *et al.*, 1988) and it has been demonstrated that sodium fluoride in sub lethal doses is toxic to testis of mice (Chinoy, *et al.*, 2005). Cytotoxicity of sodium fluoride in human cell culture studies has been observed by Sivikova and Dianovsky (1995), He *et al.* (1983), Hayashi and Tsutsui (1993) and Nair *et al.* (2004).

The sex ratio is an important factor for any sexually reproducing species. A stable population is one, which has enough number of males and females to breed and produce the offspring. In general, the sex ratio for most of the species or populations is 1:1 (Fischer, 1949). However; the sex ratio distortion has been noticed in certain species and populations. Even those species, which normally have equal sex ratio, at times, exhibit sex ratio distortion (Fischer, 1949; Hegde and Krishnamurthy, 1979). In the present study, the sex ratio is not uniform in treated groups. The sex ratio distortion was noticed in higher concentrations of sodium fluoride treated groups (Table 1.3). It is also be possible that the sex ratio imbalance may be due to both genetic and environmental factors. Even though there is sex ratio distortion, which is in favor of females it would not affect the productivity of that population.

Factors such as differential mortality between sexes due to lethal genes or due to chromosomal anomalies may also tilt the balance and can produce sex ratio imbalance. Experiments have also demonstrated that restricted nutrition, hyperactivity of one sex and differential utilization of habitat by two sexes to have influence on sex ratio distortion. In the present investigations in some concentrations males are preferred and in some females (Table 1.3).

In recent years, repeated male mating has been well documented in many species of *Drosophila* (Aspi and Lankinen, 1992; Sharathchandra and Hegde, 2002). Since a male can inseminate more than one female present in the population, a few males could inseminate most of the females of the population and hence it is not disadvantageous to have less number of males than females. Having more number of females ensures greater productivity of the population than those having equal number of males and females. Thus, the natural selection is favoring the females to produce more offsprings. The reason for the imbalance also could be the meiotic drive, during which the X or Y bearing sperms is either less active or lethal so that such pairs produce more sons or daughters.

Conclusions

This work has shown the toxic effect of sodium fluoride to *D. melanogaster*, which is a non – target organism similar to man, and hence warrants further thorough investigations on cytogenotoxic and reproductive effects using different test systems.

Acknowledgements

We thank Chairman Dept. of P.G. Studies and Research in Environmental Science and Prof. S.V. Krishnamurthy, Kuvempu University for providing laboratory facilities and also for continuous encouragement.

References

Aspi, J., Lankinen, P., 1992. Frequency of multiple insemination in a natural population of *D. montana*. *Hereditas*, 117: 169-177.

Basheer, S., Vasudev, V., Venu, R., Guruprasad, K.P., Harish, S.K., 1999. Toxic effects of a recently introduced Carbamate pesticide, Dunet (methomyl) on *Drosophila melanogaster*. *J. Environ. Biol.*, 20:135 -139.

Budnik, M., Korep–Santibanez, S., Brancic, D., 1971. Rate of development and inversion polymorphism in *Drosophila pavani* at two different temperatures. *Genetics*, 69: 227–233.

Chinoy, N.J., Mehta, D., Jhala, D.D., 2005. Beneficial effects of a protein rich diet on fluoride induced free radical toxicity in the liver of male mice. *Fluoride*, 38: 276–283.

Delcour, J., 1969. A rapid and efficient method of egg collection. Drosophila inform. *Ser.*, 44:133-134.

Fischer, A.W., 1949. The design of experiment, Oliver and Boyd, London

Hayashi, N., Tsutsui, T., 1993. Cell cycle dependence of cytotoxicity and clastogenicity induced by treatment of synchronized human diploid fibroblasts with sodium fluoride. *Mutat. Res.*, 290: 293 – 302.

He, W., Liu, A., Bao, H., Wang, Y., Cao, W., 1983. Effects of sodium fluoride and fluroacetamide on sister chromatid exchanges and chromosomal aberrations in cultured Red Muntjac (*Muntjacus muntjak*) cells. *Acta. Scient. circumst.*, 3: 94-100.

Hegde, S.N., Krishnamurthy, N.B., 1979. Studies of mating behaviour in *Drosophila bipectinata* complex. *Aust. J. Zool.*, 27: 421-431.

Krishnamurthy, N.B., Nagaraj, H.J., Vasudev, V., 1993. Pre – adult competition studies in three sympatric species of *Drosophila. Biol. Zent. Bl.*, 112: 300 – 311.

Laamanen, I., Sorsa, M., Bamfold, D., Gripenberg, U., Meretoja, T., 1976. Mutagenecity and toxicity of Amitrole, *Drosophila* testis. *Mut. Res.*, 40: 443-449.

Luning, K.G., 1966. *Drosophila* tests in Pharmacology. *Nature*, 209: 84-86.

Meenakshi, G., Kavita, V.K., Renuka, Malik, A., 2004. Groundwater quality in some villages of Haryana, India: focus on fluoride and fluorosis. *J. Hazard Mater.*, 106: 55-60.

Meenakshi, G., Maheshwari, R.C., 2006. Fluoride in drinking water and its removal. *J Hazard Mater.*, 137: 456-463.

Nair, S.B., Jhala, D.D., Chinoy, N.J., 2004. Mitigation of genotoxic effects of fluoride and arsenic by ascorbic acid in human lymphocyte cultures. *Fluoride*, 37: 249–256.

Pillai S.K., Stanley V.A., 2002. Implications of fluoride–an endless uncertainty. *J. Environ. Boil.*, 32: 81-87.

Pillai, S.K., Mathai, A.T., Deshmukh, P.B., 1988. Effect of sub acute dosage of fluoride on male mice. *Toxicol. Lett.*, 44: 21-29.

Rajasekarashetty, M.R., Gayathri, M.V., Krishnamurthy, N.B., 1978. Effects of Ceresan–a mercurial fungicide on *Drosophila*. Intr. Symp. Environ. Agents and their boil effects, Hyderabad Pp. 44.

Sharathchandra, Y., Hegde, S.N., 2002. Remating in *Drosophilid Phorticella striata*. *Korean J. Genetics*, 24: 113-118.

Sivikova, K., Dianovsky, J., 1995. Sister–chromatid exchanges after exposure to metal- containing emissions. *Mutat. Res.*, 327: 17-22.

Sorsa, M., Pfeifer, S., 1973. Response of puffing pattern in vitro treatments with organomercurials in *Drosophila melanogaster*. *Hereditas*, 74: 89-102.

Vasudev, V., Krishnamurthy, N.B., 1979a. Toxicity of Dithane M-45 on *Drosophila melanogaster*. *Experientia*, 35: 528-529.

Vasudev, V., Krishnamurthy, N.B., 1979b. Induction of dominant lethals by cadmium chloride in *Drosophila melanogaster*. *Curr. Sci.*, 48: 1007-1008.

Vasudev, V., Krishnamurthy, N.B., 1982 – 83. Effect of Dithane M-45 on the rate of development, viability, morphology and fecundity in *Drosophila melanogaster J. Mys. Univ.*, 29:79-86.

Vasudev, V., Krishnamurthy, N.B., 1991. Utilization of *Drosophila* to understand toxicity and mutagenecity of Baygon. In environmental pollution and resources of land and water (Eds: R.C. Dalela *et al.*) *The Acad. Environ. Biol. Lucknow*, 205-213.

Vogel, E., Sobels, F.H., 1976. The function of *Drosophila* in genetic toxicology testing in chemical mutagens; Principles and methods for their detection (Ed: A Hollaender). Plenum Publ. Co. New York 93-142.

Chapter 2

Does Predation Affect the Life Style of Freshwater Copepoda?

H.H. Mohammed[1], S.D. Salman[1]* and A.A.M. Abdullah[2]

[1]Department of Marine Biology, Marine Science Centre, Basrah University, Iraq

[2]Department of Fisheries and Marine resources, Colllege of Agriculture, Basrah University, Iraq

ABSTRACT

Quantitative water samples were collected from a pool at the University Campus of Garmat-Ali from August 1998 to July 1999. The diapause in *Apocyclops dengizicus* extended from mid August 1998 to the beginning of February 1999. While that of *Mesocyclops isabellae* occurred from January to the beginning of April 1999. The presence of *M. isabellae* in the water column was synchronized with the absence of *A. dengizicus*, which suggested a strategy of avoiding predation by *M. isabellae*. The diapause stage in *A. dengizicus* was CIV and individuals were found at 5 cm deep in the sediments whereas the diapause stages of *M. isabellae* were CIV and CV and were found at a

* Corresponding author: E-mail: dr_salmands@yahoo.com

depth of 20 cm in the mud. Quiescence is only exhibited by the last naupliar stage and all the copepodite stages including the adult of *M. isabellae*.

Keywords: *Diapause, Apocyclops dengizicus, Mesocyclops isabellae, Predation, Life cycle, Quiescence, Basrah.*

Introduction

The ecosystem of ponds differs from lakes, rivers and any other aquatic habitat because it is rather small and shallow and there is a slight difference in temperature between the surface and the bottom, and is subjected to a complete dryness during summer when the temperature rises up to 35°C or it may be freezed when the temperature drops to -5 °C, thus, the organisms living in these aquatic habitats should be ecophysiologically adapted to the surrounding factors as well as having special strategies for growth, reproduction and life cycles enabling them to pass the unsuitable environmental conditions (Thompson and Coldrey, 1985).

The life cycles of many species of freshwater cyclopoid had been studied in details in various localities in the world and represented complex types including diapause and relatively long life cycles. It is well known that many zooplankton communities both in freshwater and in marine habitats are usually having short lives extending for one year at the most, for instance Protozoa, Rotifera and Cladocera are having a life span varying from a few days to one year (Elgmork, 1981). Longer generation times are found among Copepoda, for instance, in the temporary pools, they usually have a one year life cycle, whereas in some other species the life cycle may extends for two years or more as in *Cyclops scutifer* (Sars) of Lake Hazen in Iceland (McLaren, 1961), and in Kuril Lake (Nosova, 1970a,b),these localities are arctic or sub-arctic and the lakes are exposed to very low temperatures even during summer, for the same species, a three years life span was recorded in the sub-arctic lakes and cold high mountains of Norway (Halvorson, 1973) and in the Swidish sub-arctic lake, Latnjajaure (Nauwerck *et al.*, 1980), apparently without diapause.

The main reason for the prolonged life span in these localities is the low temperatures which in turn causes lowering of the rate of development, and many species exhibit one period of diapause or sometimes two consecutive periods of diapause (Elgmork, 1981). The first report of diapause in freshwater Cyclopoida was that of Brige and Juday (1908) on *Cyclops bicospedatus* which stimulated the interest in investigating this phenomenon in other species of Cyclopoida and several hypotheses attempting to explain the causes of the presence of the resting stages in these species, were put foreword. In this respect many studies concerning the resting stage of *Mesocyclops leuckarti* Claus in Russia (Monakov, 1958), and of *Cyclops strenuus strenuus* Fisher in Norway (Elgmork, 1955) were carried out, followed by those of Smyly (1961) and Fryer and Smyly (1954) on *Mesocyclops leuckarti* (Claus) and those of Wierzbeeka (1960, 1962) on *Cyclops bohater* Kezminski and *Cyclops vicinus vicinus* Uljanin. According to Elgmork (1980), "diapause" evolved to optimize reproduction and growth and to avoid food shortages and increased competition and predation.

The present article is aimed at understanding the tactics exhibited by the cyclopoids *Apocyclops dengizicus* and *Mesocyclops isabellae* to cope with each other and with the critical conditions imposed by a pool at Basrah, south of Iraq, an investigation conducted for the first time in such subtropical area.

Materials and Methods

Study Area

The sampling site is a shallow pool at the University Campus of Garmat-Ali. It represents a draining water surrounded by agricultural area and covered with water throughout the study period. The width of the pond is 1.5 m., the length is about 100 m and the depth is nearly 1m. The sediments of the pool are soft mud with sand and organic material there is no aquatic plant except a few *Phragmites australis* and two species of green algae *Cladophora* sp. and *Oscillatoria* spp. which covered a large area of the pond during winter and spring and considered as a good food for the nauplius stages of Cyclopoda. In addition there are some crustaceans and benthic animals like Ostracoda and Cladocera and the snail *Lymnaea tenera euphratica* (Mousson) and aquatic insects which represented the naiads and adults of Notonecta (Hemiptera).

In the sediment samples, meiofauna were found represented by species of Harpacticoida and larvae of *Chironomus* (Diptera).

Sampling Methods

Quantitative water samples were collected early in the morning, every two weeks, from the pool for the period from August 1998 to July 1999. A plastic cylinder of a diameter of 13.5 cm and a height of 10 cm with a capacity of 1 liter, was used for sampling. The sampler was rinsed in the water until fullness and quickly pulled back. Water samples were fixed with 4 per cent Formalin. One liter of water was collected every time.

Resting stages were collected by a metal container with a length of 30 cm and a width of 10 cm. Mud samples were taken by complete insertion of the frame into the sediment and collecting the mud block which was cut into parts of 5 cm each. Each section was filtered by washing with water through sieves of mesh sizes of 0.30, 1, 1.53 mm, after filtration each sample was placed into a Petri dish and examined under a dissecting microscope. The resting individuals of *A. dengizicus* were obtained at a depth of 5 cm, whereas, those of *M. isabellae* were found at a depth reaching 20 cm. The samples were repeated for several days to obtain appreciable numbers of diapausing individuals.

Results

Figures 2.1 and 2.2 showed the percentages of the naupliar, copepodite stages and adult males and females of *Apocyclops dengizicus* and *Mesocyclops isabellae*, respectively. *A. dengizicus* were represented by all the stages in August 1998. The nauplii and copepodites were forming 50 per cent and 43 per cent of the population, whereas the adults were 5 per cent females and 2 per cent males (Figure 2.1). There was a complete absence of the population from the water column during September 1998 – January 1999. In February 1999, no nauplii were encountered in the water column, whereas the advanced copepodites and adult males and females constituted 24.5, 53 and 22.5 per cent, respectively. However, in March 1999, the nauplii formed about 76 per cent of the population, and their numbers dropped to 57 per cent in April, followed by 30 per cent copepodites, and few adult males and females. In May to the cease of sampling in July 1999, no individual of any stage of life of *A. dengizicus* were encountered in the water column (Figure 2.1).

M. isabellae, on the other hand, dominated the plankton of the pool from August 1998 to December of the same year, disappeared

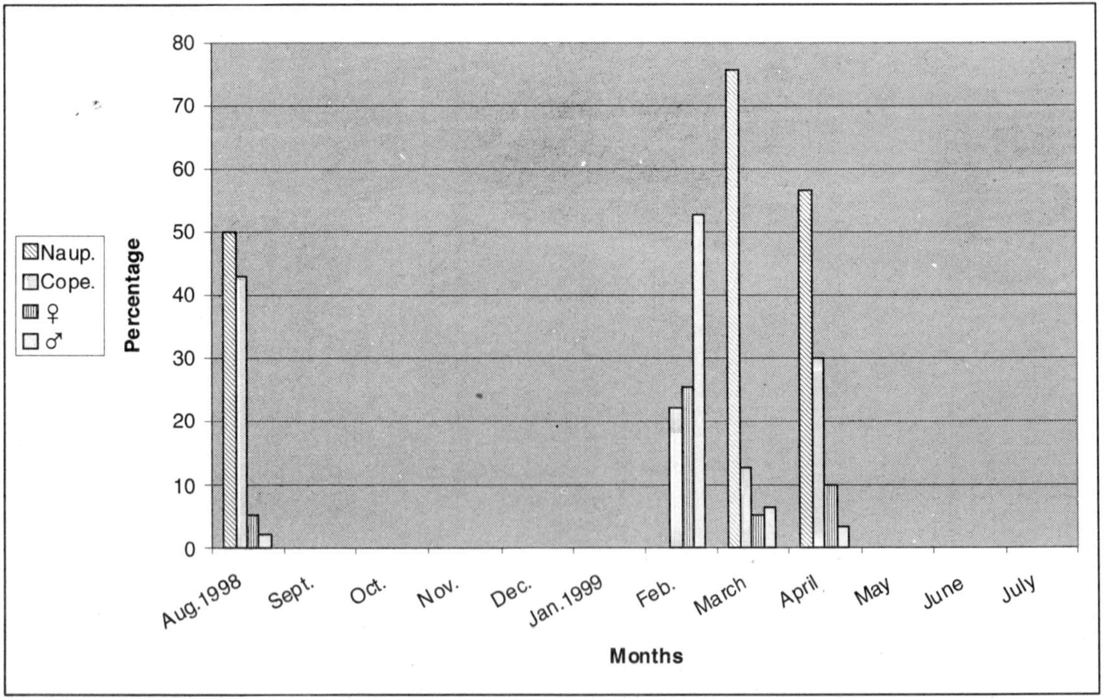

Figure 2.1: Percentage (per cent) of Nauplii Instars, Copepodite and Adults of *Apocyclops dengizicus* during August 1998–July 1999

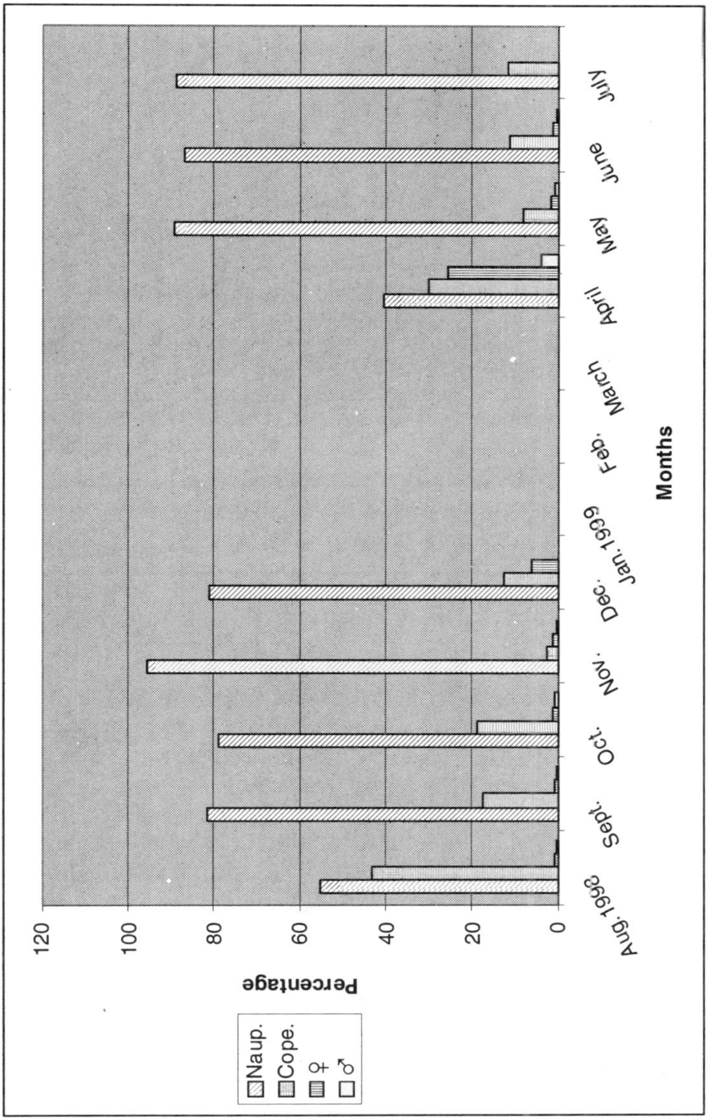

Figure 2.2: Percentage (per cent) of Nauplii Instars, Copepodite and Adults of *Mesocyclops Isabellae* during August 1998–July 1999

in January, February and March 1999, and reappeared again from April through the end of sampling in July of the same year (Figure 2.2). Although, higher percentages of 96 and 76 per cent were recorded in October and November, but these are because lower numbers of copepodites were encountered, however, the highest actual density was reported in September (82 per cent).

Diapause

Table 2.1, shows the resting stages of both species where the diapause period of *A. dengizicus* is extended for 6 months, from mid August 1998 to the beginning of February 1999. There was another diapause period starting from the beginning of May 1999.

Table 2.1: Resting Stages of *A. dengizicus* and *M. isabellae* Together with the Depth and Period

Species	*Diapause Instars*	*Depth (cm)*	*The period of Diapause (month)*	*Quiescence Instars*
A. dengizicus	C.IV	5	6	–
M. isabellae	C.IV, C.V	20	2.5	N.VI-C.VI

The resting stage was the copepodite IV which was obtained from the sediments of 5 cm deep.

The period of diapause of *M. isabellae* was extending from mid December 1998 to the beginning of April 1999. The temperature during this period was 12-14°C, the diapause stages were the copepodite IV and V which were found at a depth of 10-20 cm.

Through the microscopic investigations of the resting stages of both species, the following characters were found, diagnosing the resting individuals from the active ones present in the water column:

1. Body colour light grey.
2. The animal looks still and immovable but it responds to some effective stimuli like a fine needle sting or on increasing light intensity of the microscope which may lead to a weak movement of the appendages (the swimming legs and the antennules).
3. The intestine was empty of food particles.

4. The presence in *M. isabellae* of numerous oil droplets of varying sizes all over the body of the animal but were more concentrated in the cephalothrax, and pale yellow in colour, whereas, they were small in size and in addition to the pale yellow droplets there were bright red ones in *A. dengizicus*. However, these droplets can be observed in active individuals of both species, but they were small in size and few in numbers.
5. Some individuals of *A. dengizicus* were found with debris on their body, especially in the jointed parts, but in *M. isabellae* the body was clean.
6. The abdomen appeared bent underneath the cephalothorax, with the antennules extending to the body laterals.

Quiescence

This type of dormancy was obtained for a short period, about a few days before the diapause period, during which the population started gradual decrease in numbers from the water column from mid December 1998 to mid January 1999. The individuals of this type were found near the bottom, and had the same features of diapausing individuals but the body was straight and the movement was weak but the animal was not completely immovable as in the case of diapause. The quiescence was observed only in *M. isabellae* and it includes the larval stages from N VI (in small numbers) to C VI (in large numbers).

The Relationship Between the Two Species

Monthly plankton samples indicate that *A. dengizicus* was only present in the water column in August 1998, disappeared from September 1998 to January 1999 and appeared again from February to April 1999 (Figure 2.1). Nauplii were dominant in August 1998, March and April 1999. The copepodites were present in these three months and in February, so as the males and females. The males dominated the sample in February 1999.

M. isabellae, was encountered in the plankton from August – December 1998, disappeared from January – March 1999, and appeared again from April – the end of sampling in July 1999 (Figure 2.2). The nauplii dominated the plankton throughout the entire sampling period, followed by the copepodites, the females and the males.

An obvious strong predator –prey relationship was observed in a laboratory experiments when putting the two species together in the same dish. It was noticed that *M. isabellae* is predating upon various stages of development of *A. dengizicus*. The predatory stages were C IV – C V of the former species, whereas the preys were the naupliar stages and the first three copepodite stages of the latter. Moreover, the predatory stages of *M. isabellae* were found attacking the advanced copepodites and adults of *A. dengizicus*, but were unable to ingest them. They captured them and released them again. All adults of the latter species were found dead after being attacked by *M. isabellae.*

Discussion

The adaptive significance of diapause in the freshwater Cyclopoida is centered on two aspects, the escape from unfavourable environmental conditions, and the timing of the important events in the life cycle. The diapause is considered as the most tolerant stage to extreme environmental conditions like low temperatures, lack of oxygen and shortage of food. It is the only means of survival and may be regarded as a regulatory mechanism in the life history to secures survival during critical periods and catastrophes (Elgmork, 1980).

However, the influence of the abiotic factors on the diapause may be different, as it was found in certain species like *Cyclops vicinus* which can enter diapause in some lakes but, remains in the water column in others, although the environmental conditions are similar especially temperature (Maier, 1989; Hansen and Jappesen, 1992).

Danks (1987) generally defined dormancy as a "state of suppressed development" which is represented either by quiescence or diapause, and defined quiescence as " an immediate direct response to limiting factors, such as cessation of development if temperature falls below the developmental threshold, but immediate resumption of development if temperature rises above the developmental threshold ". He also defined diapause as "a more profound interruption that routes the metabolic program of the organisms away from direct developmental pathway and into much clearly organized break development that not controlled simply by the direct action of developmental factors.

Most studies of dormancy in cyclopoids have not attempted to distinguish quiescence from diapause. These two forms of dormancy are some times confused with one another which may create problems in interpretation of the life histories. However, a distinction can be made between the two phenomena, as quiescence is characterized by being short and irregular and directly imposed by adverse environmental conditions, and is not limited to a special ontogenetic instar and may be repeated in the same individual, whereas, diapause is a response to predictable cyclic changes in the environment that occurs regularly in the seasonal cycle and manifests itself to a definite ontogenetic instar (Andrwartha, 1952; Elgmork, 1959; Mansingh, 1971).

Dormancy in cyclopoids may includes prolonged duration of juvenile instars (Smyly, 1962), cessation of feeding (Williamson, 1984), settlement to the bottom mud (Elgmork, 1962, 1996; Santer and Lampert, 1995), encystment (Cole, 1953) and reduced oxygen consumption (Watson and Smallman, 1971).

The diapause did not occur only in Cyclopoida but, also in other orders of Copepoda, Williamson and Coull (1992) and Fryer and Smyly (1954) reported the occurrence of diapause in the adult stage of Harpacticoida. Whereas, females of Calanoida produced resting eggs as cysts which tolerate and survive a long period of unfavourable conditions (Brewer, 1964).

The diapause may occur in summer (summer resting stage) initiated during the beginning of summer, or there may be a winter resting stage initiated in the autumn. In both cases the resting periods may extend to the next spring, thus, it may last for 10 months, often under severe abiotic conditions (Elgmork, 1967).

There are many reasons to cause diapause to occur in summer. It may be a response to avoid high temperatures or it may be behavioural, exhibited by species living in temporary ponds (Maier, 1989; Einsle, 1987; Hunt and Robertson, 1977; Munro, 1974), or it may be an escape from predation by fish during the winter (Nilssen and Elgmork, 1977).

The present results showed obvious fluctuations in the population densities of both *A. dengizicus* and *M. isabellae* during the study period, for when a sharp decline in numbers of the first species was reported, there was a gradual increase of the second species which reached a high density in September 1998 (371 ind./l) in which time there was a complete absence of individuals of the first species from the water column.

The results obtained from the mud sediments showed the presence of *A. dengizicus* in a resting state at the copepodite IV, which is characterized by pale colour, empty gut and spreading of oil droplets in various parts of the body, these demonstrated in the literatures in different species of cyclopoids (Elgmork, 1959, 1962 1998; Vijverberg, 1977). Moreover, clay particles and detritus were observed adhered to the body of the individuals. These were also observed by Elgmork (1981) in *Cyclops scutifer*, but were absent in other species or in individuals of the same species (Elgmork, 1998). Wierzbicka (1972) demonstrated physiologically that the gut is isolated from the environment by the formation of bungs which were considered as a metabolic products taking definite shapes like star, crystal or without a definite shape depending on the species. The chemical analysis of these bodies illustrates that they were derived from uric acid and they cast off through the vent after the end of the diapause period (Wierzbicka, 1972).

The results of the examination of the sediments illustrated that *M. isabellae* during the period of dormancy is represented by C IV and C V. This result is partly coincided with the result of Elgmork (1980, 1998) who indicated that the diapause is most frequently observed in C IV which in many species seems to be the only diapause stage, whereas, C V is the next frequent stage, however the diapause may also occurred occasionally in other instars.

It was found that the diapause instars in *Mesocyclops* were C IV and C V (Papinska, 1984; Elgmork, 1964; Elgmork *et al.*, 1990; Nauwerck *et al.*, 1980; Smyly, 1961). Moreover, the diapause instar may not be the same in every year like in *Acanthocyclops robustus* for instance, as in one year it may be C III and C IV, whereas in several other years the dormant stages were C IV and C V. This may be caused by the ice cover which may fluctuates from year to year by about 16 – 38 days (Vijverberg, 1977).

The present results indicate that both *M. isabellae* and *A. dengizicus* were present as a resting stage in the bottom of the pool, but there were no individuals in the slop of the pool. The resting individuals didn't penetrate to greater depth, but they are in relatively restricted areas of the pool's bottom. However, there were species present in the deepest part of the pond or lake, and in some other species there seems a tendency to concentrate in the deepest part of the lake leading to tremendous numbers in restricted areas like in *Cyclops scutifer* which was found in a density of about 4 million individuals per m^2 in Norway (Elgmork, 1962).

The horizontal distribution of Cyclopoida may be affected by the environmental factors of which the oxygen may be the most important factor (Elgmork, 1967). In Esthwaite waters in England the resting stage of *M. leuckarti* was found in the deepest basin (Smyly, 1961), while in a lake in Poland the same species was confined to the slope of the basin (Szlauer, 1963). These differences may be due to the fact that the diapause in the lake in England started after the autumn turnover whereas, in Poland it starts before. Apparently the oxygen deficiency in the deepest areas is the key factor in the escape of the animals from these areas of the lake or pond (Szlauer, 1963).

The present results showed that the resting copepodite instars of *A. dengizicus* were found in depth of not more than 5 cm, whereas in *M. isabellae* the depth was 20 cm. However, Elgmork (1959) demonstrated that the resting stage of Cyclopoda have been found as deep as 30 cm. Generally, the majority of the resting individuals were found in the upper layer of the mud. An important aspect of copepods is the possible factors terminating and initiating the resting period. In the present study, it seems that the change in temperatures may be considered as an important factor especially in *M. isabellae*, but changes in other environmental conditions are usually important as reviving factors, and it seems that changes in temperature, especially rising temperature, act as arousing factor in the field (Elgmork, 1959; Smyly, 1961). Wierzbicka (1962) states that temperature has no significant effect in the emergence from a resting to an active state in the laboratory and surmises, as Szlauer (1963), that a rise in the oxygen pressure may have reviving effect. It is apparent that the resting conditions in *C. strenuus strenuus* terminated by internal physiological changes in a constant environment, there thus seems to be an internal clock that can awake the animals in the absence of environmental fluctuations (Elgmork, 1959).

Moreover cannibalism was observed to occur in the population of *M. isabellae*, whereby, individuals at stage C IV predating on individuals of C I and the naupliar stages of the same species. The intensity of predation was maximal when the temperature increases, and a repetitive incidence of the females predating on males was recorded.

Cannibalism was also noticed to occur at a very lesser extent in *A. dengizicus*, whereby adults were found attacking the naupliar stages, but at certain environmental stresses like the scarcity of food and increase of temperature.

Generally, *A. dengizicus* can not persist for long and reproduce successfully in the presence of *M. isabellae*, therefore, it develops the strategy of diapause to disappear from the water column while the latter is in abundance and reappeared again in the absence of *M. isabellae* (Figures 2.1 and 2.2).

The disappearance of *A. dengizicus* may be regarded as an escape from predation by *M. isabellae* during the presence of the latter, this phenomenon was quite apparent through a laboratory experiment done here demonstrating this relation between the two species. Nilssen and Elgmork (1977) presented some evidence that diapause in *C. abyssorum* may be regarded as an escape from predation by fish during the winter. Also in insects, diapause is considered to minimize the risk of predation (Southwood, 1978).

Acknowledgements

We are grateful to Dr. M. Holynska of the Museum and Institution of Zoology, Warsaw, Poland for the identification of *M. isabellae.* H.H.M. would like to thank Prof. K. Elgmork of the Univ. Oslo, Norway for help with some important references.

References

Andrewartha, H.G., 1952. Diapause in relation to the ecology of insects. *Bil. Rev.,* 27: 50–107.

Brewer, R.H., 1964. The phenology of *Diaptomus stagnalis* (Copepoda: Calanoida). The development and the hatching of the egg stage. *Physiol. Zool.,* 37: 1–20.

Brige, E.A. and Juday, C., 1908. A summer resting stage in the development of the *Cyclops bicuspidatus* Claus. Trans. *Wis. Acad. Sci. Arts. Lett.,* 16: 1-9.

Cole, G.A., 1953. Arret du developpement chez les copepods. *Bull. Biol.,* 67: 276-287.

Danks, H.V., 1987. Insects dormancy: an ecological perspective. *Biol. Surv. Canada,* 1: 439.

Einsle, U., 1987. Zur Vertikae wan derung planktischer Copepoden m Bodensee – Obersee. *Schweizerische Zeitschift fur. Hydrologie*, 49: 303-315.

Elgmork, K., 1955. A resting stage without encystment in the annual cycle of the freshwater copepod *Cyclops strenuus strenuous*. *Ecology*, 36: 739-743.

Elgmork, K., 1959. Seasonal occurrence of *Cyclops strenuus strenuus* in relation to environment in small water bodies in Southern Norway. *Folia limnol. Scand.*, 11: 196 p.

Elgmork, K., 1962. A bottom resting stage in the planktonic freshwater copepod *Cyclops scutifer* Sars. *Oikos*, 13: 306-310.

Elgmork, K., 1964. Dynamics of Zooplankton communities in some small inundated ponds. *Folia limnol Scand.*, 12: 1-83.

Elgmork, K., 1967. On the distribution and ecology of *Cyclops scutifer* Sars in New England (Copepoda, Crustacea). *Ecology*, 48: 967-971.

Elgmork, K., 1980. Evolutionary aspects of diapause in freshwater copepods. In Kerfoot, W.C. (ed.), Evolution and Ecology of Zooplankton Communities. *Univ. Press, New England*, p. 411-417.

Elgmork, K., 1981. Extraordinary prolongation of life cycle in a freshwater planktonic copepod. *Holaric. Ecol.*, 4: 278-290.

Elgmork, K., 1996. Variation in torpidity of diapause in freshwater cyclopoids. *Hydrobiologia*, 320: 63-70

Elgmork, K., 1998. Diapause in the life cycle of *Cyclops scutifer* (Copepoda) in a meromictic lake and the problem of termination by an internal clock. *Arch. Hydrobiol. Spec. Issues. Advanc. Limnol.*, 52: 371-381.

Elgmork, K., Halvorsen, G., Eie, J. and Longland, A., 1990. Coexistence with similar life cycles in two species of freshwater copepods (Crustacea). *Hydrobiologia*, 208: 187-199.

Fryer, G. and Smyly, W., 1954. Some remarks on the resting stages of some freshwater cyclopoid and harpacticoid copepods. *Ann. Mag. nat. Hist.*, 7(12): 65-72.

Halvorsen, G., 1973. Crustacean from the high mountain area Haradangervidda, South Norway. *Rapp. Hoyfjellsokol. Forsk. Stn Finse, Norge*, 2: 1-17.

Hansen, A.M. and Jeppesen, E., 1992. Life cycle of *Cyclops vicinus* in relation to food availability, predation, diapause and temperature. *J. Plank. Res.*, 14: 591-605.

Hunt, G.W. and Robertson, A., 1977. The effect of temperature on the development time and brood size of *Diaptomus pallidus* Herrick. *Hydrobiologia,* 61: 75-80.

Maier, G., 1989. Variable life cycles in the freshwater copepod *Cyclops vicinus* (Uljanin 1875), support for the predator avoidance hypothesis? *Archiv. Hydrobiologie,* 115: 203-219.

Mansingh, A., 1971. Physiological classification of dormancies in insects. *Can. Entomol.*, 103: 983-1009.

McLaren, I.A., 1961. A biennial copepod from Lake Hazen, Ellesmere Island. *Nature,* 189: 7 74-779.

Monakov, A.V., 1958. Some data on the biology of development and reproduction of *Acanthocyclops viridis. Dokl. Acad. Nauk. SSSR* (*Tran. Am. Inst. Biol. Sci.*), 119: 613-616.

Munro, I. G., 1974. The effect of temperature on the development of egg, naupliar and copepodite stages of two species of copepods *Cyclops vicinus* (Uljanin) and *Eudiaptomus gracilis* (Sars). *Oecologia,* 16: 355-367.

Nauwerck, A., Duncan, A. Hillbricht-Ilkowska, A. and Larsson, P., 1980. Zooplankton. In: Le Cren E. D. and Lowe McConnell, R.H. (eds.). The functioning of freshwater ecosystems. *Cambridge Univ. Press. Cambridge*, p. 251-285.

Nilssen, J.P. and Elgmork, K., 1977. *Cyclops abyssorum,* life cycle dynamics and habitat selection. *Mem. Idrobio.*, 34: 197-238.

Nosova, I.A., 1970a. Life cycle of *Cyclops scutifer* Sars (Copepoda: Cyclopoida) from Kuril Lake (South Kamchatka) Instomosok. ryb. Knoz. Okeanogr., 3: 82-92 (Russian with English summary).

Nosova, I.A., 1970_b. Data on the reproduction and development of *Cyclops scutifer* Sars in Lake Kuril *Inst. morok. Ryb. Khoz. Okeanogr.*, 78: 171-185. (Russian with English summary). Izv. Tikhookean. Nauchno.

Papinska, K., 1984. The life cycle and the zones of occurrence of *Mesocyclops leuckarti* Claus (Cyclopoida, Copepoda). *Eol. Pol.*, 32: 493-531.

Santer, B. and Lampert, W., 1995. Summer diapause in cyclopoid copepods: adaptive response to a food bottleneck? *J. Anim. Ecol.*, 64: 600-613.

Smyly, W.J., 1961. The life cycle of the freshwater copepod *Mesccyclops leuckarti* Claus, in Esthwaite water. *J. Anim. Ecol.*, 30: 153-169.

Smyly, W.J., 1962. Laboratory experiments with stage V copepods of the freshwater copepod *Cyclops leuckarti* Claus, from Windermere and Esthwaite water. *Crustaceana*, 4(4): 273-280.

Southwood, T.R.E., 1978. Habitat, the templet for ecological strategies. *J. Anim. Ecol.*, 46: 337-365.

Szlauer, L., 1963. The resting stages of Cyclopoida in Stary Dwor Lake. *Polk. Arch. Hydrobiol.*, 1(24): 385-394.

Thompson, G. and Coldrey, J., 1985. The pond. Toppan Priting Company: 256 pp.

Vijverberg, J., 1977. Population structure, life histories and abundance of copepods in Tjeukemeer, the Netherlands. *Freshwater Biol.*, 7: 579-597.

Watson, N.H. and Smallman, B.N., 1971. The role of photoperiod and temperature in the induction and termination of an arrested development in two species of freshwater cyclopoid copepods. *Can. J. Zool.*, 49: 855-862.

Wierzbicka, M., 1960. *Cyclops bohater* Kozm dans le birtope. *Pol. Arch. Hydrobiol.*, 7: 143-156.

Wierzbicka, M., 1962. On the resting stage and mode of life of some species of Cyclopoida. *Pol. Arch. Hydrobiol.*, 10: 215-229.

Wierzbicka, M., 1972. The metabolic products of copepodites of various Cyclopoida species during their resting stage. *Pol. Arch. Hydrobiol.*, 19: 279-290.

Williams-Howze, J. and Coull, B.C., 1992. Are temperature and photoperiod necessary cues for encystment in the marine benthic harpacticoida copepod *Heteropsyllus nunni* Coull. *Biol. Bull.*, 182: 109-116.

Williamson, C.E., 1984. Laboratory and field experiment of feeding ecology of the cyclopoid copepode *Mesocyclops edax*. *Freshwater Biol.*, 14: 575-585.

Chapter 3

Integration of Botanicals and Microbial Pesticides for the Control of Dengue Vector, *Aedes aegypti* (Insecta : Diptera : Culicidae)

K. Murugan[1]*, *A. Naresh Kumar*[1], *K. Kovendan*[1], *K. Prasanna Kumar*[1], *Jiang-Shiou Hwang*[2] *and Donald R. Barnard*[3]

[1]*Division of Entomology, Department of Zoology, Bharathiar University, Coimbatore – 641 046, Tamil Nadu, India*

[2]*Institute of Marine Biology, National Taiwan Ocean University, Keelung 20224, Taiwan*

[3]*USDA-ARS-CMAVE, Gainesville, FL 32608, USA*

ABSTRACT

Mosquitoes are the most single group of insects in terms of public health significance and causing diseases such as malaria, filariasis, dengue fever, Japanese encephalitis and other fevers. There has been an outbreak of Chikungunya and dengue all over the India from 2006 – 2009. *Aedes aegypti*, commonly known as the Yellow Fever Mosquito, is a mosquito that can host the dengue fever, Chikungunya and yellow fever viruses. Moreover, chemical insecticides to control mosquitoes were

* Corresponding author: E-mail: kmvvk@yahoo.com

favored so far. But they are nonselective harmful to other beneficial organisms. Some of the insecticides are carcinogenic agents and are positively dangerous and even carried through food chain in turn affect the non- target organism. Therefore alternative pest control strategies, especially effective and low cost are thus needed. Hence, in the present investigation an attempt has been made to evaluate the impact of neem active principle, Azadiracthin with other microbial insecticides (*Bacillus thuringiensis, Bacillus sphaericus, Beauveria bassiana,* spinosad, nanomaterials and copepods) on dengue vector, *Aedes aegypti.* Lethal concentrations were also worked out for the neem active principal and its combination with microbial insecticides against mosquito larvae. Field trials were also conducted at the breeding sites of different agro-climatic zone of Tamil Nadu. Predatory efficacy of copepod was also tested on immature stages of dengue vector. The results are correlated and discussed on the effect of neem active principal and microbial pesticides on the mosquito vectors and changing efficacy of biopesticides against mosquito vectors management.

Keywords: *Azadiracta indica, Bacillus thuringiensis, Bacillus sphaericus, Beauveria bassiana, Spinosad, Nanomaterials, Copepods, Aedes aegypti, Larvicidal and control.*

Introduction

Mosquitoes are insects that have been around us for more than 30 million years. And it seems that, during those millions of years, mosquitoes have been honing their skills so that they are now experts at finding people to bite. Mosquitoes are common flying insects in the family Culicidae that are found around the world. There are about 3,500 species. There are three main mosquito vectors namely *Anopheles, Culex* and *Aedes* which are responsible millions of death worldwide.

A single female can layover 200 eggs at a time. Mosquito eggs can survive for more than five years. All mosquitoes need water to complete their life cycle. Not all species bite humans; some prefer birds, others prefer horses, and some will even bite frogs and turtles. Only females take blood; males feed only on plant nectar. Mosquitoes can fly considerable distances; some species remain close to their larval habitats while others can fly 20 miles or more. Mosquitoes do not develop in grass or shrubbery, although adults frequently rest in these areas during daylight hours. Mosquitoes are responsible for more human death than any other living creature.

Mosquitoes are flies with slender bodies, delicate legs, and scaled wings. The mosquito life cycle is an example of complete metamorphosis. There are four distinct stages in the life of a mosquito; egg, larva, pupa and adult. Mosquitoes are one of the most important insect pests that affect the health and well being of humans and domestic animals worldwide. If environmental conditions are favorable vast populations can occur. Female mosquitoes require a blood meal for egg production, and they produce a painful bite as they feed. While feeding, they can transmit a number of disease-causing organisms to humans and animals.

Mosquitoes are known to perceive visual, thermal and olfactory stimuli which enable them to detect light source, odour and several other volatile chemicals emanating from the skin, breath and waste products of their hosts (Takken, 1991; Davis and Bowen, 1994). Few genera of mosquitoes are major vectors of human diseases such as malaria, filariasis and viral diseases like Japanese encephalitis, dengue, dengue haemorrhagic fever, yellow fever, chikungunya, etc. Mosquitoes breed in varied habitats such as ponds, marshes, ditches, pools, drains, water containers and other similar water collections (Rozendaal, 1997). Different genera have shown specific breeding preferences. *Anopheles* sp. are associated with freshwater habitats whereas *Culex* sp. and *Mansonia* sp. may also be found in polluted conditions, including septic tanks and *Aedes* breeds in domestic, peri-domestic and other small water collection including desert coolers (Parthiban *et al.*, 2007; Rozendaal, 1997).

Dengue is transmitted to humans by the *Aedes aegypti* or more rarely the *Aedes albopictus* mosquito, which feed during the day (WHO, 2006). The WHO says some 2.5 billion people, two fifths of the world's population, are now at risk from dengue and estimates that there may be 50 million cases of dengue infection worldwide every year. The disease is now epidemic in more than 100 countries. The yellow fever mosquito, *Aedes aegypti* (*Stegomyia aegypti*, *Aedes* (*Stegomyia*) *aegypti*), is a mosquito that can spread the dengue fever, Chikungunya and yellow fever viruses, and other diseases as well. The mosquito can be recognized by white markings on legs and a marking of the form of a lyre on the thorax. It is now found in the tropics worldwide (Womack, 1993).

Yellow fever is a mosquito born viral illness that causes hemorrhagic fever in tropical Africa and South America. From April 1995 through November 1997 a dengue epidemic occurred in Ibagué (400,000 population), Colombia, where 3,419 cases were reported and DEN 2 virus was isolated from seven patients. A sero-survey conducted in 1996 found evidence of previous dengue infection in 9.6 per cent of the population, indicating that many infections had not been reported. The dengue infections occurred in all age groups, but children under five years of age were most frequently infected. Forty-five percent of this Ibagué population were born after the re-appearance of dengue in Colombia in 1972, but have never been infected with dengue virus. Most of the cases reported as dengue hemorrhagic fever did not fulfill the current case definition. *Aedes aegypti* larvae were found in 19 per cent of dwellings surveyed, most often in uncovered low tanks used for water storage. Many residents were not acquainted with the domestic nature of the mosquito vector (Camacho *et al.*, 2004).

Aedes aegypti, the primary carrier for viruses that cause dengue and dengue hemorrhagic fever and yellow fever, are widespread over large areas of the tropic and subtropics. At present, no effective vaccine is available for dengue; therefore, the only way of reducing the incidence of their disease is by mosquito control, which is frequently dependent on applications of conventional synthetic insecticides (Malavige *et al.*, 2004) chemical measures in public health programs were initially considered likely to decrease mosquito population, but these have failed because the constant use of chemical insecticides has often led to disruption of natural biological control system and outbreaks of insect species. Moreover problems created by using synthetic insecticides.

The harmful effects of chemicals on non-target populations and the development of resistance to these chemicals in mosquitoes along with the recent resurgence of different mosquito-borne diseases (Milam *et al.*, 2000) have prompted us to explore alternative, simple, sustainable methods of mosquito control.

Major drawback with the use of chemical insecticides is that they are non-selective and could be harmful to other organisms in the environment. It has also provoked undesirable effects, including toxicity to nontarget organisms, and fostered environmental and human health concerns (Lee *et al.*, 2001). The toxicity problem, together with the growing incidence of insect resistance, has called attention to the need for novel insecticides (Macedo *et al.*, 1997) and for more detailed studies of naturally occurring insecticides (Ansari *et al.*, 2000).

In the last few years, there was an increase of public concern on the safety of many chemical products that instigated a renewed interest on the use of natural products from plant origin for vector management. New botanical natural products are effective, environment-friendly, easily biodegradable, inexpensive, and readily available in many areas of the world, no ill effect on non-target organisms and have novel modes of action (Su and Mulla, 1999).

Neem (*Azadirachta indica*) is a tree in the mahogany family Meliaceae. It is one of two species in the genus *Azadirachtin*, and is native to India, Myanmar, Bangladesh, Sri Lanka, Malaysia and Pakistan, growing in tropical and semi-tropical regions. The neem tree is noted for its drought resistance. Normally it thrives in areas with sub-arid to sub-humid conditions, with an annual rainfall between 400 and 1200 mm. It can grow in regions with an annual rainfall below 400 mm, but in such cases it depends largely on ground water levels. Neem can grow in many different types of soil, but it thrives best on well drained deep and sandy soils. It is a typical tropical to subtropical tree and exists at annual mean temperatures between 21-32°C. It can tolerate high to very high temperatures and does not tolerate temperature below 4°C.

Larvicidal effect of neem (*Azadirachta indica*) and karanja (*Pongamia glabra*) oil cakes (individuals and combination) was studied against mosquito species. Both the oil cakes showed larvicidal activity against the mosquito species tested. The combination of neem and karanja oil cakes in equal proportion proved to have better effect than the individual treatments (Shanmugasundaram *et al.*, 2008).

Bacillus sphaericus is a naturally occurring soil bacterium that can effectively kill mosquito larvae present in water. *B. sphaericus* has the unique property of being able to control mosquito larvae in water that is rich in organic matter. *B. sphaericus* is effective against *Culex* spp. but is less effective against some other mosquito species. Commercially available formulations of *B. sphaericus* are sold under the trade name Vectolex. When community mosquito control is needed to reduce mosquito-borne disease, the Department of Health favors use of larvicide applications targeted to the breeding source of mosquitoes. Larvicides are more effective and less toxic than adult mosquito sprays, and the applications are unlikely to result in human exposure.

B. sphaericus is typically applied to water with high organic content where mosquito larvae live. Areas where *B. sphaericus* is often the preferred choice for mosquito control includes waste lagoons (where animal wastes are treated) and storm water catch basins. Application of *B. sphaericus* is not permitted in reservoirs that contain drinking water. *B. sphaericus* formulations must be applied by licensed pesticide applicators. The interference of the phytochemicals in combination with the microbial insecticide *Bacillus sphaericus* on the growth, development and reproduction mechanism in relation to biochemical changes are poorly understood. The plant extracts are active only at high concentrations, which h made them uneconomical for field use (Kalyanasundaram and Das, 1985). However, synthetic insecticides have been used widely in mosquito control programmes. It is suggested that the combined use of both natural and synthetic insecticides would reduce the economic environmental constrains.

Microbial larvicides such as *Bacillus thuringiensis israelensis* (Bti) and *Bacillus sphaericus* (*B. sphaericus*) are gram-positive, aerobic (facultative anaerobic) entomopathogenic soil bacteria (Johnson *et al.*, 1995; de Maagd *et al.*, 1999; Bobrowski *et al.*, 2002). Lower numbers of egg rafts have been recorded in ovitraps treated with Bti and *B. sphaericus* than in controls, and furthermore, an adverse relationship was found between the *Bacillus* product concentration and oviposition (Zahiri and Mulla, 2005).

Earlier, Murugan *et al.* (2002, 2003, 2007) investigated the interactive effect of Botanicals and bacterial insecticides (*Bacillus thuringiensis* Subsp. Israelensis, *Bacillus sphaericus*) on different species of mosquito species. Moreover, vector control is an essential and effective means for controlling transmission of vector-borne diseases, especially in areas where resistance in parasite to drugs is growing. Unlike insecticides, bio-control agents are host specific, safer to the environment, find easy application in the field, are cost-effective in production, lack infectivity and pathogenicity in mammals including man and has little evidence of resistance development in target mosquito species. Many populations of mosquito vectors of diseases have developed resistance to synthetic organic insecticides, used mostly during the last half of the 20th century. Thus interest in alternate strategies as well as in integrated control grew increased (WHO, 1982 a, b; 1986).

Beauveria bassiana is a fungus that grows naturally in soils throughout the world and acts as a parasite on various arthropod species, causing white muscardine disease; it thus belongs to the entomopathogenic fungi. It is being used as a biological insecticide to control a number of pests such as termites, whitefly, and different beetles. Its use in the control of the malaria-transmitting mosquitoes is under investigation. *Beauveria bassiana* can be used as a biological insecticide to control a number of pests such as termites, whitefly, and many other insects. Its use in the control of the malaria-transmitting mosquitoes is under investigation. As an insecticide, the spores are sprayed on affected crops as an emulsified suspension or wet table powder or applied to mosquito nets as a malaria control agent. *Beauveria bassiana* parasitizes a very wide range of arthropod hosts, and so should be considered a nonselective biological insecticide. It should not be applied to flowers visited by pollinating insects.

Spinosad (spinosyn A and spinosyn D) are a new chemical class of insecticides that are registered by the United States Environmental Protection Agency (EPA) to control a variety of insects. The active ingredient is derived from a naturally occurring soil dwelling bacterium çalled *Saccharopolyspora spinosa*. Spinosad kills susceptible species by causing rapid excitation of the insect nervous system. Due to this unique mode of action, Spinosad is valued in resistance management programs. Spinosad must be ingested by the insect, therefore it has little effect on sucking insects and non-target predatory insects. Spinosad is relatively fast acting. The insect dies within 1 to 2 days after ingesting the active ingredient. There appears to be 100 per cent mortality.

Spinosad is relatively low in toxicity to mammals and birds, and, although moderately toxic to fish, this toxicity represents a reduced risk to fish when compared with many synthetic insecticides in use. In addition, 70-90 per cent of beneficial insects and predatory wasps are left unharmed by spinosad. The unique mode of action of spinosad, coupled with a high degree of activity on targeted pests, low toxicity to non-target organisms (including many beneficial arthropods), and resistance management properties make spinosad an excellent new tool for integrated pest management.

The nanoparticles are defined as a small object that behaves as a whole unit in terms of its transport and properties. It is further classified according to size: In terms of diameter, fine particles cover a range between 100 and 2500 nanometers, while ultra fine particles, on the other hand, are sized between 1 and 100 nanometers. Similarly to ultra fine particles, nanoparticles are sized between 1 and 100 nanometers, though the size limitation can be restricted to two dimensions. Nanoparticles may or may not exhibit size-related properties that differ significantly from those observed in fine particles or bulk materials (Cristina Buzea, 2007).

Human beings have been exposed to air borne nano sized particles throughout their evolutionary stages, and such exposures have increased dramatically over the last century. The rapidly developing field of nanotechnology will result in new sources of this exposure, through inhalation, ingestion, and injection. Although nanomaterials are currently being widely used in modern technology, there is a serious lack of information concerning the human health and environmental implications of manufactured nanomaterials. Since these are relatively new particles, it is necessary to investigate their toxicological behaviour. The objective of this review was to trace the cellular response to nanosized particle exposure. Therapeutic application of selected nanoparticles together with their range of toxic doses was also reviewed. Effect of therapeutically used nanoparticles on cell membrane, mitochondrial function, prooxidant/antioxidant status, enzyme leakage, DNA, and other biochemical endpoints was elucidated. This chapter highlights the need for caution during the use and disposal of such manufactured nanomaterials to prevent unintended environmental impacts (Ansary and -Daihan, 2009).

Oxidative stress caused by free radicals generated by the interaction of particles with cells may result in cell death. Evidence of mitochondrial distribution and oxidative stress response after endocytosis of nanoparticles was noted. It was suggested that nanoparticles, because of their small sizes, could act like haptens to modify protein structures, either by altering their function or rendering them antigenic, thus raising their potential for autoimmune effects (Klimuk, 2000).

Copepods are a group of small crustaceans found in the sea and nearly every freshwater habitat. Many species are planktonic (drifting in sea waters), but more are benthic (living on the ocean floor), and some continental species may live in limno-terrestrial habitats and other wet terrestrial places, such as swamps, under leaf fall in wet forests, bogs, springs, ephemeral ponds and puddles, damp moss, or water-filled recesses (phytotelmata) of plants such as bromeliads and pitcher plants. Many live underground in marine and freshwater caves, sinkholes, or stream beds. Copepods are sometimes used as bioindicators.

Jorge *et al*. (2004), studied the Laboratory and field studies of *Macrocyclops albidus* (Crustacea: Copepoda) for biological control of mosquitoes in artificial containers in a subtropical environment. Since then, various species of predacious copepods have been tested for their potential to control mosquitoes. The exceptional potential of copepods for mosquito control was first recognized by Riviere and Thirel (1981), who observed in Tahiti that the number of *Ae. aegypti* and *Ae. polynesiensis* larvae was greatly reduced in ovitraps that contained *Mesocyclops aspericornis* accidentally introduced with creek water. Marten (1984a) independently discovered the same for *M. aspericornis* with *Ae. albopictus* larvae in artificial containers in Hawaii, and Suarez *et al*. (1984) did the same for *Ae. aegypti* larvae in water storage tanks in Colombia.

Larvivorous copepods such as *Macrocyclops albidus, Mesocyclops longisetus* and *Mesocyclops aspericornis* are highly effective for controlling *Aedes* ssp. larvae in discarded tires (Marten, 1990a; Riviere *et al*., 1987). If cyclopoids are to be an operational part of mosquito control, it is highly desirable for them to survive and function alongside other mosquito control activities such as the use of larvicides and adulticides. There is an additional reason that it would be desirable for cyclopoids to be compatible with larvicides. These tiny crustaceans prey on first instar mosquito larvae (Marten, 1989). Even if they kill all new larvae that come along, the cyclopoids will not kill larger larvae already on site when they are introduced. Mosquito larvae can take many weeks to reach the adult stage if temperatures are low or their food supply is poor (Service, 1985).

Cyclopoid copepods (planktonic microcrustaceans) have been extensively used as biocontrol agents in the South-East Asian countries for containerbreeding mosquito species like *Ae. aegypti*

(Marco *et al.*, 1992). The copepod, *Mesocyclops aspericornis*, is an effective predator of *Ae. aegypti*. It is known for its wide distribution and predatory efficiency against several species of mosquito larvae.

Hence, in the present investigations an attempt has been made to evaluate the impact of neem active principle, Azadiracthin with other microbial insecticides (*Bacillus thuringiensis, Bacillus sphaericus, Beauveria bassiana*, spinosad, nanomaterials and copepods) on the larvicidal, pupicidal toxicity effect of dengue vectors, such as *Aedes aegypti*. Studies have also included on the combined effect of neem and *Bacillus thuringiensis, Bacillus sphaericus, Beauveria bassiana* and *Spinosad* on the dengue vector of *Aedes aegypti*.

Materials and Methods

Systematic Position of *Aedes aegypti* Liston

Classification (Linnaeus, 1762)

Phylum	:	Arthropoda
Class	:	Insecta
Order	:	Diptera
Sub order	:	Namatocera
Family	:	Culicidae
Subfamily	:	Culicinae
Genus	:	*Aedes*
Species	:	*aegypti*

Collection of Eggs and Mosquitoes

The eggs of *Aedes aegypti* were collected from National Institute for Communicable Diseases (NICD), Mettupalayam, Coimbatore, Tamil Nadu, India without exposure to any insecticide, the egg rafts were then brought to the laboratory and transferred to 18 × 13 × 4 cm size enamel trays containing 500 ml water and kept for larval hatching.

Maintenance of Larvae

The mosquito larval culture will be maintained in our laboratory at 27±2°C, 75-85 per cent RH, under14L: 10D photoperiod cycles. The mosquito larvae will be fed with dog biscuits and yeast at

3:1ratio. The feeding will be continued till the larvae are transformed into the pupa stage.

Maintenance of Pupae and Adult

The pupae will be collected from the culture trays and will be now transferred to plastic containers (12 × 12 cm) containing 500 ml of water with the help of a dipper. The plastic jars will be kept in 90 × 90 × 90 cm size mosquito cage for adult emergence. The cage is made up of wooden frames and covered with polythene sheets on four sides (two laterals, one back and other one upper) and the front part as covered with a muslin cloth bottom of the cage is fitted with 10 per cent sugar solution for a period of three days before they will be provided with animal for blood feeding.

Blood Feeding of Adult *Aedes aegypti*

The adult female mosquitoes will be allowed to feed on the blood of a rabbit (exposed on the dorsal side) for two days, to ensure adequate blood feeding for 5 days. After blood feeding enamel trays with water from the culture trays will be placed in the cage for the adults to lay eggs.

Collection of Plant Materials

Neem leaves were collected from in and around Bharathiar University Campus, Coimbatore, Tamil Nadu, India. The plants were authentified at BSI (Botanical Survey of India) and the specimens were deposited at Zoology Department, Bharathiar University, Coimbatore, India.

Azadirachtin and its Preparations

Samples of AZA was obtained from Sigma Aldrich Chemical Company, USA (95 per cent pure) and diluted with distilled water to get the desired concentrations ranging from 0.05 to 1.0 ppm.

Collection and Culture of Copepod

Copepod, *Mesocyclops aspericornis* was collected from pond (Muthanamkulam, Coimbatore-641 046, India). Copepods were collected during early morning before sunrise by using 100μm mesh net.

Culture techniques are followed by methods used by Kosiyachinda *et al.* (2003) Isofemale lines were established from gravid females and maintained at the Department of Zoology, School of Life Sciences, Bharathiar University, Coimbatore, India. All the collected samples were identified and confirmed by Dr. Y. Ranga Reddy, Department of Zoology, Acharya Nagarjuna University, Andhra Pradesh, India to be *Mesocyclops aspericornis*. Once identified, gravid female *M. aspericornis* from different isofemale lines were pooled and mass-reared in dechlorinated water (pH 7) in a 15-liter fish tank at 27 ± 2°C (mean ± SD). *Paramecium* spp. prepared from boiled rice straw water extract and commercial powdered fish foods were used to support the copepod cultures. We sampled 100 copepods to apply as the initial number to each treatment that contained copepods as a control agent.

Larval/Pupal Toxicity Test of Biopesticides (Azadirachtin, Microbial Insecticides, Gold Nanoparticle)

Laboratory colonies of mosquito larvae/pupae were used for the larvicidal and pupicidal activity. Twenty-five numbers of first, second, third and fourth instar larvae and pupae were introduce into the 500 ml glass beaker containing 249 ml of de-chlorinated water and 1ml of desired concentrations of biopesticides were added separately. Larval food was given for the test larvae. At each tested concentration 2 to 5 trials were made and each trial consisted of three replicates. Mixing 1ml of acetone with 249 ml of de-chlorinated water set up the control. The control mortalities were corrected by using Abbott's formula (Abbott's, 1925).

$$\text{Corrected mortality} = \frac{\text{Observed mortality in treatment} - \text{Observed mortality in control}}{\text{100-Control mortality}} \times 100$$

$$\text{Percentage mortality} = \frac{\text{Number of dead larvae/pupae}}{\text{Number of larvae/pupae introduced}} \times 100$$

LC_{50}, LC_{90}, regression equation and 95 per cent confidence limit of lower confidence of limit (LCL) and Upper Confidence Limit (UCL) were calculated from toxicity data by using probit analysis (Finney, 1971).

LC_{50} and LC_{90} were calculated from toxicity data by using probit analysis (Finney,1971).

Predatory Efficiency Test

Adult copepods were used for the predatory activity towards the second instar mosquito larvae. Hundred numbers of mosquito larvae (I to IV instars) and ten numbers of adult copepods were introduced into the 500ml glass beaker containing 250 ml of de-chlorinated water. The mosquito larvae were replaced daily with the new ones. The experiment was held up with 3 trials and each trial consisted of three replicates. The glass beakers were checked after 24, 48, 72, 96 and 120 hours and the number of prey consumed by the predator was recorded. Predatory efficiency of a copepod was calculated by the following formula:

$$\text{Predatory efficiency a copepod} = \frac{\text{No. of fed prey / No. of predator introduced}}{\text{Total number of prey introduced}} \times 100$$

Field Trial

For the field trial the quantity of plant residues required (Based on laboratory LC_{90} values) for each treatment was determined by calculating the total surface area of the water in each habitat. The required quantities of neem were mixed thoroughly with water in a bucket with constant agitation. Teepol was used as emulsifying agent (0.05 per cent). Field applications of the neem, were done with the help of a knapsack sprayer and uniformly on the surface of the water in each habitat. Dipper sampling and counting of larvae monitored the larval density before 24 hrs, 48 hrs and 72 hrs after the treatment. A separate sample was taken to determine the species composition of each larval habitat. Twelve trails were conducted for neem combined treatment. The percentage of reduction was calculated by the following formula:

$$= \frac{C - T}{C} \times 100$$

where,

C: The total number of Mosquitoes in control

T: The total number of Mosquitoes in treatment

Statistical Analysis

All data were subjected to analysis of variance means were separated using Duncan's multiple range test DMRT by (Alder and Rossler, 1977). The average larval mortality data were subjected to probit analysis for calculating LC_{50} and LC_{90} values were calculated by using Finney's Method (1971). SPSS 18.00 versions were used.

Results

Larval and pupal toxicity effect of neem active compound, Azadirachtin on *Aedes aegypti* is shown in the Table 3.1. Greater mortality rate of larvae and pupae of *Aedes aegyti* was noticed after treated with Azadirachtin at different concentrations (25, 50, 100, 200 and 400 ppm). The maximum mortality rate was 89 per cent at 400 ppm concentration in the I instar larvae. The minimal mortality rate was 13 per cent at 25 ppm concentration in the IV instar larvae. Azadirachtin at 25ppm showed 23 per cent mortality in the I instars larvae. Similar trend has been noted for all the instars of *Aedes aegypti* at different concentration of Azadirachtin. The LC_{50} Values and LC_{90} values were represented as follows: LC_{50} value of I instar was 46.83 per cent, II instar was 52.25 per cent, III instar was 56.68 per cent, and IV instar was 62.41 per cent, respectively. LC_{90} value of I instar was 57.39 per cent, II instar was 63.15 per cent, III instar was 67.59 per cent, and IV instar was 73.07 per cent, respectively. At 25 ppm of treatment the pupal mortality was 22 per cent, where as it has been increased at 80 per cent at 400 ppm of Azadirachtin treatment. The LC_{50} value of pupal stage after the treatment of Azadirachtin was 52.95 per cent, and LC_{90} value was 65.15 per cent, respectively.

Larval and pupal toxicity effect of gold nanoparticles on *Aedes aegypti* is shown in the Table 3.2.The percentage of mortality of *Aedes aegypti* after the treatment of gold nanoparticle on I to IV instar larvae and pupal from 20,40,60,80, and 100 ppm were carried out higher mortality rate was 100 per cent at 100 ppm concentration in the I instar larvae and the minimal mortality rate was 18 per cent at 20 ppm concentration in the IV instar larvae similar trant has been noted for all the instar of Gold nanoparticles at 20 ppm showed 30 per cent mortality in the I instar larva similar trend has been noted for all the instars of *Aedes aegypti* at different concentration of gold nanoparticles treatment. The LC_{50} values and LC_{90} values were represented as follows: LC_{50} value of I instar was 20.56 per cent, II

Table 3.1: Larval and Pupal Toxicity Effect of Azadirachtin on Dengue Vector, *Aedes aegypti*

Larval and Pupal Stages	*Per cent of Larval and Pupal Mortality*					*LC_{50} and LC_{90} (per cent)*	*Regression Equation*	*95% Confidence Limit*		*Chi Square Value χ^2*
	Concentration (ppm)							*LCL*	*UCL*	
	25	*50*	*100*	*200*	*400*			*LC_{50} LC_{90} (per cent)*	*LC_{50} LC_{90} (per cent)*	
I	23[a]	39[b]	57[c]	71[d]	89[e]	52.31920 (106.92527)	0.2347	46.83849 (97.71909)	57.39602 (199.88661)	0.970
II	20[a]	37[b]	51[c]	65[d]	85[ef]	57.76461 (116.83517)	0.02207	52.25123 (105.24007)	63.15041 (131.10845)	1.397
III	18[a]	34[b]	46[c]	60[d]	84[ef]	62.06951 (120.13736)	0.02207	56.68956 (109.5587)	67.59311 (136.17150)	2.875
IV	13[a]	31[b]	39[bc]	56[d]	82[ef]	67.53251 (122.58849)	0.02328	62.41997 (111.71424)	73.07663 (138.14784)	4.332
Pupa	22	37	50	64	80	59.8748 (124.83643)	0.01949	52.95534 (111.94240)	65.15086 (144.30365)	0.367

LCL: 95 per cent Lower Confidence Limit; UCL: 95 per cent Upper Confidence Limit.

Within a column means followed by the same letter(s) are not significantly different at 5 per cent level by DMRT.

Table 3.2: Larval and Pupal Toxicity Effect of Gold Nano Particle on Dengue Vector, *Aedes aegypti*

Larval and Pupal Stages	Per cent of Larval and Pupal Mortality – Concentration (ppm)					LC_{50} and LC_{90} (per cent)	Regression Equation	95% Confidence Limit		Chi Square Value χ^2
	25	50	100	200	400			LCL LC_{50} LC_{90} (per cent)	UCL LC_{50} LC_{90} (per cent)	
I	30	48	60	82	100	42.90008 (88.01228)	0.02841	20.56055 (70.89094)	56.84703 (136.57502)	10.933
II	26	45	56	78	100	46.62834 (91.24806)	0.02872	23.33538 (72.69789)	62.23326 (150.26529)	13.157
III	24	40	52	74	100	50.16329 (94.60977)	0.02883	25.13294 (74.31660)	68.39853 (170.02407)	15.964
IV	18	36	46	66	97	56.53727 (102.11230)	0.02812	36.40152 (81.23301)	75.13421 (121.58631)	14.262
Pupa	30	48	56	75	90	46.01531 (106.66222)	0.02113	39.36579 (96.53883)	57.57194 (121.42506)	2.511

LCL: 95 per cent Lower Confidence Limit; UCL: 95 per cent Upper Confidence Limit.

Within a column means followed by the same letter(s) are not significantly different at 5 per cent level by DMRT.

instar was 23.33 per cent, III instar was 25.13 per cent, and IV instar was 36.40 per cent, respectively. LC_{90} value of I instar was 56.84 per cent, II instar was 62.23 per cent, III instar was 68.39 per cent, and IV instar was 75.13 per cent, respectively. Similar trend has been noted for all the instar of *Aedes aegypti* at different concentration of gold nanoparticles treatment. At 20 ppm of gold nanoparticles, treatment the pupal mortality rate was 30 per cent, where as it has been increased at 90 per cent at 100 ppm of gold nanoparticles treatment. The LC_{50} value of pupal stage after the treatment of gold nanoparticles was 39.36 per cent, and LC_{90} value was 57.57 per cent, respectively.

Combined effect of larval and pupal toxicity study after the treatment of Azadirachtin and gold nanoparticle is provided in the Table 3.3. The mortality was high at 2.5 ppm + 7.5 ppm concentration of Azadirachtin and gold Nanoparticles was 100 per cent mortality in the I instar larva. Similar trend has been noted for all the instar of *Aedes ageypti*. The LC_{50} values and LC_{90} values were represented as follows: LC_{50} value of I instar was -0.093 per cent, II instar was 0.47 per cent, III instar was 0.52 per cent, and IV instar was 0.46 per cent respectively. At 0.5 pm + 1.5 ppm of Azadirachtin and gold nanoparticle treatment, the pupal mortality was 50 per cent, were as it has been increased at 99 per cent at 2.5 ppm + 7.5 ppm of Azadirachtin and gold Nanoparticles treatment. The LC_{50} value of pupal stages after the treatment of Azadirachtin and gold nanoparticle was-0.004 per cent and LC_{90} value was 3.87 per cent respectively. Value of I instar was 40 per cent, II instar was 35 per cent, III instar was 32 per cent, and IV instar was 30 per cent, respectively. Similar trend has been noted for all the instar of *Aedes aegypti* at different concentration of gold nanoparticle treatment. At 0.5+1.5 ppm of gold nanoparticle, treatment the pupal mortality rate was 50 per cent, where as it has been increased at 99 per cent at 2.5+7.5 ppm of gold nanoparticle treatment. The LC_{50} value of pupal stage after the treatment of gold nanoparticle, was-0.004 per cent and LC_{90} value was 3.87 per cent, respectively.

Larval and pupal toxicity effect of *Bacillus thuringiensis* var. *israelensis* (Bti) on *Aedes aegypti* is shown in the Table 3.4. At 20 ppm of *Bacillus thuringiensis* var. *israelensis* (Bti), mortality 25 per cent in the I instar larvae. Similar trend has been noted for all the instars of *Aedes aegypti* at different concentration of *Bacillus thuringiensis* var.

Table 3.3: Larval and Pupal Toxicity Effect of Azadirachtin and Gold Nano Particle on Dengue Vector, *Aedes aegypti*

Larval and Pupal Stages	Per cent of Larval and Pupal Mortality					LC_{50} and LC_{90} (per cent)	Regression Equation	95% Confidence Limit		Chi Square Value χ^2
	Concentration (ppm)							LCL	UCL	
	0.5+1.5	1+3	1.5+4.5	2+6	2.5+7.5			LC_{50} LC_{90} (per cent)	LC_{50} LC_{90} (per cent)	
I	40	52	70	80	100	3.55465 (8.75629)	0.24637	-0.09334 (6.85900)	5.13349 (15.23275)	10.985
II	35	50	68	77	100	3.75629 (8.97126)	0.25409	0.47941 (7.00777)	5.55345 (16.02895)	12.399
III	32	48	65	74	100	4.22490 (9.23902)	0.25559	0.52195 (7.12949)	6.00946 (18.01574)	14.587
IV	30	45	60	71	100	4.55522 (9.57844)	0.25513	0.46358 (7.27943	6.60697 (21.34926)	17.328
Pupa	50	59	75	90	99	2.59859 (7.90819)	0.24136	-0.00440 (6.51540)	3.87096 (11.01288)	5.369

LCL: 95 per cent Lower Confidence Limit; UCL: 95 per cent Upper Confidence Limit.

Within a column means followed by the same letter(s) are not significantly different at 5 per cent level by DMRT.

Table 3.4: Larval and Pupal Toxicity Effect of *Bacillus thuringiensis* var. *israelensis* (Bti) on Dengue Vector, *Aedes aegypti*

Larval and Pupal Stages	Per cent of Larval and Pupal Mortality — Concentration (ppm)					LC_{50} and LC_{90} (per cent)	Regression Equation	95% Confidence Limit		Chi Square Value χ^2
	20	40	60	80	100			LCL LC_{50} LC_{90} (per cent)	UCL LC_{50} LC_{90} (per cent)	
I	25[e]	42[d]	58[e]	72[e]	89[e]	50.24 (106.99)	Y = -1.13445 + 0.2258X	44.40 (97.45)	55.5 (120.57)	0.907
II	23[c]	39[c]	53[d]	67[c]	87[d]	54.70 (113.33)	Y = -1.19542 + 0.02186 X	48.98 (102.89)	160.09 (128.41)	1.720
III	21[b]	36[b]	48[b]	62[b]	86[c]	59.03 (118.04)	Y = -1.28125 + 0.02172 X	53.50 (107.03)	64.53 (134.03)	3.444
IV	16[a]	33[a]	41[a]	58[a]	85[b]	64.33 (119.94)	Y = -1.48252 +0.02305 X	52.55 (99.96)	77.60 (165.64)	5.436
Pupa	24[d]	39[c]	52[c]	69[d]	83[a]	55.07 (117.89)	Y= -1.12346 + 0.02040X	48.99 (106.32)	60.81 (135.01)	0.288

Chi-square value significant at < 0.05 level.

Within a column means followed by the same letter(s) are not significantly different at 5 per cent level by DMRT.

israelensis. The LC_{50} Values and LC_{90} values were represented as follows: LC_{50} value of I instar was 44.40 per cent, II instar was 48.98 per cent, III instar was 53.50 per cent, and IV instar was 52.55 per cent respectively. LC_{90} value of I instar was 55.51 per cent, II instar was 60.09 per cent, III instar was 64.53 per cent, and IV instar was 77.60 per cent, respectively. At 20 ppm of *Bacillus thuringiensis* var. *israelensis* treatment the pupal mortality was 24 per cent, where as it has been increased at 83 per cent at 100 ppm of *Bacillus thuringiensis* var. *israelensis* treatment. The LC_{50} value of pupal stage after the treatment of *Bacillus thuringiensis* var. *israelensis* was 48.99 per cent. and LC_{90} value was 60.81 per cent, respectively.

Combined effect of larval and pupal toxicity study after the treatment of Azadirachtin and *Bacillus thuringiensis* var. *israelensis* (Bti) is provided in the Table 3.5. The mortality was high at 2.0 ppm + 2.0 ppm concentration of Azadirachtin and *Bacillus thuringiensis* var. *israelensis* (Bti) was 84 per cent mortality in the II instar larva. Similar trend has been noted for all the instar of *Aedes ageypti*. The LC_{50} values and LC_{90} values were represented as follows: LC_{50} value of I instar was 0.88 per cent, II instar was 0.73 per cent, III instar was 1.34 per cent, and IV instar was 1.56 per cent respectively. LC_{90} Value of I instar was 2.73 per cent, II instar was 2.43 per cent, III instar was 3.03 per cent, and IV instar was 3.21 per cent, respectively. The LC_{50} value of pupal stages after the treatment of Azadirachtin and *Bacillus thuringiensis* var. *israelensis* (Bti) was 1.71 per cent and LC_{90} value was 3.23 per cent respectively. Toxicological study as the Azadirachtin and *Bacillus thuringiensis* var. *israelensis* (Bti) showed larvicidal and pupicidal agent *Aedes aegypti*.

Larval and pupal toxicity effect of *Bacillus sphaericus* (*Bs*) on *Aedes aegypti* is shown in the Table 3.6. The percentage of mortality of *Aedes aegypti* after the treatment of *Bacillus sphaericus* (*Bs*) on I to IV instar larvae and pupal from 0.5, 1.0, 1.5, 2.0, and 2.5 ppm were carried out higher mortality rate was 77 per cent at 2.5 ppm concentration in the II instar larvae and the minimal mortality rate was 10 per cent at 0.5 ppm concentration in the IV instar larvae similar trend has been noted for all the instar of *Aedes aegypti* at different concentration of *Bacillus sphaericus* (*Bs*) treatment. The LC_{50} values and LC_{90} values were represented as follows: LC_{50} value of I instar was 1.633 per cent, II instar was 1.44 per cent, III instar was 1.93 per cent, and IV instar was 2.106 per cent respectively. LC_{90}

Table 3.5: Larval and Pupal Toxicity Effect of Azadirachtin and *Bacillus thuringiensis* var. *israelensis* (Bti) on Dengue Vector, *Aedes aegypti*

Larva and Pupa	*Per cent of Larval and Pupal Mortality*					*LC_{50} (ppm) (LCL – UCL)*	*LC_{90} (ppm) (LCL – UCL)*	*Chi Square Value (χ^2)*
	Concentration of NSKE + Bti (ppm)							
	2.0+0.25	*2.0+0.50*	*2.0+1.00*	*2.0+1.50*	*2.0+2.00*			
I	29^{b}	43^{ab}	58^{ab}	62^{b}	79^{b}	0.88 (0.69 – 1.04)	2.73 (2.34 – 3.37)	3.137
II	34^{a}	45^{a}	60^{a}	69^{a}	84^{a}	0.73 (0.54 – 0.89)	2.43 (2.11 – 2.94)	0.933
III	20^{c}	28^{b}	39^{b}	54^{c}	70^{c}	1.34 (1.18 – 1.52)	3.03 (2.63 – 3.68)	0.261
IV	14	22^{c}	34^{c}	46^{d}	64^{d}	1.56 (1.40 – 1.78)	3.21 (2.78 – 3.90)	0.523
Pupa	9^{c}	17^{d}	28^{d}	39^{e}	59^{e}	1.71 (1.52 – 1.99)	3.23 (2.78 – 3.94)	0.612

LCL: 95 per cent Lower Confidence Limit; UCL: 95 per cent Upper Confidence Limit.

Within a column means followed by the same letter(s) are not significantly different at 5 per cent level by DMRT.

Table 3.6: Larval and Pupal Toxicity Effect of *Bacillus sphaericus* (*Bs*) on Dengue Vector, *Aedes aegypti*

Larva and Pupa	*Per cent of Larval and Pupal Mortality*					*LC_{50} (ppm) (LCL – UCL)*	*LC_{90} (ppm) (LCL – UCL)*	*Chi Square Value (χ^2)*
	Concentration of Bs (ppm)							
	0.5	*1.0*	*1.5*	*2.0*	*2.5*			
I	20^{e}	31^{d}	47^{e}	63^{e}	72^{e}	1.633 (1.476 – 1.802)	3.373 (3.000 – 3.951)	0.493
II	25^{c}	37^{c}	51^{d}	67^{c}	77^{d}	1.445 (1.278 – 1.607)	3.222 (2.864 – 3.780)	0.142
III	13^{b}	25^{b}	32^{b}	49^{b}	71^{c}	1.939 (1.786 – 2.127)	3.529 (3.157 – 4.096)	2.098
IV	10^{a}	19^{a}	26^{a}	45^{a}	66^{b}	2.106 (1.947 – 2.310)	3.626 (3.249 – 4.198)	1.737
Pupa	6^{d}	15^{c}	20^{c}	38^{d}	61^{a}	2.279 (2.113 – 2.501)	3.707 (3.329 – 4.282)	2.152

LCL: 95 per cent Lower Confidence Limit; UCL: 95 per cent Upper Confidence Limit.

Within a column means followed by tho same letter(s) are not significantly different at 5 per cent level by DMRT.

value of I instar was 3.373 per cent, II instar was 3.222 per cent, III instar was 3.529 per cent, and IV instar was 3.626 per cent, respectively. Similar trend has been noted for all the instar of *Aedes aegypti* at different concentration of *Bacillus sphaericus* (*Bs*) treatment. At 0.5 ppm of *Bacillus sphaericus* (*Bs*) treatment the pupal mortality rate was 6 per cent, where as it has been increased at 61 per cent at 2.5 ppm of *Bacillus sphaericus* (*Bs*) treatment. The LC_{50} value of pupal stage after the treatment of *Bacillus sphaericus* (*Bs*) was 2.279 per cent, and LC_{90} value was 3.707 per cent, respectively.

Combined effect of larval and pupal toxicity study after the treatment of Azadirachtin and *Bacillus sphaericus* (*Bs*) is provided in the Table 3.7. The mortality was high at 2.0 ppm + 2.0 ppm concentration of Azadirachtin and *Bacillus sphaericus* (*Bs*) was 96 per cent mortality in the I instar larva. Similar trend has been noted for all the instar of *Aedes ageypti*. The LC_{50} values and LC_{90} values were represented as follows: LC_{50} value of I instar was 2.61 per cent, II instar was 3.53 per cent, III instar was 4.57 per cent, and IV instar was 5.23 per cent respectively. LC_{90} Value of I instar was 8.25 per cent, II instar was 9.26 per cent, III instar was 10.80 per cent, and IV instar was 11.94 per cent respectively. The LC_{50} value of pupal stages after the treatment of Azadirachtin and *Bacillus sphaericus* (*Bs*) was 6.38 per cent and LC_{90} value was 13.17 per cent, respectively.

Larval and pupal toxicity effect of Spinosad on *Aedes aegypti* is shown in the Table 3.8. The percentage of mortality of *Aedes aegypti* after the treatment of Spinosad on I to IV instar larvae and pupal from 0.01, 0.02, 0.04, 0.06 and 0.08 ppm were carried out higher mortality rate was 80 per cent at 0.08 ppm concentration in the I instar larvae and the minimal mortality rate was 28 per cent at 0.01 ppm concentration in the III instar larvae. Similar trend has been noted for all the instar of *Aedes aegypti* at different concentration of Spinosad treatment. The LC_{50} values and LC_{90} values were represented as follows: LC_{50} value of I instar was 0.15 per cent, II instar was 0.21 per cent, III instar was 0.27 per cent, and IV instar was 0.26 per cent respectively. LC_{90} value of I instar was 0.32 per cent, II instar was 0.36 per cent, III instar was 0.41 per cent, and IV instar was 0.04 per cent respectively. Similar trend has been noted for all the instar of *Aedes aegypti* at different concentration of Spinosad treatment. At 0.01 ppm of Spinosad, treatment the pupal mortality rate was 35 per cent, where as it has been increased at 79 per cent at 0.08 ppm of Spinosad treatment. The LC_{50} value of pupal stage after

Table 3.7: Larval and Pupal Toxicity Effect of Azadirachtin and *Bacillus sphaericus* (*Bs*) on Dengue Vector, *Aedes aegypti*

Larva and Pupa	*Per cent of Larval and Pupal Mortality*					*LC_{50} (ppm) (LCL – UCL)*	*LC_{90} (ppm) (LCL – UCL)*	*Chi Square Value (χ^2)*
	Concentration of NSKE + Bs (ppm)							
	2.0+0.25	*2.0+0.25*	*2.0+0.25*	*2.0+0.25*	*2.0+0.2*			
I	45[e]	62[d]	78[e]	88[e]	96[e]	2.612 (1.677 – 3.298)	8.253 (7.478 – 9.354)	0.209
II	38[c]	55[c]	68[d]	82[c]	95[d]	3.536 (2.767 – 4.139)	9.266 (8.413 – 10.811)	1.710
III	31[b]	47[b]	57[b]	75[b]	89[c]	4.577 (3.890 – 5.160)	10.806 (9.757 – 12.351)	1.530
IV	29[a]	41[a]	52[a]	68[a]	85[b]	5.232 (4.562 – 5.840)	11.948 (10.697 – 13.847)	1.711
Pupa	22[d]	35[c]	41[c]	60[d]	79[a]	6.383 (5.767 – 7.034)	13.171 (11.749 – 15.354)	2.831

LCL: 95 per cent Lower Confidence Limit; UCL: 95 per cent Upper Confidence Limit.

Within a column means followed by the same letter(s) are not significantly difforont at 5 per cent level by DMRT.

Table 3.8: Larval and Pupal Toxicity Effect of Spinosad on Dengue Vector, *Aedes aegypti*

Larval and Pupal Stages	*Per cent of Larval and Pupal Mortality*					*Value of LC_{50} and LC_{90} (per cent)*	*Regression Equation*	*95% Confidence Limit*		*Chi Square Value χ^2*
	Concentration (ppm)							*LCL*	*UCL*	
	0.01	*0.02*	*0.04*	*0.06*	*0.08*			*LC_{50} LC_{90} (per cent)*	*LC_{50} LC_{90} (per cent)*	
I	37	49	61	74	80	0.2496 (0.1018)	16.46855	0.1530 (0.0870)	0.3216 (0.1271)	1.153
II	34	44	59	73	79	0.2964 (0.1018)	17.75401	0.2160 (0.8779)	0.3618 (0.1248)	1.078
III	28	43	57	69	76	0.3471 (0.1070)	17.71390	0.2739 (0.9225)	0.4115 (0.1313)	2.674
IV	31	42	55	70	73	0.3484 (0.1141)	16.16937	0.2677 (0.9693)	0.0418 (0.4371)	2.284
Pupa	35	59	59	75	79	0.2746 (0.1042)	17.32660	0.1877 (0.1871)	0.0325 (0.0125)	1.0125

LCL: 95 per cent Lower Confidence Limit; UCL: 95 per cent Upper Confidence Limit.

Within a column means followed by the same letter(s) are not significantly different at 5 per cent level by DMRT.

Table 3.9: Larval and Pupal Toxicity Effect of Azadirachtin and Spinosad on Dengue Vector, *Aedes aegypti*

Larval and Pupal Stages	Per cent of Larval and Pupal Mortality – Concentration (ppm)					Value of LC_{50} and LC_{90} (per cent)	Regression Equation	95% Confidence Limit		Chi Square Value χ^2
	0.01+2	0.02+4	0.04+6	0.06+8	0.08+10			LCL LC_{50} LC_{90} (per cent)	UCL LC_{50} LC_{90} (per cent)	
I	40	44	50	66	69	5.0658 (17.6052)	0.10220	3.6490 (14.2292)	6.1616 (25.0796)	1.661
II	35	37	47	50	65	6.9335 (20.7535)	0.0927	5.299 (16.2640)	8.5209 (31.7005)	1.765
III	32	34	43	47	61	7.9255 (22.0073)	0.09101	6.6743 (17.0924)	10.3755 (34.2894)	1.405
IV	28	33	42	46	59	7.3587 (21.4678)	0.09735	7.0887 (16.9227)	10.3755 (32.1462)	0.662
Pupa	34	36	45	49	63	7.3587 (21.5391)	0.09037	6.1253 (16.7401)	9.1840 (33.5457)	1.449

LCL: 95 per cent Lower Confidence Limit; UCL: 95 per cent Upper Confidence Limit.

Within a column means followed by the same letter(s) are not significantly different at 5 per cent level by DMRT.

the treatment of Spinosad was 0.18 per cent, and LC_{90} value was 0.03 per cent, respectively.

Combined effect of larval and pupal toxicity study after the treatment of Azadirachtin and Spinosad is provided in the Table 3.9. The mortality was high at 0.08 ppm + 10 ppm concentration of Azadirachtin and Spinosad was 69 per cent mortality in the I instar larva. Similar trend has been noted for all the instar of *Aedes ageypti*. The LC_{50} values and LC_{90} values were represented as follows: LC_{50} value of I instar was 3.64 per cent, II instar was 5.29 per cent, III instar was 6.67 per cent, and IV instar was 7.08 per cent respectively. LC_{90} Value of I instar was 6.16 per cent, II instar was 8.52 per cent, III instar was 10.37 per cent, and IV instar was 10.37 per cent respectively. The LC_{50} value of pupal stages after the treatment of Azadirachtin and Spinosad was 6.12 per cent and LC_{90} value was 9.18 per cent, respectively.

Combined effect of larval and pupal toxicity study after the treatment of Azadirachtin and *Beauveria bassiana* is provided in the Table 3.10. The mortality was high at 0.08 ppm + 10 ppm concentration of Azadirachtin and *Beauveria bassiana* was 69 per cent mortality in the I instar larva. Similar trend has been noted for all the instar of *Aedes ageypti*. The LC_{50} values and LC_{90} values were represented as follows: LC_{50} value of I instar was 3.64 per cent, II instar was 5.29 per cent, III instar was 6.67 per cent, and IV instar was 7.08 per cent respectively. LC_{90} Value of I instar was 6.16 per cent, II instar was 8.52 per cent, III instar was 10.37 per cent, and IV instar was 10.37 per cent respectively. The LC_{50} value of pupal stages after the treatment of Azadirachtin and *Beauveria bassiana* was 6.12 per cent and LC_{90} value was 9.18 per cent, respectively. Toxicological study as the Azadirachtin and *Beauveria bassiana* showed larvicidal and pupicidal agent *Aedes aegypti*.

Larval and pupal toxicity effect of *Beauveria bassiana* on *Aedes aegypti* is shown in the Table 3.11.The percentage of mortality of *Aedes aegypti* after the treatment of *Beauveria bassiana* on I to IV instar larvae and pupal from 0.5, 1.0, 1.5, 2.0 and 2.5 ppm were carried out higher mortality rate was 80 per cent at 2.5 ppm concentration in the II instar larvae and the minimal mortality rate was 10 per cent at 0.5 ppm concentration in the IV instar larvae. Similar trend has been noted for all the instar of *Aedes aegypti* at different concentration of *Beauveria bassiana* treatment. The LC_{50} values and LC_{90} values were

Table 3.10: Larval and Pupal Toxicity Effect of Azadirachtin and *Beauveria bassiana* on Dengue Vector, *Aedes aegypti*

Larval and Pupal Stages	Per cent of Larval and Pupal Mortality — Concentration (ppm)					Value of LC_{50} and LC_{90} (per cent)	Regression Equation	95% Confidence Limit		Chi Square Value χ^2
	0.01+2	0.02+4	0.04+6	0.06+8	0.08+10			LCL LC_{50} LC_{90} (per cent)	UCL LC_{50} LC_{90} (per cent)	
I	40	44	50	66	69	5.0658 (17.6052)	0.10220	3.6490 (14.2292)	6.1616 (25.0796)	1.661
II	35	37	47	50	65	6.9335 (20.7535)	0.0927	5.299 (16.2640)	8.5209 (31.7005)	1.765
III	32	34	43	47	61	7.9255 (22.0073)	0.09101	6.6743 (17.0924)	10.3755 (34.2894)	1.405
IV	28	33	42	46	59	7.3587 (21.4678)	0.09735	7.0887 (16.9227)	10.3755 (32.1462)	0.662
Pupa	34	36	45	49	63	7.3587 (21.5391)	0.09037	6.1253 (16.7401)	9.1840 (33.5457)	1.449

LCL: 95 per cent Lower Confidence Limit; UCL: 95 per cent Upper Confidence Limit.

Within a column means followed by the same letter(s) are not significantly different at 5 per cent level by DMRT.

Table 3.11: Larval and Pupal Toxicity Effect of *Beauveria bassiana* on Dengue Vector, *Aedes aegypti*

Larva and Pupa	*Per cent of Larval and Pupal Mortality*					*LC_{50} (ppm) (LCL – UCL)*	*LC_{90} (ppm) (LCL – UCL)*	*Chi Square Value (χ^2)*
	Concentration of Baveria bassiana (per cent)							
	0.5	*1.0*	*1.5*	*2.0*	*2.5*			
I	22^{ab}	34^{ab}	49^{ab}	65^{ab}	76^{ab}	1.53 (1.37 – 1.69)	3.23 (2.89 – 3.77)	1.102
II	24^{b}	37^{a}	53^{c}	68^{a}	80^{a}	1.41 (1.25 – 1.56)	3.05 (2.74 – 3.53)	0.018
III	14^{b}	26^{b}	34^{c}	51^{b}	76^{b}	1.84 (1.70 – 2.01)	3.35 (3.02 – 3.84)	3.208
IV	10^{c}	22^{b}	29^{d}	46^{c}	72^{bc}	1.99 (1.85 – 2.17)	3.43 (3.10 – 3.93)	3.135
Pupae	8^{c}	18^{cd}	24^{d}	42^{cd}	68^{c}	2.12 (1.97 – 2.31)	3.53 (3.19 – 4.04)	3.110

LCL: 95 per cent Lower Confidence Limit; UCL: 95 per cent Upper Confidence Limit.

Within a column means followed by the same letter(s) are not significantly different at 5 per cent level by DMRT.

represented as follows: LC_{50} value of I instar was 1.53 per cent, II instar was 1.41 per cent, III instar was 1.84 per cent, and IV instar was 1.99 per cent respectively. LC_{90} value of I instar was 3.23 per cent, II instar was 3.05 per cent, III instar was 3.35 per cent, and IV instar was 3.43 per cent respectively. Similar trend has been noted for all the instar of *Aedes aegypti* at different concentration of *Beauveria bassiana* treatment. At 0.5 ppm of *Beauveria bassiana*, treatment the pupal mortality rate was 8 per cent, where as it has been increased at 68 per cent at 2.5 ppm of *Beauveria bassiana* treatment. The LC_{50} value of pupal stage after the treatment of *Beauveria bassiana* was 2.12 per cent, and LC_{90} value was 3.53 per cent, respectively.

Table 3.12 showing the copepod, *Mesocyclops aspericornis* showed effective predation against the larval instars of *Aedes aegypti*. It provides the percentage of predatory efficiency of copepods towards the differe nt larval instars of *Aedes aegypti*. The percentage predatory efficiency of a single adult copepod, *Mesocyclops aspericornis* against the I instars larvae of the *Aedes aegypti* was 6.80 per cent and percentage predatory efficiency of copepod against II, III, IV instars larvae were 3.81 per cent, 1.20 per cent, and 0.33 per cent, respectively.

Table 3.13 showing the copepod, *Mesocyclops aspericornis* showed effective predation against the larval instars of *Aedes aegypti* after the treatment of Azadirachtin. It provides the percentage of predatory efficiency of copepods towards the different larval instars of *Aedes aegypti*. The percentage predatory efficiency of a single adult copepod, *Mesocyclops aspericornis* against the I instars larvae of the *Aedes aegypti* was 8.40 per cent and percentage predatory efficiency of copepod against II, III, IV instars larvae were 4.28 per cent, 1.63 per cent, and 0.43 per cent, respectively.

Table 3.14 provides field trial after using Neem extract of against malarial vector, *Aedes aegypti* at breeding habitats (Bharathiar University Campus) Coimbatore, India. Field trial has been conducted by using the Neem extract of dengue vector, *Aedes aegypti* (overhead tank). Neem extract were prepared at required concentrations and sprayed by using knapsack sprayer. Bio-efficacy of plant extract have been noted. Based on the lethal concentrations of plants the LC_{90} value has been doubled for Neem extract and sprayed individually at different breeding sites of dengue vector. The percentage of larval reduction was noticed during 24 hrs, 48 hrs

Table 3.12: Predatory Efficiency of Copepods, *Mesocyclops aspericornis* on Dengue Vector, *Aedes aegypti*

Mosquito Larval Instars	*No. of Copepod Introduced*	*Predation*					*Average Predation*	*Percentage Predatory Efficiency*
		Time (in hr)						
		Day-1	*Day-2*	*Day-3*	*Day-4*	*Day-5*		
I	10	152±9.2	144±7.9	140±8.6	139±8.0	110±6.8	137[a]	6.80[a]
II	10	93±8.1	79±7.1	76±6.9	68±5.6	65±7.0	76.2[b]	3.81[b]
III	10	36±3.6	29±3.1	18±2.7	16±3.0	21±1.9	24[c]	1.20[c]
IV	10	9±1.6	5±1.1	8±0.9	6±0.6	5±0.5	6.6[d]	0.33[d]

Within Column means followed by the same letter(s) are not significantly different at 5 per cent level by DMRT.

Table 3.13: Predatory Efficiency of Copepods, *Mesocyclops aspericornis* on Dengue Vector, *Aedes aegypti* After the Treatment Azadirachtin

Mosquito Larval Instars	*No. of Copepod Introduced*	*Predation*					*Average Predation*	*Percentage Predatory Efficiency*
		Time (in hr)						
		Day-1	*Day-2*	*Day-3*	*Day-4*	*Day-5*		
I	10	182±8.09	171±7.6	166±4.6	159±6.04	162±8.6	168[a]	8.40[a]
II	10	102±7.1	88±8.3	83±8.0	76±5.7	79±7.0	85.6[b]	4.28[b]
III	10	39±3.5	33±3.5	36±4.4	27±4.06	28±2.2	32.6[c]	1.63[c]
IV	10	10±0.9	9±0.7	7±1.6	9±0.5	8±1.8	8.6[d]	0.43[d]

Within Column means followed by the same letter(s) are not significantly different at 5 per cent level by DMRT.

and 72 hrs at the breeding sites. There was complete reduction of larval density was noted after the treatment of plant extracts. Similarly, larval reduction was also noted after the treatment of plant extract at the different breeding habitats of dengue vector, *Aedes aegypti*.

Table 3.14: Field Trail by Using Neem (*Azadiracta indica*) Extract of Against Dengue Vector, *Aedes aegypti*

Place:	Bharathiar University Campus, Coimbatore
Habitat:	Water Tank
Size:	3x2 m
Depth:	1 cm
Species:	*Aedes aegypti*
Stage:	Larvae
Calculation:	$3 \times 2 = 6 \times 1.34 \times 10 = 80.4$
Required Concentration:	80.4 percentage

Sl.No.	*Larval Density*			
	Before Treatment	*After Treatment*		
		24 hrs	*48 hrs*	*72 hrs*
1.	298	19	3	—
2.	307	25	9	—
3.	193	13	4	—
4.	187	11	2	—
5.	164	21	6	—
6.	276	14	3	—
Total	1425	103	27	—
Average	237.5	17.17	4.5	—
Reduction	—	92.8 per cent	98.1 per cent	100 per cent

Discussion

Mosquitoes cause more human suffering than any other organism. Over one million people die from mosquito-borne diseases every year. Not only can mosquitoes carry diseases that afflict humans, they also transmit several diseases and parasites that dogs and horses are very susceptible to. Dengue is a serious arborvitae disease of the Americas, Asia and Africa. Although it has a low mortality, dengue has very uncomfortable symptoms and has become more serious, both in frequency and mortality, in recent years. *Aedes aegypti* and *Ae. albopictus* are the vectors of dengue and chikungunya. During the 1950s, chemicals such as DDT were the main weapons used in this battle (Breakley *et al.*, 1984), and whose apparent success was evident 30 years ago with the eradication of *Aedes aegypti* from 18 countries of the American continent (Kuno, 1995; Guzman and Kouri, 2002). Recently, the outbreak of chikungunya was happened during 2006-2007 in the Asia pacific region (www.mongpalatino.motime.com).

Mosquitoes can be an annoying, serious problem in man's domains. They interfere with work and spoil hours of leisure time. Their attacks on farm animal can cause loss of weight and decreased milk production. Some mosquitoes are capable of transmitting disease such as malaria, Yellow fever, dengue, filariasis, etc. There are three main mosquito vectors namely Anopheles, Culex and Aedes which are responsible for million of death worldwide. The medical importance of mosquitoes as vectors for the transmission of serious diseases that cause morbidity, mortality, economical loss and social distribution (Becker *et al.*, 2003).

At present effective vaccine is not available for dengue; therefore, the only way of reducing the incidents of their disease in by mosquito control, which is frequently dependent applications of conventional synthetic insecticides (Malavige *et al.*, 2004). Use of chemical insecticide has often led to disruption on natural biological control system and outbreaks of insect species. Moreover problem created by using synthetic insecticides.

Neem-based pesticides are now extensively used in agriculture practices all over the world. It contains azadirachtin, which is a predominant insecticidal active ingredient, having antifeedant, ovipositional deterrence repellency, growth disruption, sterility and larvicidal action against insects (Schmutterer, 1990). In the present study different concentrations of Neem Seed Kernel Extract showed appreciable mortality against the different larval instars of *Aedes aegytpi*. The earlier instars were more susceptible than the late instars. The active compounds of NSKE were seemed to interrupt the developmental hormones and arrest the moulting process. Hence, the treated larvae showed no moulting or very late moulting which leads to death of the larvae. As corroborate to our present study there are various reports on control of mosquito breeding under laboratory and field conditions. An emulsion of neem oil in water was found to be effective in controlling breeding of *Cx. quinquefasciatus*, *An. stephensi* and *Ae. aegypti* in pools, tanks and coolers up to 2 to 3 weeks (Batra *et al.*, 1998) whereas an application of neem cake powder resulted in drastic reduction in the late instar larvae and pupae of culicine mosquitoes in paddy field (Rao *et al.*, 1992). Murugan *et al.* (1996) established the neem seed kernel extract possess antipupational property for mosquito species. Murugan and Jeyabalan (1999) studied the effect of some indigenous plants on the larvicide and ovipositional properties on *Anopheles stephensi*. Babu and Murugan (2000) investigated that the larvicidal effect of resinous extracts from the tender leaves of *Azadirachta indica*.

In the present study, the larvicidal activity against *Aedes aegypti* was more pronounced with the neem, *Bacillus thuringiensis*, *Bacillus sphaericus*, *Beauveria bassiana*, Spinosad and nanomaterial. These results suggest that neem acts as best interpreter with the microbial pesticides for the production of greater toxicity rate in the immature stages of mosquitoes. Sukumar *et al.* (1991) has pointed out the most promising botanical mosquito control agents are in the families' Astraceae, Cladophoraceae, Lamiaceae, Meliaceae, Oocystaceae and Rutaceae.

In the present study, neem, *Bacillus thuringiensis*, *Bacillus sphaericus*, *Beauveria bassiana*, Spinosad and nanomaterial have been brought out toxicity on different larval instars of *Aedes aegypti* and moreover complete reduction of larval and pupal moratlity was noticed after combination of neem with *Bacillus thuringiensis*, *Bacillus sphaericus*, *Beauveria bassiana*, Spinosad and nanomaterial. At the highest concentration tested (*i.e.* 100ppm) the mortality 100 per cent was higher in I instar larva. The 22 plant samples were extracted in acetone and petroleum ether separately. The xtracts were tested for their activity against larval of *Cluex quinquefasciatus*. The extract was studied further with pyrethrum for its synergistic and the synergistic factor was 0.81 at 5mg/l (Thangam and Kathiresan, 1992). The extracts for the prolongation of developmental period and induction of morphogenetic abnormalities of mosquito larval treated with plant extracts are generally attributed to the extracts with the endocrine system (Zebitz, 1984; 1986). Further studies to understand the chemical nature of the extracts and field trials were required.

Various organisms, known as natural biological control agents, can be utilized to control mosquito populations, thus avoiding the use of chemicals and harm to the environment in the process. It is desirable to use biological control agents that can adapt to mosquito breeding habitats, are found naturally, and pose no danger to people (Rishikesh *et al.*, 1988; Spielman *et al.*, 1993). We have already established by integrating plant products with Bacterial larvicide's such as *Bacillus thuringiensis* israelensis (Bti) and *Bacillus sphaericus* as well as fungal pathogen, *Beauveria bassiana* for the control of mosquito vectors (Murugan *et al.*, 2003).

In the present study copepods are very much booming as predators with first and second instar larvae but are not effective against the late instars. Hence, a combined approach have been made to increase the predatory efficiency of copepods against the late instars. In conjunction with neem the copepods showed higher predation against *A. aegypti* larvae when compared with individual treatment. Azadirachtin and other Allelochemicals such as azadirachtin, nimbin, nimbidin, nimbolides, nimolic acid, salanin, meliantriol, azadirachtol present in Azadirachtin interrupted the development and active movement of early and late instar larvae, which increased the predatory efficacy of copepod on the early and also late instars. The active chemicals compounds in neem also showed no effect on the development of copepod. Similar investigations have also done on the *M. aspericornis* in conjunction with other controlling methods resulted in the eradication of *Ae. aegypti* (Locantoni *et al.*, 2006; Lardeux *et al.*, 1992; Nam *et al.*, 2000; Russell *et al.*, 1996; Kay *et al.*, 1992). *Bacillus thuringiensis* var. *israelensis* has been used in conjunction with *M. aspericornis* because of its high toxicity and high specificity to mosquito larvae. (Riviere *et al.*, 1987; Tietze *et al.*, 1994).

Biological control, using the natural enemies of *Aedes*, appears to be an alternative approach to the systematic failure of use of insecticides (Lardeux *et al.*, 2002). Employing the copepods for the mosquito control is another option and the acquired result shows that copepods and other predators can be the best alternative to synthetic insecticides. The development of resistance to botanical insecticides may also be compromised by the predatory copepods.

Among the microbial pesticides, bacterial insecticide belonging to *Bacillus thuringiensis* constitutes a dominant group. *Bacillus thuringiensis* produces many parasporal crystal toxins during sporulation that on proteolysis bind on the specialized midgut receptors, thereby causing disruption of gut epithelium, gut paralysis, toxemia and eventual death of the host insect. Considerable mortality was evident after the treatment of Bt and there was significant mortality after the combined treatment with Bt toxins and it implies that the Bt toxins might have affected on the midgut of mosquito and brought such a toxicity. The gram-positive endospore forming bacterium *Bacillus thuringiensis* produces parasporal crystalline inclusion that contain polypeptides (δ-endotoxin) that are toxic to a variety of insect species. The toxin induces the formation of a lytic pore in the midgut epithelial membrane that results in cell lysis, cessation of feeding and death of the larva (Charles and de Barjac, 1983; Singh *et al.*, 1986; Daniel *et al.*, 1995). In the present study, Bti treated larvae showed mortality as well as lower growth rate suggested that, *Bt* toxins might have interfered the gut system and brought out higher mortality at high dose treatment and also inhibited growth after the treatment of Bt toxin at lower dose.

Addition of Bti with the plant extracts had adverse effect upon the larval mortality. When combined with plant extracts, Bti increased the percentage of larval mortality and decreased the time to kill when compared with treatment contain only Bti. The addition of Bti with plant extracts caused a significant mortality due to avoidance of treated diet and may be due to increased toxicity (Gould *et al.*, 1991). In the present study, the results showed higher mortality in the combined treatment of Bti and neem. It can therefore be concluded that Bti and plant compounds caused swelling of the gut epithelial cells (Nasiruddin and Mordue (Luntz), 1993). At naturally occurring concentrations, allelochemicals produce midgut lesions, reduce feeding, growth and increase mortality (Lindroth *et al.*, 1988). Larvae of *Culex quinquefasciatus* treated with *Bacillus thuringiensis* var. *israelensis* exhibited reduced weight gain and delayed development compared with control and result in a delayed (or) inhibition of moulting (Sieber and Rembold, 1983). In the present study also at lower dose level caused growth regulatory activities. Mortality of *Culex quinquefasciatus* after the treatment of Bti at different dose level showed considerable effect on the various larval instars and dose dependent mortality were evident at Bt toxin treatment. Larval feeding behaviour of these two strains was different when they were exposed to potato foliage treated with Cry IIIA (Alter *et al.*, 1996).

The fast ecological changes of the environment and the emergence of vector-borne diseases and morphological variation in vector species are warranted to plane innovative strategy to use *B. sphaericus* as a sustainable mosquito control in semi-arid zone of India (Singh and Prakash, 2008). For the control of mosquito larvae, research on the larvicidal potential of microbial particular fungi has been extensively carried out but with varied results (Vyas *et al.*, 2007). Moreover, resistance to *B. sphaericus* can be readily induced in the laboratory, and resistance has developed in the field population of mosquitoes in several parts of the world. *Bacillus sphaericus*, a spore-forming, entomopathogenic bacterium, has been shown to possess potent larvicidal activity against several species of mosquito larvae (Davidson, 1983).

In the present study *Bacillus sphaericus* the bacterial pesticide was isolated from the soil samples and used to control the Dengue vector, *Aedes aegypti*. *Bacillus sphaericus* showed a good control over *Aedes aegypti* which may be due to the presence of binary toxin (Bin) and mosquitocidal toxins (Mtxs). As a consequence of the specific toxicity to mosquito larvae of binary toxin (Bin) and mosquitocidal toxins (Mtxs) produced during the sporulation and vegetative stages, respectively, some toxic strains have been widely used for many years as biopesticides in the field in mosquito control programs. The soil bacterium showed varied mortality rate related to the larval stages and concentrations. The younger larval stages were much susceptible than the later ones. Active strains of *B. sphaericus* are known to produce considerable quantities of at least two sets of proteinaceous mosquito larvicidal factors (MLF) at the onset of stationary phase (Souza *et al.*, 1988; Baumann *et al.*, 1991).

Beauveria bassiana is one of the frequently isolated entmopathogenic fungal genera and has a cosmopolitan distribution. Although the genus has a very broad host ranges (Roberts, 1974). The natural occurrence of *Beauveria* on mosquitoes has been reported only four times (Clarak *et al.*, 1968). Besides infecting larvae, the fungus proved to be virulent to adult mosquito as well, although no *Beauveria* infected adult mosquito have been reported for results.

In the present study, Laboratory test against adult *Culex tarsalis*, *Culex pipens*, *Aedes aegypti* and *Anopheles albimanus*, conidia of

Beauveria bassiana produced 100 per cent mortality within 5 days after exposure, while less than 50 per cent occurred in corresponding control (Clark *et al.*, 1968). In laboratory rests 82 per cent of *Anopheles gambiae* were infected, with an LT_{50} of 3.85 days from the control group (Scholte *et al.*, 2003). Later studies confirmed the existence of toxins produced by species of this genus; Beauverician, Bassianin, Bassianolide, Beauverolides and Tenellin form *B. bassiana* and Oospoerin from *B. brogniartii* (Ferron, 1981; Grove and Pople, 1980; Strasser *et al.*, 2000). A dicholoromethane extract form mycelium showed acitivity when assayed against *Aedes aegypti* larvae at 100ppm (Gupta *et al.*, 1995). This extract contained Beauverian and two analogous (Beauverian A and B). The larvicidal properties of Beauvericin had already been reported by Grove and Pople (1980), who found 86 per cent mortality with *Aedes aegypti* larvae after 48 hrs (Strasser *et al.*, 2000). In the present investigation, *Beauveria bassiana* have been brought out mosquitocidal toxicity on different larval instars of against dengue vector, *Aedes aegypti*.

Spinosad proved to be highly toxic to larvae of both species of mosquitoes in laboratory assays. Laboratory assays on *C. capitata* indicated LC_{50} values of 0.013 ppm. for neonate larvae continuously exposed in diet (Ada´n *et al.*, 1996), Spinosad is slower acting than many conventional chemical insecticides, such that observations of mortality shortly after exposure may not accurately reflect the proportion of the population that have acquired a lethal dose of the compound (Williams *et al.*, 2003). In demographic studies on *Daphnia pulex*, continuous exposure to spinosad resulted in population extinction at >0.01 ppm. However, spinosad was at least five times less toxic than the organophosphate diazinon during continuous exposure studies.

Human beings have been exposed to airborne nanosized particles throughout their evolutionary stages, and such exposures have increased dramatically over the last century. The rapidly developing field of nanotechnology will result in new sources of this exposure, through inhalation, ingestion, and injection. Although nanomaterials are currently being widely used in modern technology, there is a serious lack of information concerning the human health and environmental implications of manufactured nanomaterials. Since these are relatively new particles, it is necessary to investigate their toxicological behaviour. The objective of this review was to trace the cellular response to nanosized particle exposure. Therapeutic application of selected nanoparticles together with their range of toxic doses was also reviewed. Effect of therapeutically used nanoparticles on cell membrane, mitochondrial function, prooxidant/antioxidant status, enzyme leakage, DNA, and other biochemical endpoints was elucidated. This chapter highlights the need for caution during the use and disposal of such manufactured nanomaterials to prevent unintended environmental impacts (Ansary and Daihan, 2009). In the present study it is also evident that the percentage of mortality of *Aedes aegypti* against Gold Nanoparticles was increased as the concentration was increased and the mortality was high in early instar when compared with the later ones. This is the first time nanoparticles have been used for the control of mosquito vectors and it showed a good result.

Mesocyclops is one of the genus of copepods that has most been studied as an antagonist of mosquito larvae and whose effectiveness has been demonstrated in different countries, including the United States (Marten, 1990), Honduras (Marten *et al.*, 1994a), The present work acquaints that the predatory efficacy of *Mesocyclops aspericornis* is substantial against the different larval instars of *Ae. aegypti*. The predator *Mesocyclops aspericornis* preferred maximum on the first and second instar larvae. This may be due to the active movements showed by the late larval instars and the increased size in third and fourth larval stages. Though there was no sustainable predation on the late instars, punctures and injures are seen on the late instars, which lead to constrained development and death. This shows the approach of *Mesocyclops aspericornis* towards the late instars in starvation. As a support reports from earlier work states that, *Mesocyclops thermocyclopoides* is a very common species in Costa Rica (Collado *et al.*, 1984, Hernández-Chavarría and Schaper, 2000) and was evaluated as a biological control agent against *Aedes*. This copepod feeds on the 1st and 2nd instars of the mosquito larvae, fatally wounding about seven individuals per day (Shaper and Hernández, 1998).

In the present study, the field trials were conducted by using *Azadiracta indica* (neem) treatment in Coimbatore city, India. The percentage reduction of larval mortality of impact of geographical affect and environmental pollution of *Aedes agepti*. Field have been conducted to test on the efficacy to neem seed kernel extract, pogamia seed kernel extract lecuas leaves extract with Bti toxin at different breeding habitats of *Culex quinquefaciatus* in and around Bharathiar university campus, Coimbatore for the field trial the quantity of plant residues and Bti required (Based on the laboratory of LC_{90} values). For each treatment was determined by calculating the total surface area of the each habitat. Piper sampling and counting of larvae as been monitored on the larval density before 24 hours, 48 hours and 72 hours after treatment. Among the plant extract treatment the neem and pongamia seed extracts, pongamia seed kernel extract, leucas leaves and Bti broth our higher mortality within shorter span of time suggest the interactive effect of plant extract with Bti toxins. The thin film of oiling layer of plant extracts spread on the water surface which cuts of oxygen supply to mosquito larvae come up to the water surface, which cuts of oxygen supply to the mosquito larvae come up to the water surface to breathe. Further plant principle dissolved into the water and penetrates the larvae through the respiratory table and kills it either by suffocation or by poisoning (Murugan *et al.*, 2003). The Nanoparticle and nanotechnology field is a fast growing research niche (Artken *et al.*, 2004). It is further classified according to size. In terms of diameter, fine particle cover a range between 100 and 2500 nm. While ultra fine particle 1 and 100 nm. Similarly too ultra fine particle, 1 and 100 nm, through the size limitations can be restricted to two dimensions (Cristian Buzer *et al.*, 2007).

The finding of the present of investigation revealed that *Azadiracta indica* good larvicidal and pupicidal activity against *Aedes aegypti* at different breeding sites. Their mode of action and effect on non target organism are presently under the investigations. To evaluate the impact of neem active principle, Azadiracthin with other microbial insecticides (*Bacillus thuringiensis, Bacillus sphaericus, Beauveria bassiana,* spinosad, nanomaterials and copepods) on the larvicidal, pupicidal toxicity effect of dengue vectors, such as *Aedes aegypti*. It is an obligate aerobe bacterium showed that has good effective mosquito control properties and also can act as an ecofriendly, biopesticide for further vector control programs.

References

Abbott, W.S., 1925. A method of computing the effectiveness of insecticides. *J. Econ. Enotomol.*, 18: 267-269.

Alder, H.L. and Rossler, E.B., 1977. *Introduction to Probability and Statistics*. WH Freeman Company, San Francisco p. 246.

Ansary, Daihan, 2004. On the Toxicity of Therapeutically Used Nanoparticles: An Overview. *Journal of Toxicology* Volume 2009 (2009), Article ID 754810, 9 pages doi: 10.1155/2009/754810.

Babu, R. and Murugan, K., 2000. Larvicidal effect of resinous exudates from the tender leaves of *Azadirachta indica*. *Neem Newsl.*, 17(1).

Batra, C.P., Mittal, P.K., Adak, T. and Sharma, V.P., 1998. Efficacy of neem-water emulsion against mosquito immatures. *Indian Journal of Malariol.*, 35: 15–21.

Baumann, P., Underman, B.M., Baumann, L., Broadwell, A.H. and Abebene, S.J., 1985. Purification of the larvicial toxin of *Bacillus spaericus* and evidence for high molecular weight precursors. *J. Bacteriol.*, 163: 738-741.

Breakley, C.J., Crampton, P.L., Ricket, F.E. and Chadwick, P.R., 1984. Resistance mechanisms to DDT and Transpermethrin in *Aedes aegypti*. *Pesticide Science.*, 15: 121-133.

Becker, N., Petric, D., Zgomba, M., Boase, C., Dahl, C., Lane, J. and Kaiser, A., 2003. *Mosquitoes and their Control*. Kluwer Academic/ Plenum Publishers, New York.

Bobrowski, V.L., Pasquali, G., Bodanese-Zanettini, M.H., Pinto, L.M.N. and Fiuza, L.M., 2002. Characterization of two *Bacillus thuringiensis* isolates from South Brazil and their toxicity against *Anticarsia gemmatalis* (Lepidoptera: Noctuidae). *Biol. Control*, 25: 129-135.

Clark, T.B., Kellen, W., Fukuda, T. and Lindgren, J.E., 1968. Field and laboratory studies on the pathogenicity of the fungus *Beauveria bassiana* to three genera of mosquitoes. *J. Invertbr. Path.*, 11: 1-7.

Camacho, T., de la Hoz, F., Cárdenas, V., Sánchez, C., de Calderón, L., Pérez, L. and Bermúdez, A. 2004. Jun, Incomplete surveillance of a dengue-2 epidemic in Ibagué, Colombia, 1995-1997. *Biomedica.*, 4: 174-82.

Charles, J.F. and de Barjac, H., 1983. Action des cristaux de *Bacillus thuringiensis* var. *israelensis* Su 1′ intestin moyen des larves de *Aedes aegypti* L. en microscopic electronique. *Ann. Microbiol. Ins. Pasteur.*, 134: 197–218.

Collado, C.D., Defaye, D., Dussart, B.H. and Fernando, C.H., 1984. The freshwater Copepoda of Costa Rica with notes on some species. *Hydrobiologia,* 119: 89-99.

Cristina Buzea, Ivan Pacheco. and Kevin Robbie, 2007. "Nanomaterials and Nanoparticles: Sources and Toxicity". *Biointerphases,* 2(1007) MR17-MR71.

Daniel, T., Umarani, S. and Sakthivadivel, M., 1995. Insecticidal action of *Ervatamia divaricata* L. and *Acalypha indica* L. against *Culex quinquefasciatus* Say. *Geobias,* 14: 95–98.

Davis and Bowen, 1994. Sensory physiological basis for attraction in mosquitoes. 10: 316–25.

Davidson, E.W., 1983. Alkaline extraction of toxin from spores of the mosquito pathogen. *Bacillus sphaericus* strain 1593. *Canadian Journal of Microbiology,* 29: 271-275.

de Maagd, R.A., Bosch, D. and Stiekema, W., 1999. *Bacillus thuringiensis* toxin-mediated insect resistance in plants. *Trends Plant Sci.,* 4: 9-13.

Ferron, P., 1981. Pest control by the fungi Beauveria and Metarhizium. In: *Microbial Control of Pests and Plant Diseases,* (Ed.) H.D. Burgess. 1970-1980, London, Academic Press, 24: 465-482.

Finney, D.J. 1971. *Probit Analysis.* Cambridge University, London. pp. 68–78.

Grove, J.F. and Pople, M., 1980. The insecticidal activity of Beauverian and the enniatin complex. *Mycopathologia,* 70: 103-105.

Gould, F., Anderson, A., Landis, D. and Van Mellaert, J., 1991. Feeding behaviour and growth of *Heliothis virescens* larvae on diets containing *Bacillus thuringiensis* formulations or endotoxins. *Entomol. Exp. Appl.,* 58: 199–210.

Gupta, S., Montllor, C. and Hwang, Y.S., 1995. Isolation of novel Beauverian analogous form the fungus *Beauveria bassiana. J. Nat. Products,* 58: 733-738.

Guzman, M.G. and Kouri, G., 2002. Dengue: an update. *Lancet Infectious Diseases,* 2: 33–42.

Johnson, K.S., Scriber, J.K., Nitao, J.K. and Smitley, D.R., 1995. Toxicity of *Bacillus thuringiensis* var. *kurstaki* to three non-target Lepidoptera in field studies. *Environ Entomol.*, 24: 288-297.

Kalyanasundaram, M. and Das, P.K., 1985. Larvicidal and synergistic activity of plant extracts for mosquito control. *Indian J. Med. Res.*, 82: 19–23.

Kay, B.H., Cabral, C.P., Sleigh, A.C., Brown, M.D., Ribeiro, Z.M. and Vasconcelos, A.W., 1992. Laboratory evaluation of Brazilian *Mesocyclops* (Copepoda: Cyclopidae) for mosquito control. *Journal of Medical Entomology*, 29: 599–602.

Klimuk, Semple and Nahirney, 2000. "Enhanced anti-inflammatory activity of a liposomal intercellular adhesion molecule-1 antisense oligodeoxynucleotide in an acute model of contact hypersensitivity." *Journal of Pharmacology and Experimental Therapeutics*, 292: 480–488.

Kosiyachinda, P., Bhumiratana, A. and Kittayapong, P., 2003. Enhancement of the efficacy of a combination of *Mesocyclops aspericornis* and *Bacillus thuringiensis* var. *israelensis* by community-based products in controlling *Aedes aegypti* larvae in Thailand. *Am. J. Trop. Med. Hyg.*, 69: 206–212.

Kuno, G., 1995. Review of the factors modulating dengue transmission. *Epidemiology Reviews*, 17: 321-335.

Lardeux, F.J.R., Séchan, Y., Rivière, F. and Kay, B.H., 1992. Release of *Mesocyclops aspericornis* (Copepoda) for control of larval *Aedes polynesiensis* (Diptera: Culicidae) in land crab burrows on an atoll of French Polynesia. *J. Med. Entomol.*, 29: 371–376.

Lindroth, R.L., Scriber, J.M. and Hsia, M.T.S., 1988. Chemical ecology of the tiger swallowtail: mediation of host use by phenolic glycosides. *Ecology*, 69: 814-822.

Lucantoni, L., Giusti, F., Cristofaro, M., Pasqualini, L., Esposito, F., Lupetti, P. and Habluetzel, A., 2006. Effects of neem extract on blood feeding, oviposition and oocyte ultrastructure in *Anopheles stephensi* Liston (Diptera: Culicidae). *Tissue Cell*, 38: 361-371.

Malavige, G.N., Fernando, S., Fernando, D.J. and Seneviratne, S.L., 2004. Dengue viral infections. *Postgrad.*

Marten, G.G., 1984. Impact of the copepod *Mesocyclops leuckarti pilosa* and the green alga *Kirchneriella irregularis* upon larval *Aedes albopictus* (Diptera: Culicidae). *Bull. Soc. Vector Ecol.*, 9: 1–5.

Marten, G.G., 1990a. Evaluation of cyclopoid copepods for *Aedes albopictus* control in tires. *J. Am. Mosquito Contr.*, 6: 681-688.

Marten, G.G., 1990b. Elimination of *Aedes albopictus* from tire piles by introducing *Macrocyclops albidus* (Copepoda, Cyclopidae). *J. Am. Mosq. Control Assoc.*, 6: 689–693.

Marten, G.G., Bordes, E.S. and Nguyen, M., 1994a. Use of cyclopoid copepods for mosquito control. *Hydrobiologia*, 292/293: 491–496.

Marten, G.G., Astaiza, R., Suárez, M.F., Monje, C. and Reid, J.W., 1989. Natural control of larval *Anopheles albimanus* (Diptera: Culicidae) by the predator *Mesocyclops* (Copepoda: Cyclopoida). *J. Med. Entomol.*, 26: 624–627.

Mousson, L., Dauga, C., Garrigues, T. and Schaffner, F., 2005. Phylogeography of *Aedes* (*Stegomyia*) *aegypti* (L.) and *Aedes* (*Stegomyia*) *albopictus* (Skuse) (Diptera: Culicidae) based on mitochondrial DNA variations. *Genet. Res.*, 86: 1-11.

Murugan, K., Babu, R., Jeyabalan, D., Senthilkumar, N. and Sivaramakrishnan, S., 1996. Antipupational effect of neem oil and neem seed kernel extract against mosquito larvae of *Anopheles stephensi* Liston. *J. Ent. Res.*, 20: 137–139.

Murugan, K. and Jeyabalan, D., 1999. Effect of certain plant extracts against the mosquito, *Anopheles stephensi* Liston. *Current Science*, 76(5): 631-633.

Murugan, K., Thankamathi, P. and Jayabalan, D., 2002. Interactive effect of Botanical and *Bacillus thuringiensis subsp.* Israelensis on *Culex quinquefasciatus* say. *Journal of Scientific and Industrial Research*, 61: 1068-1076.

Murugan, K., Vahitha, R., Baruah, I. and Das, S.C., 2003. Interaction of botanical and microbial pesticides for the control of filarial vector, *Culex quinquefasciatus*. *Ann. of Med. Entomol.*, 12: 11-23.

Murugan, K., Murugan, P. and Noortheen, A., 2007. Larvicidal and repellent potential of *Albizzia amara* Boivin and *Ocimum basilicum* Linn against dengue vector, *Aedes aegypti* (Insecta: Diptera: Culicidae). *Bioresource Technology*, 98: 198-201.

Nam, V.S., Nguyen, T.Y., Hoyñska, M., Reid, J.W. and Kay, B.H., 2000. National progress in dengue vector control in Vietnam: survey for *Mesocyclops* (Copepoda), *Micronecta* (Corixidae), and fish as biological control agents. *Am. J. Trop. Med. Hyg.*, 62: 5–10.

Nathan, S.S., Kalaivani, K. and Murugan, K., 2001. Effects of neem limonoids on the malaria vector, *Anopheles stephensi* Liston (Diptera: Culicidae). *Acta Trop.*, 96: 47-55.

Nasiruddin, M. and Mordue (Luntz), A.J., 1993. the effect of azadirachtin on the midgut histology of the locusts *Schistocerca gregaria* and *Locusta migratoria*. *Tissue Cell*, 25: 875–884.

Rao, D.R., Reuben, R., Venugopal, M.S., Nagasampgi, B.A. and Schmutterer, H., 1992. Evaluation of neem – *Azadirachta indica* with and without water management for the control of culicine mosquito larvae in rice field. *Medical Veterinary Entomology*, 6: 318–324..

Rivière, F. and Thirel, R., 1981. La prédation du copépode *Mesocyclops leuckarti pilosa* (Crustacea) sur les larves de *Aedes* (*Stegomyia*) *aegypti* et *Ae.* (*St.*) *polynesiensis* (Dip.: Culicidae): essais préliminaires d'utilisation comme agent de lutte biologique. [Predation of the copepod *Mesocyclops leuckarti pilosa* (Crustacea) on the larvae of *Aedes* (*Stegomyia*) *aegypti* and *Ae.* (*St.*) *polynesiensis* (Dip.: Culicidae): preliminary trials of its use as a biological control agent. *Entomophaga*, 26: 427–439.

Rivière, F., Kay, B.H., Klein, J.M. and Séchan, Y., 1987. *Mesocyclops aspericornis* (Copepoda) and *Bacillus thuringiensis* var. *israelensis* for biological control of *Aedes* and *Culex* vectors (Diptera: Culicidae) breeding in crab holes, tree holes, and artificial containers. *J. Med. Entomol.*, 24: 425–430.

Russell, B.M., Muir, L.E., Weinstein, P. and Kay, B.H., 1996. Surveillance of the mosquito *Aedes aegypti* and its biocontrol with copepod *Mesocyclops aspericornis* in Australian wells and gold mines. *Med. Vet. Entomol.*, 10: 155–160.

Schaper, S., 1999. Evaluation of Costa Rican copepods (Crustacea: Eudecapoda) for larval *Aedes aegypti* control with special reference to *Mesocyclops thermocyclopoides*. *J. Am. Mosq. Control Assoc.*, 15: 510–519.

Scholte, E.J., Takken, W., Knols, B.G.J., 2003. Pathogenicity of six east African entomopathogenic fungi to adult Anopheles gambiae s.s (Diptera: Culicidae) mosquitoes. *Pro. Exp. Appl. Entomol. NEV*, Amsterdam 14: 25-29.

Schmutterer, H., 1990. Properties of natural pesticides from the neem tree, *Azadirachta indica. Annual Review of Entomology*, 35: 271–297..

Service, M.W., 1985. Population dynamics and mortalities of mosquito preadults, pp. 185-201. *In: Ecology of Mosquitoes*, (Eds.) L. P. Lounibos, J. R. Rey and J. H. Frank. Florida Medical Entomology Laboratory, Vero Beach, FL.

Singh, G.J.P., Schouest, L.P. and Jr Gill, S.S., 1986. The toxic action of *Bacillus thuringiensis* var. *israelensis* on *Aedes aegypti* in vivo I. The relevance of midgut lesions to its poisoning syndrome. *Pest. Biochem. Phy.*, 26: 36–46.

Singh, G. and Prakash, S., 2008. Ultrastructure of wing scales in adult mammophilic vector *Culex* (*Culex*) *quinquefasciatus* (Say) in a semi-arid zone. *J. Entomol. Res. Soc.*, 10: 1–12.

Sieber, K.P. and Rembold, H., 1983. The effects of Azadirachtin on the endocrine control of moulting in *Locusta migratoria. J. Insect. Physiol.*, 29: 523-527.

Shanmugasundaram, R., Jeyalakshmi, T., Dutt, M.S. and Murthy, P.B., 2008. Jan, Larvicidal activity of neem and karanja oil cakes against mosquito vectors, *Culex quinquefasciatus* (say), *Aedes aegypti* (L.) and *Anopheles stephensi* (L.). *J. Environ. Biol.*, 29: 43-5.

Spielman, A., Kitron, U. and Pollack, R.J., 1993. Time limitation and the role of research in the worldwide attempt to eradicate malaria. *Journal of Medical Entomology*, 30: 6-19.

Strasser, H., Vey, A. and Butt, T., 2000. Are there any risks in using entomopathogenic fungi for pest control, with particular reference to bio-active metabolites, *Tolypocladium* and *Beauveria* species. *Bio. Sci. and Tech.*, 10: 717-715..

Suárez, M.F., Ayala, D., Nelson, M.J. and Reid, J.W., 1984. Hallazgo de *Mesocyclops aspericornis* (Daday) (Copepoda: Cyclopidae) depredador de larvas de *Aedes aegypti* en Anapoima-Colombia. [Finding of *Mesocyclops aspericornis* (Daday) (Copepoda:

Cyclopidae) a predator of larvae of *Aedes aegypti* in Anapoima-Colombia. *Biomedica*, 4: 74–76.

Su, T. and Mulla, M.S., 1998. Ovicidal activity of neem products (Azadirachtin) against *Culex tarsalis* and *Culex quinquefasciatus* (Diptera: Culicidae). *J. Am. Mosq. Control Assoc.*, 14: 204-209.

Sukumar, K., Perich, M.J. and Boobar, L.R., 1991. botanical derivatives in mosquito control: A review. *J. Am. Mos. Control Assoc.*, 7: 210-217.

Takken, 1991. The role of olfaction in host-seeking of mosquitoes: a review. *Insect Sci. Appl.*, 12: 287–95.

Tietze, N.S., Hester, P.G., Shaffer, K.R., Prescott, S.J. and Schreiber, E.T., 1994. Integrated management of waste tire mosquitoes utilizing *Mesocyclops longisetus* (Copepoda: Cyclopidae), *Bacillus thuringiensis* var. *israelensis, Bacillus sphaericus* and methoprene. *J. Am. Mosq. Control Assoc.*, 10: 363–373.

WHO, 1982a. The role of biological agents in integrated vector control and the formulation of protocols for field-testing of biological agents. Report of the sixth meeting of the scientific working group on biological control of vectors. WHO/TDR/VEC-SWG (6)82: 46.

WHO, 1982b. Biological control of vectors of disease. Sixth report of WHO expert committee, Vector Biology and Control. *WHO Tech. Rep.*, Ser No. 679: 39.

WHO, 1986. Resistance of vectors and reservoirs of disease to pesticides. Tenth report of the Expert Committee on Vector Biology and Control. *Technical Report* Series, p. 737, 87.

Williamson, C.E. and Reid, J.W., 2001. Copepoda. In: *Ecology and Classification of North American Freshwater Invertebrates*, (Eds.) J.H. Thorp and A.P. Covich. San Diego, CA Academic Press. p. 915–954.

Womack, M., 1993. "The yellow fever mosquito, *Aedes aegypti*". *Wing Beats*, 5: 4.

Zahiri, N.S. and Mulla, M.S., 2002. Strategies for the management of resistance in mosquitoes to the microbial control agent *Bacillus sphaericus*. *J. Med. Entomol.*, 39: 513-520.

Zahiri, N.S. and Mulla, M.S., 2005. Non larvicidal effects of *Bacillus thuringiensis israelensis* and *Bacillus sphaericus* on oviposition and adult mortality of *Culex quinquefasciatus* Say (Diptera: Culicidae). *J Vector Ecol.*, 30: 155-162.

Zebitz, C.P.W., 1984. Effects of some crude and Azadirachtin enriched neem *Azadirachta indica.* Seed Kernel extracts on larvae of *Aedes aegypti. Entomologia Experimentalis et Applicata.*, 35: 11–16.

Zebitz, C.P.W., 1986. Effects of three different neem seed kernel extracts and Azadirachtin on the larvae of different mosquito species. *J. Appl. Entomol.*, 102: 455-463.

Chapter 4

Body Metric Variation in Populations of the Giant African Snail, *Achatina fulica* (Bowdich) from two Different Environ

M. Jayashankar[1]*, *M.S. Reddy*[1], *P. Marimuthu*[2] and *Katre Shankuntala*[3]

[1]*Department of Zoology, Bangalore University, Jnana Bharathi, Bangalore – 560 056, Karnataka, India*
[2]*Assistant Professor, Department of Biostatistics, NIMHANS, Bangalore, Karnataka, India*
[3]*Former Professor of Zoology, Department of Zoology, Bangalore University, Bangalore, Karnataka, India*

ABSTRACT

A pilot study has been undertaken to analyse the impact of immediate environ on the giant African snail *Achatina fulica* (Bowdich) populations in two different areas of Bangalore region.

Significant variations are observed confirming the microhabitat influence but further work and larger sample sizes

* Corresponding author: E-mail: jay_zoology@rediffmail.com

need to be assessed to establish eco-morphological or eco-phenotypical relevance.

Keywords: *Body metric variation, Giant African snail, Achatina fulica, populations, Microhabitat, Eco-morphological, Eco-phenotypical.*

Introduction

The Giant African snail *Achatina fulica* (Bowdich) is a global pest and has reached from east Africa to different parts of the world because of inadequate quarantine arrangements. In India it was introduced in Calcutta in 1847, by a British Conchologist William Henry Benson and from there it has reached many states of the country in course of time (Mead, 1961). Although Benson had got the snail to India from Mauritius, probably from his old school friend Sir David Barclay, he had handed them to a friend and neighbour before leaving India and it was the friend who released them in his garden (Naggs, 1997). It is today established in different parts of India, the Giant African snail was first reported as a serious pest of ornamental crops in Bangalore by Veeresh *et al.* (1979). The shell of *A. fulica* (Bowdich) can grow up to 20 cm in length and 10 cm in maximum diameter. The brownish shell with darker brown vertical stripes covers at least half of the length of the snail. The shell consists of 7 to 9 whorls.

Shells of land snails often provide relevant morphometric data used in taxonomy and phylogenetic inference as well as in population biology. Shell morphology, which preserves the ontogenic record of growth, is a principal subject of a subfield of morphometrics, namely theoretical morphology, which has led, since the initial mathematical modelling of Raup (1966), to convincing studies on the formal and historical determinants of shell forms, as well as functional interpretations of their observed distributions in theoretical morphospaces (Stone, 1996, 1999; Mc Ghee, 1999; Samadi *et al.*, 2000).

Population biologists have long appreciated that an animal's morphology reflects its ecology. A defensible method of predicting habitat use may be derived from mechanistic approaches to ecology. According to Schoener (1986) "mechanistic approaches to community ecology are those which employ individual-ecological concepts-those of behavioural ecology, physiological ecology, and ecomorphology-as theoretical bases." Such approaches have been successful in understanding resource use at the individual level (microhabitat scale). Werner and Hall (1988) have successfully predicted habitat shifts related to changes in feeding strategy. Sagnes *et al.* (1997) demonstrated that ontogenetic shifts in habitat (water velocities) were related to improved hydrodynamic shape with growth. Further, individual-based models of resource use have already been successful at describing population level ecology of fisheries (Van Winkle *et al.,* 1998; Rose *et al.,* 1999). Such models illustrate that mechanistic approaches at the level of individuals can be used to infer population and community level ecology.

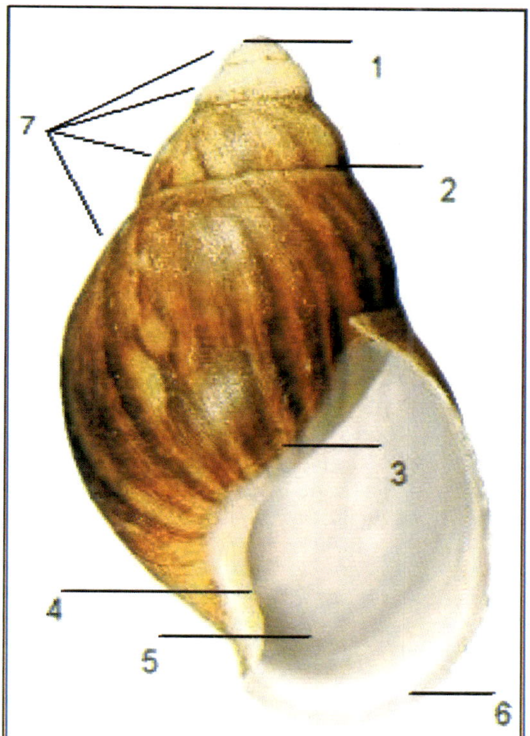

Figure 4.1: External Morphology of the Giant African Snail, *Achatina fulica*

1: Apex; 2: Suture; 3: Parietal wall; 4: Columella; 5: Aperture; 6: Lip; 7: Whorls

The shape of molluscan shells has been characterized, in more traditional approaches, by the use of simpler measurements, such as the ratio of width to height (Goodfriend, 1986), or by the plotting of these two measurements in order to create a 'size/shape space' (Cain, 1981; Cameron and Cook, 1989). Multivariate morphometrics have also been extensively used to separate size and shape components of the shell. The aim of the present study is based on similar approach to investigate the body metric variations in snail populations from two different localities of different environ.

Materials and Methods

A thorough survey of Bangalore region was undertaken during 2005-2009 confirming the distribution of the snail and their occurrence in different parts of the region. For the present study the

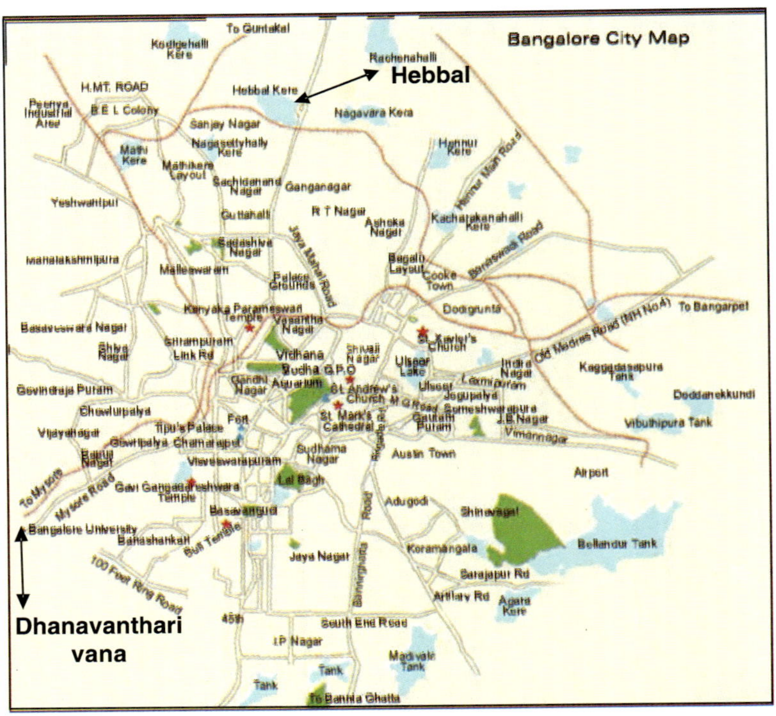

Map 4.1: Bangalore Map Showing the Study Sites of Hebbal and Dhanavanthri vana

(Courtesy: www.thisismyindia.com)

eastern environ of Hebbal lake (150 acres) in Bangalore north taluk and the Dhanavanthari vana nursery (32 acres) in Bangalore south taluk areas (Map 4.1) were selected for the following reasons:

- Easy accessibility
- Perennial habitat
- More human activities – Solid waste dumping, fishing, small scale agriculture and horticulture.

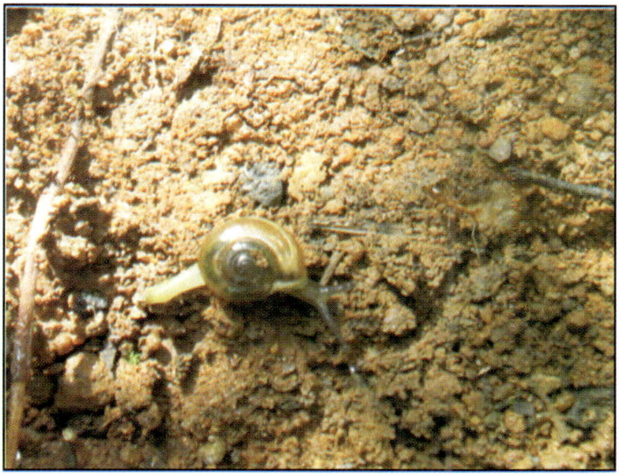

Figure 4.2: ***Macrochlamys indica***

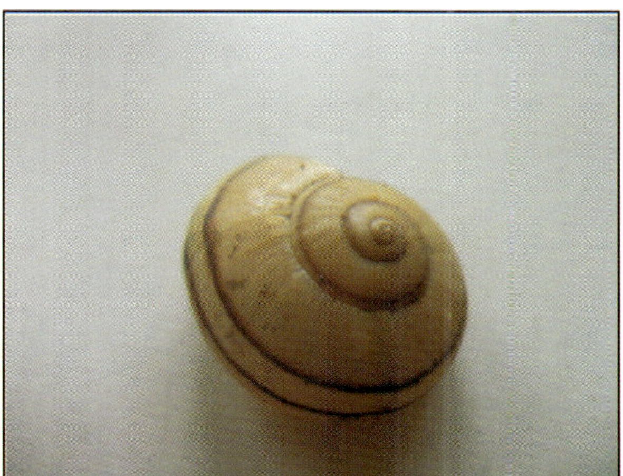

Figure 4.3*:* ***Ariophanta solata***

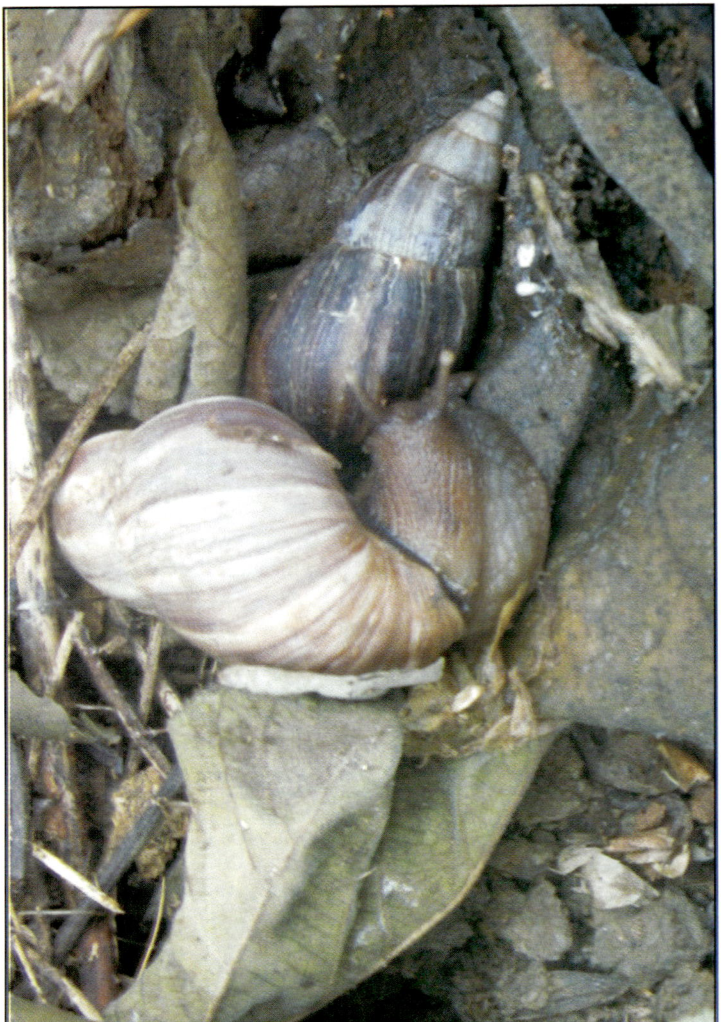

Figure 4.4: ***Achatina fulica***

A periodic survey of giant African snails found in the chosen habitats was undertaken. Snail samples comprising of twenty five snails were collected randomly within the habitat from Hebbal and Dhanavanthari vana nursery. Samples comprising of different shell size, were collected during early hours of the day in polythene bags and transported to the laboratory for morphometric measurements.

A large shell is measured with a ruler, vertically, but for smaller shells vernier callipers are more accurate. The most accurate method for measuring very small shells is to use a microscope fitted with either a vernier scale on the stage or an eye-piece graticule. When counting the whorls on a shell which is taller than it is wide, it is probably easier to count from the body whorl up towards the apex. Measurements for the maximum height and the maximum width is expressed in centimetres. The total length (Apex- distal part of lip) and total breadth (Broadest width of first whorl) of each snail was measured to the nearest millimetre, using a thread and a centimetre scale. Using an electronic balance, the mass of each individual was measured.

The data obtained was analysed by multiple linear regression method to establish the relationship of snails' length with weight and width and further statistical analysis were carried out for comparing body metric parameters using the t-test.

Results

In both habitats in the present study were also present other snail species, *Macrochlamys indica* in Hebbal (Figure 4.2) and *Ariophanta solata* in Dhanavanthari vana (Figure 4.3), along with *A. fulica* populations (Figure 4.4).

Multiple linear regression analysis (Tables 4.1–4.3) to establish snails' length as dependent variable, with width and weight as independent variables was carried out separately for Hebbal and Dhanavanthari vana.

Weight was excluded from the linear model by the stepwise regression analysis for Hebbal, therefore the model turned out be a simple regression analysis between snails' length and width. The ANOVA (Table 4.2) indicates significant (p=0.000) linear relationship between length and the width. The Figure 4.5 shows the highly significant positive correlation 0.956 (p=0.00).

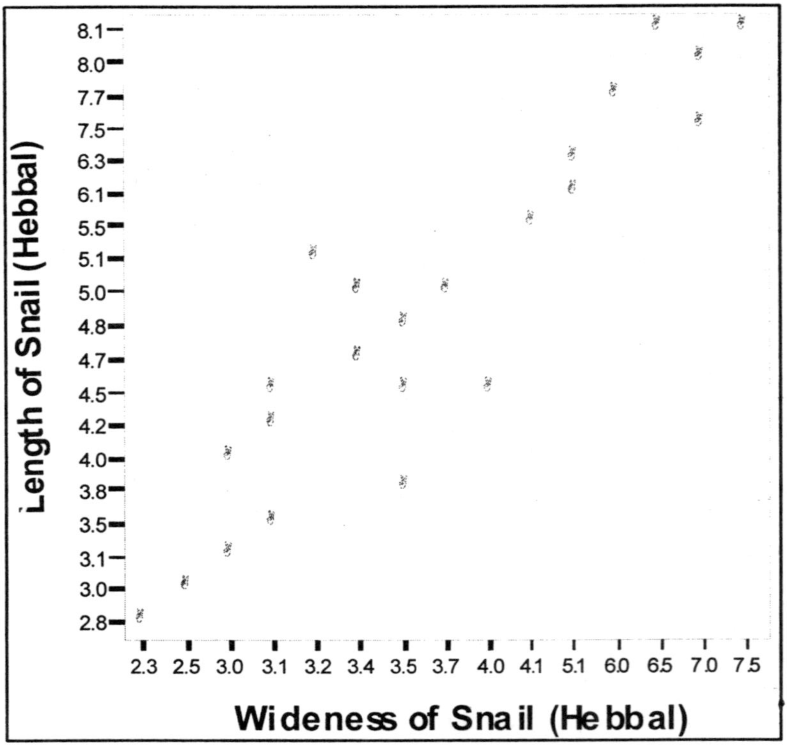

Figure 4.5: Body Metric Characters of Snails (Hebbal)

The regression line (Table 4.1) for Hebbal is:

Snails' length = 0.894+1.028 × snails' width

Ninety four percentage of snails' length was explained by the snails' width. The regression coefficient for width as well as constant in the equation are significant at p=0.006 and p=0.000 respectively (Table 4.3).

Regression Analysis (Hebbal-Sample Site-1)

Table 4.1: Model Summary

Model	*R*	*R Square*	*Adjusted R Square*	*Std. Error of the Estimate*
1.	0.956(a)	0.914	0.910	0.4973

a Predictors: (Constant), Wideness of Snail (Hebbal).

Table 4.2: ANOVA

Model	*Sum of Squares*	*df*	*Mean Square*	*F*	*Sig.*
Regression	58.112	1	58.112	234.935	0.000(a)
Residual	5.442	22	0.247		
Total	63.553	23			

a Predictors: (Constant), Wideness of Snail (Hebbal)

b Dependent Variable: Length of Snail (Hebbal)

Table 4.3: Coefficients

	Unstandardized Coefficients		*Standardized Coefficients*		
Model	*B*	*S.E*	*Beta*	*t*	*P*
(Constant)	0.894	0.297		3.015	0.006
Wideness of Snail (Hebbal)	1.028	0.067	0.956	15.323	0.000

a: Dependent Variable: Length of Snail (Hebbal).

Multiple linear regression analysis (Tables 4.4–4.8) for the Dhanavanthari vana site by considering the length, width, weight and length as dependent variable was carried out by the stepwise method, both independent variables *viz.*, weight and width had significant contribution (p=0.000) on the snails' length. Figure 4.6 explains the three dimensional relationships among length, width and weight; it is evident that all the 3 variables have positive correlation.

It is observed from the ANOVA (Tables 4.4–4.6) that the linear relationship is significant (p=0.000).The regression equation for Dhanavanthari vana is:

$$\textit{Snails' length} = 0.0334 + 0.006 \times \textit{snails' width} + \textit{snails weight} \times 0.0027$$

Ninety nine percentage of snails' length was explained by the snails' width and weight. The regression coefficient for width, weight and as well as constant in the equation are significant at p=0.000.

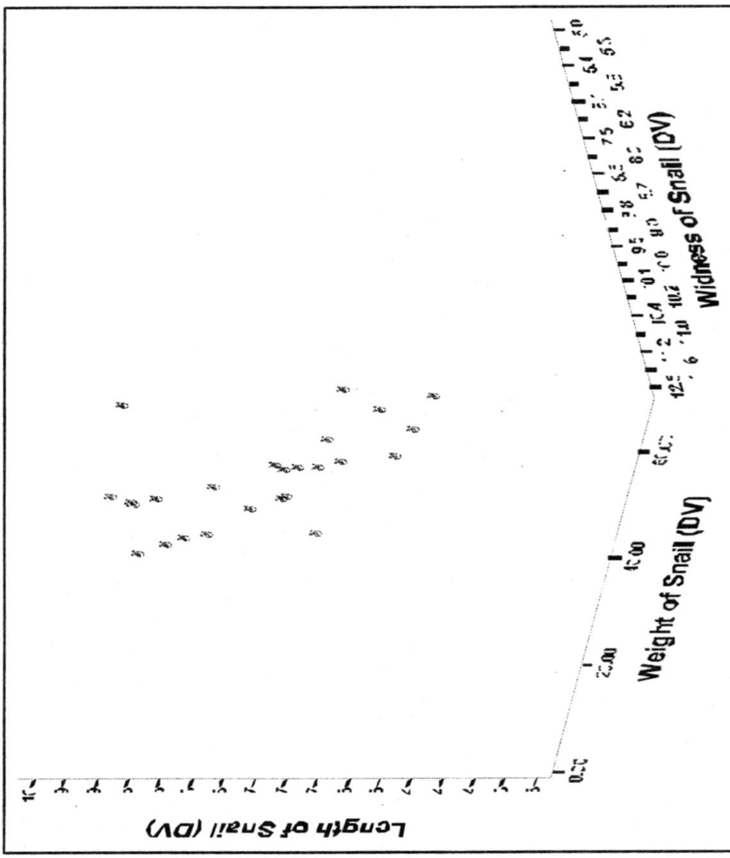

Figure 4.6: Body Metric Characters of Snails at Dhanavanthathari Vana (Sample site 2)

Regression Analysis (Dhanavanthari Vana(DV)-Sample Site 2

Table 4.4: Model Summary

Model	*R*	*R Square (a)*	*Adjusted R Square*	*Std. Error of the Estimate*
1	0.997(b)	0.994	0.994	0.509
2	0.999(c)	0.997	0.997	0.358

a: For regression through the origin (the no-intercept model), R Square measures the proportion of the variability in the dependent variable about the origin explained by regression. This CANNOT be compared to R Square for models which include an intercept.

b: Predictors: Wideness of Snail (DV)

c: Predictors: Wideness of Snail (DV), Weight of Snail (DV)

Table 4.5: ANOVA

Model	*Sum of Squares*	*df*	*Mean Square*	*F*	*Sig.*
Regression	1121.130	2	560.565	4385.345	0.000(c)
Residual	2.940	23	0.128		
Total	1124.070(b)	25			

a: Predictors: Wideness of Snail (DV)

b: This total sum of squares is not corrected for the constant because the constant is zero for regression through the origin.

c: Predictors: Wideness of Snail (DV), Weight of Snail (DV)

d: Dependent Variable: Length of Snail (DV)

e: Linear Regression through the Origin

Table 4.6: Coefficients

	Unstandardized Coefficients		*Standardized Coefficients*		
Model	*B*	*S.E*	*Beta*	*t*	*P*
Wideness of Snail (DV)	0.660	0.019	0.881	34.857	0.000
Weight of Snail (DV)	0.03335	0.007	0.128	5.061	0.000

Dependent Variable: Length of Snail (DV).

Linear Regression through the Origin.

The variation between the body metric characters of snails from the two sites is significant (Tables 4.7and 4.8) as established by the t-test.

Table 4.7: Group Statistics

	Place	N	Mean	S.D	S. E of Mean
Length of snails	Hebbal	25	5.27	1.70	0.341
	Dv	25	6.39	2.08	0.416
Weight of Snail	Hebbal	25	8.33	8.39	1.678
	Dv	25	20.30	16.13	3.227
Wideness of Snail	Hebbal	25	8.66	2.31	0.461
	Dv	24	4.15	1.55	0.316

Conclusions

Morphometric methods have been instrumental in advancing the study of how organismal shape covaries with size (allometry), time (evolution), environ (ecophenotyphy), geography (morphological biogeography), ecology (ecomorphology), development (heterochrony) (Quentin, 2008). *Ecomorphology or Ecological Morphology* is the study of relationships of form and environmental factors as an attempt to isolate the contribution of one on the other (Motta *et al.*, 1995), *i.e.* it attempts "to understand the interrelationships between morphological variation among individuals, populations, species and higher taxa, and communities and the corresponding variation in their ecology"(Liesler and Winkler, 1985).while, *Ecophenotypy* is the divergence of phenotypes due to developmental changes induced by local environmental conditions, producing distinct ecophenotypes. Such divergence is not heritable, but when found in the fossil record can be mistaken for speciation.

The main approach of the present work has been to realise the influence between snail morphology and their habitat. The variations observed could perhaps be attributed to the environment of the selected areas; Hebbal is subject to stressful situation (anthropogenic pollution), also has a perennial water source next to it, while the Dhanavanthari vana nursery is adjacent to a scrub forest.

Table 4.8: Test of Significance Between Hebbal and DV on Body Metric Parameters

	t	*df*	*P*	*Mean Difference*	*S.E Difference*	*95% Confidence Interval of the Difference*	
Length of Snai	–2.08	48	0.043	–1.120	0.538	–2.201	–0.038
Weight of Snail	–3.29	48	0.002	–11.966	3.637	–19.278	–4.653
Widness of Snail	8.00	47	0.000	4.506	0.563	3.373	5.639

Form constrains the use of resources through performance of important tasks and resource availability helps construct the form (via evolution) by determining which tasks are most important for increased fitness. In land snails, limited dispersal capacity and restricted habitat requirements may enhance the process of adaptation to local conditions and as a consequence, reproductive isolation may develop between distant populations which are exposed to different selection pressures (Bruno and Anette, 1992.). Ecotypic variation in the shell maybe widespread in malacofauna of the region, and shell characters should therefore be used with caution in studies of taxonomy, phylogeny and adaptation.

The present ecological approach perhaps serves as a probe into the underlying phenomena like ecomorphology or ecophenotypy, these analyses need further work and larger sample sizes to confirm and consequently describe the relationships of morphology to habitat preference and other life style performance.

Acknowledgements

The authors gratefully acknowledge the staff of Dhanavanthari vana for permitting to collect the samples and to carry out the field experiments.

References

Bruno Baur and Anette Baur, 1992. Reduced reproductive compatibility in *Arianta arbustorum* (Gastropoda) from distant populations. *Heredity,* 69: 65-72.

Cain, A.J., 1981. Variation in shell shape and size of helicid snails in relation to other Pulmonates in faunas of the Palaeartic region. *Malacologia,* 21: 149–176.

Cameron, R.A.D and Cook, L.M., 1989. Shell size and shape in Madeiran land snails: do niches remain unfilled? *Biol. J. Linn Soc.,* 36: 79–96.

Goodfriend, G.A., 1986. Variation in land snail shell form and size and its causes: a review. *Syst Zool.,* 35: 204–223.

Leisler, B., and Winkler, H., 1985. Ecomorphology, p. 155-186. In: *Current Ornithology,* (Ed.) R. F.Johnston. Vol. 2. Plenum Press, New York.

Mc Ghee Jr G.R., 1999. *Theoretical Morphology: The Concept and its Applications*. Columbia University Press: New York.

Mead, A.R., 1961. *The Giant African Snail: A Problem in Economic Malacology*. Chicago, U.S.A.: The University Chicago Press.

Motta, P.J., Norton, S. F. and Luczkovich, J.J., 1995. Perspectives on the ecomorphology of bony fishes. *Environ. Biol. Fishes*, 44: 11-20.

Naggs, F., 1997. William Benson and the early study of land snails in British India and Ceylon. *Archives of Natural History*, 24: 37-88.

Quentin, Wheeler. 2008. *The New Taxonomy*. CRC Press, 237 pp.

Raup, D.M. 1966. Geometric analysis of shell coiling: General problems. *J. Paleontol.*, 40: 1178–1190.

Rose, K. A., Rutherford, E.S., McDermot, D.S., Forney, J.L., Mills, E.L., 1999. Individual-based model of yellow perch and walleye populations in Oneida Lake. *Ecol. Monogr.*, 69(2): 127-154.

Sagnes, P., Gaudin, P. and Statzner, B., 1997. Shifts in morphometrics and their relation to hydrodynamic potential and habitat use during grayling ontogenesis. *J. Fish Biol.*, 50: 846-858.

Samadi, S., David, P. and Jarne, P., 2000. Variation of shell shape in the clonal snail *Melanoides tuberculata*, and its consequences for the interpretation of fossil series. *Evolution*, 54: 492–502.

Schoener, T.W., 1986. Mechanistic approaches to community ecology: a new reductionism. *Amer. Zool.*, 26: 81-106.

Stone, J.R., 1996. Computer-simulated shell size and shape variation in the caribbean land snail genus *Cerion:* a test of geometrical constraints. *Evolution*, 50: 341–347.

Stone, J.R., 1999. Using a mathematical model to test the null hypothesis of optimal shell construction by four marine gastropods. *Mar. Biol.*, 134: 397–403.

VanWinkle, W., Coutant, C.C., Jager, H.I., Mattice, J.S., Orth, D.J., Otto, R.G., Railsback, S.F., and Sale, M.J., 1997. Uncertainty and in stream flow standards: Perspectives based on hydropower research and assessment. *Fisheries*, 22(7): 21-22.

Veeresh, G.K., Rajgopal, D. and Puttarudraiah, M., 1979. First record of Africa giant Snail, *Achatina fulica* (Bowdich) (Mollusc: Gastropoda) as a serious pest of ornamental crops in Bangalore. *Curr. Res.*, 8: 202-204.

Werner, E.E. and Hall, D.J., 1988. Ontogenetic habitat shifts in bluegill: the foraging ratepredation risk trade-off. *Ecology*, 69(5): 1352-1366.

Chapter 5

Ionic Variability of Aquatic Environment and Osmoregulatory Adaptations in Teleost Fishes: An Ecological Perspective

Iqbal Parwez and Subuhi Abidi*

Department of Zoology, Aligarh Muslim University, Aligarh, U.P., India

ABSTRACT

While all physiological processes are intimately linked to the ambient environment, the maintenance of the body fluid salt and water balance of an organism is critical to its survival. This assumes particular significance in case of aquatic organisms where the habitat shows considerable ionic diversity. Aquatic environment occupies nearly 2/3rd of the total earth surface which makes it an extremely important component from ecological perspective. Out of the total aquatic environment, sea covers nearly 97.5 per cent and the remaining 2.5 per cent is largely occupied by freshwater with only small proportion of brackish water and virtually negligible part contributed by saline and brine waters. A freshwater teleost faces the twin problem of salt loss from its body fluid and the osmotic influx of water from permeable surfaces which, if not regulated, would

* Corresponding author: E-mail: iparwez2002@yahoo.co.in

lead to demineralization and hyper hydration of the body fluid. The seawater teleost, on the contrary, faces opposite set of osmotic challenges and are continually subjected to diffusional influx of salt and osmotic loss of water. Hence, all such organisms require a well-coordinated correctional and compensatory mechanism involving multiple target organs such as gills and kidney to maintain the osmo-ionic integrity of their body fluid. In view of the above, studies on the osmoregulatory mechanism of teleost fishes which constitute a major chunk of fish fauna has been engaging the attention of physiologists since a long time. It is, however, surprising that in India, despite its mega biodiversity of fish fauna, no detailed study, with the exception of Indian catfish *H. fossilis*, has been carried out on the teleost fishes inhabiting Indian waters. The present review will, therefore, elaborate the extreme ionic variability of the aquatic environment and summarize the existing information on the underlying osmoregulatory mechanisms of various stenohaline and euryhaline fishes. It will also focus on the hitherto unexplored facets of osmoregulatory thrust areas which need to be pursued on diverse Indian fishes. Hence, this review will serve the dual purpose of being the repository of current knowledge of osmoregulatory physiology and also act as an academic roadmap for those researchers who wish to pursue leads in this highly fascinating area.

Keywords: *Aquatic environment, Osmoregulation, Teleost fishes, Ionic diversity, Target organs.*

Introduction

Osmoregulatory control deals with the maintenance of ionic integrity of the body fluid in the face of vastly varied ambient environment. Such a regulation becomes more critical in case of aquatic organisms in which two different fluids *i.e.* the aquatic media and body fluid are separated by a biological membrane. This gives rise to more intimate interaction of physico-chemical forces such as diffusion and osmosis at the structural interface of the two fluids. Fishes are characterized by having highest number of species among vertebrates known to exist in the world. With wide variety of aquatic environment harbouring largest number of diverse species, osmoregulatory physiology of fishes has always captured the attention of the scientific community all the world over. The majority of the studies have been focused on euryhaline fishes which show remarkable ability to survive in the environment of divergent salinities. The stenohaline fishes, with only limited salinity tolerance, have been studied only sporadically. Of the existing nearly 2200 fish species inhabiting Indian waters, osmoregulatory physiology of only the catfish *Heteropneustes fossilis* has been studied comprehensively (Parwez *et al.*, 1979, 1984, 1985, 1994, 2001; Goswami *et al.*, 1983; Sherwani and Parwez, 2008). Considering the fact that India is a mega biodiversity hotspot, this existing lacuna is surprising and underlines the need for more detailed studies on larger number of fish species to understand the osmoregulatory mechanisms in the Indian fish fauna. The present review has been written to kindle the interest of the Indian scientific community, particularly fish physiologists, to take up studies in this fascinating area.

This review provides the bird's eye view of the various facets of osmoregulatory physiology in fishes with particular emphasis on its multidimensional regulatory control exercised by variety of target organs. Interestingly, the specific cellular components in these regulatory target organs mediate their response through the interplay of variety of hormones which may either act singly or in conjunction with other hormones. On the whole, the entire process, though little complex, is highly fascinating and elucidates how the homeostatic balance of salt and water metabolism in the fishes is maintained in the face of divergent ambient salinities. For the purpose of easy comprehension, the review has been split into six subsections.

Environmental Variability

Of the total earth surface, aquatic environment occupies nearly 71 per cent of the area which makes it an extremely important component from the ecological perspective. Out of the total aquatic environment sea covers nearly 97.5 per cent and the remaining 2.5 per cent is largely occupied by freshwater (FW). Only a small proportion within 2.5 per cent FW consists of brackish water or estuaries and a virtual negligible proportion by saline and brine water. Surprisingly, even saline and brine waters have some population of aquatic animals and their survival strategies in these inhospitable environments have always been a matter of great scientific curiosity. The salinity and the pH range of various types of aquatic environment has been given in Table 5.1.

Table 5.1: Salinity Range and pH of Different Aquatic Environments

	Per cent	*ppt ‰*	*ppm*	*mOsm*	*pH*	*Major Ions*
Freshwater	<0.05	<0.5	<500	15-20	6.5–7.0	Monovalent ions (Na^+, Cl^-, K^+, HCO_3^-) Divalent ions (Mg^{2+}, Ca^{2+}, SO_4^{2-}, PO_4^{2-}
Brackish Water	0.5–3	5–30	5,000-30,000	100-800	7.1–9.6	Same as in SW but lower proportion
Saline Water	3–5	35–50	35,000-50,000	900-1500	Nearly 10.5	Same as in SW but higher proportion
Sea Water	3.1–3.7 Average 3.5	35–37	35,000-37,000	1000	Alkaline in range of (7.5-8.4)	Cl^- (55), Na^+(31), SO_4^{2-} (7.6), Mg^{2+} (3.6), Ca^{2+} (1.18), K^+(1.11)in mole/kg Contribution of monovalent ions (88 per cent) and Divalent ions (12 per cent)
Brine Water	26.3 -31.5	263–315	$260x10^3$-$315x10^3$	10,000	Highly alkaline	Cl^- (181.4), Mg^{2+} (35.2), Na^+ (32.5), Ca^{2+} (14.1) in g/kg

Freshwater

A near two third proportion of FW (about 70 per cent) is frozen in glaciers and polar ice-caps, about 29.7 per cent is ground water inclusive of soil moisture, and only about 0.3 per cent is surface water in lakes and rivers. The major surface FW bodies are Lake Baikal in Russia and Great Lakes in North America and the most notable Amazon River. The above facts clearly point to the growing realization as to how precious and scarce the FW commodity is and wasteful and indiscriminate exploitation of this ecosystem will spell disaster on the entire human race.

Brackishwater

Brackish water salinity is of somewhat median value between fresh and seawater ranging between 0.05- 3 per cent. Brackish water bodies largely consist of estuaries, mangroves, swamps, brackish seas and brackish lakes in addition to lagoons, marshes and deltas. Brackish water estuaries basically result from the mixing of SW with freshwater. It essentially forms a progressively increasing salinity gradient as it traverses from FW bodies towards sea. Thus salinity can vary considerably over space and time and hence estuaries are regarded as most extensive brackish water habitat. The famous river Thames passing through London is a classical example of river estuary harbouring predominantly freshwater species in the initial strata becoming brackish in the later stretches known with the name Thamas estuary in South East England and upon reaching Gravesend adjacent to North Sea, it becomes fully marine supporting euryhaline and marine stenohaline species. A few other important rivers becoming estuary during the course of SW confluence are Amazon River, Hudson River in US, Delaware Bay and San Francisco Bay etc.

Another important brackish water habitat is mangrove swamp having endemic species like Mudskipper and Snappers. Two important mangrove forests *i.e.* Sundarbans and Pichavaram located at the coast of Bay of Bengal are worth mentioning. Some seas are brackish in nature *e.g.* the stratified Baltic Sea in proximity with the North Sea having denser sea water at the bottom supporting Cod species and the lighter freshwater atop where pike fauna thrives. Few other notable examples are Caspian Sea which is also classified as world's largest lake and Black Sea (salinity range 1.7- 1.8 per cent) which has vertical salinity gradient. Among the important brackish water lakes in India are Chilka Lake in Orissa, Pangong Tso in Ladakh, Pulicot lake Chennai and Kaliveli Lake in Pondichery.

Sea Water

Sea water is the largest component of aquatic habitat with salinity ranging between 3.1 per cent near the mouth of rivers and melting glaciers to 4.1 per cent in Red Sea. The pH is alkaline between 7.5-8.4. Interestingly, about 88 per cent of this salinity is contributed by monovalent ions in the form of chloride (55 per cent), sodium (32 per cent) and potassium (1.1 per cent) while the divalent ions principally sulphate (7.7 per cent), magnesium (3.7 per cent) and calcium (1.2 per cent) make up the total of 12 per cent of the remaining seawater. The main reason of high concentration of monovalent ions is attributed to their long residence time compared to divalent ions which tend to precipitate much faster thereby reduce their long residence time which reduces their dissolved concentration in seawater. The Red Sea lying between Africa and Asia is the most saline open sea with salinity fluctuating between 3.6 per cent in Southern part due to Gulf of Aden to 4.1 per cent in the Northern part of Gulf of Suez with average salinity of 4 per cent. This high salinity is mainly due to high evaporation coupled with low rate of precipitation and river inflow.

Despite such enormous volume, it is an irony that seawater is unfit for human consumption. The hydration achieved through SW drinking will require more water to eliminate the ingested salts thus raising NaCl concentration in the blood to toxic levels. This will ultimately result in cellular dehydration, impaired nerve conduction leading to seizure and cardiac asynchrony. Contrary to this, large fish species, whales, penguins and desert rat survive remarkably well in sea water largely due to their efficient kidney functioning.

Saline Water

Saline water is another aquatic habitat containing significant concentration of NaCl ranging from 0.1–3.5 per cent, being graded into slight (0.1–0.3 per cent), moderate (0.3–1 per cent) and highly saline water (1–3.5 per cent). In some instances such as Great Salt Lake of Utah (5–27 per cent) has also been classified as saline water body which, even though, predominantly NaCl containing, should rightly be classified into Brine water bodies. Some important examples of saline water bodies are three largest salt lakes of the world, *viz.* Caspian sea in Russian with no outflows and with approximately 1.2 per cent salinity, Aral sea in Central Asia also called "Sea of Island" has shown an alarming shrinkage in surface area and volume resulting in salinity increase from 1 per cent to 4.5 per cent during the last four decades and lake Balkhash in Central Asia is also showing shrinkage like Aral sea.

Brine Water

The brine water bodies are actually or virtually saturated with salt principally NaCl with salinity range between 5-35 per cent developing mainly due to high evaporation in arid climate coupled with the lack of outlet. It has two very notable examples- Dead Sea in Jordan with average salinity of 33.7 per cent and the Great Salt Lake of Utah, USA with salinity range of 5-27 per cent harbouring brine shrimp, *Artemia franciscana* as the only surviving aquatic animals.

The pH extremes of water bodies

The pH of the aquatic environment is one of the few important factors which affect the survival of the fish. Normally, the fish can survive in a pH range of 6.0 to 9.0 but its suited pH is between 7.0–8.0. However, in some selected water bodies, the extreme pH conditions *i.e.* highly alkaline or highly acidic may pose far greater challenge to the aquatic fauna particularly fishes than the salinity itself. Most of the alkaline lakes are in Africa mostly in Kenya such as Lake Magadi and Lake Logipi with average pH around 10.5. A few genera of Cichlids, Tilapia, Bichir are found to survive in these water bodies. Similarly few acidic lakes such as Osorezan and Usoriko in Japan with pH of 3.4 – 3.8 also harbour Japanese dace, *Tribolodon hakonesis*.

Relative Abundance of Fish Species in Different Aquatic Habitat

It is interesting to note that the seawater has the greatest number of piscine species and the brine water, understandably, has the least. The relative abundance is as follows:

SW > FW > Brackish > Saline > Brine

Also, embryonic forms are more tolerant to salinity than its own adult form in the respective environment. Few examples, nevertheless, are noteworthy. Fishes have normally been found to inhabit salinity upto 1200 mOsm and very few species thrive beyond this salinity limit. Few examples are interesting. The Desert Pupfish, *Cyprinodon macularius*, inhabiting Arizona waters of North America can survive in fresh as well as salty water of almost 3 times that of sea water (approx 10 per cent or 3000 mOsm). However, an extraordinary euryhalinity has been exhibited by sheepshead minnow, *Cyprinodon variegatus* also called pupfish which is a coastal resident of the Western Atlantic ocean and Gulf of Mexico and can survive ambient salinities from as low as 0 ‰ to more than 165‰ (4000–6000 mOsm). Invertebrates are more tolerant to higher salinities than do the vertebrates and a few of them can survive upto 5800 mOsm ambient salinity. Brine shrimp, *Atremia salina* and *Atremia franciscana* can tolerate salinity up to 50 per cent (14,500 mOsm or more) which is near saturated salt solution.

Salient Features of Osmoregulatory Mechanism in Fishes

Fishes inhabit divergent salinities ranging from highly dilute freshwater to salt-rich seawater or even much higher salinities such as saline and brine waters. Such teleost fishes which maintain the plasma osmotic pressure of their body fluid different from the environment in which they live are called osmoregulators *e.g.* majority of the teleost fishes and some of the elasmobranchs. However, such organisms which fail to maintain the osmoionic integrity of their body fluid different from the surrounding aquatic environment and simply conform to salinity changes taking place in their native environment are termed osmoconformers. Marine invertebrates and hagfishes are classified under this category. Similarly, some fishes have the ability to maintain their plasma osmotic pressure equally well both in freshwater and seawater either as part of experimental transfer or compulsory migration in divergent media to complete life cycle are termed Euryhaline. On the contrary, some fishes are osmotically more conservative and lack the ability to withstand wide fluctuation in their ambient environment and are called 'Stenohaline' fishes.

The Stenohaline Fishes

Of the total existing fish fauna, 95 per cent of them are stenohaline either endemic to freshwater or seawater thereby lacking the ability to withstand wide fluctuation in their ambient salinities.

A list of the few representative fish species which are basically stenohaline in nature is given in Table 5.2. The perusal of this table reveals the following important generalizations.

1. Most of the stenohaline fishes are able to tolerate ambient salinity which is close to isosmotic value of their body fluid *i.e.* 270 – 300 mOsm or about 30 – 35 per cent SW. This is exemplified by catfish *Heteropneustes fossilis, Clarias batrachus, Ictalurus punctatus* and many others.
2. On the contrary, some stenohaline teleost show highly variable tolerance limit towards higher side such as rainbow fish *Melanotaenia splendida* of Murray- Darling river system (upto 20.8 g/l, or 70 per cent SW) (Williams and Williams, 1991), *Carassius auratus* (1.5–1.8 per cent or 50 per cent SW) (Schofield *et al.*, 2006), *Cyprinus carpio* (1.5 per cent) (Abo Hegab and Hanke, 1982), barbel *Barbus callensis* (1.72 per cent, about 55 per cent SW) (Kraiem and Pattee, 1988), flathead catfish, *Pylodictis olivaris* (1.45 per cent–1.58 per cent) (Bringolf *et al.*, 2005).
3. In some other stenohaline teleosts, salinity tolerance is even more limited and they have been reported to survive only up to (0.95 per cent) or 15 – 20 per cent SW such as *Clarias lazera* (Chervinki 1984) and largemouth bass, *Micropterus salmoides* (0.8 per cent) (Meador and Kelso, 1990).
4. It is also interesting to note that early developmental forms such as eggs, fry and fingerlings are more tolerant to salinity compared to their adult forms. This is exemplified in the case of channel catfish *Ictalurus punctatus* in which 3 days old channel catfish egg is able to tolerate 1.6 per cent salinity whereas its adult forms do not survive beyond 1.2 per cent salinity (Allen and Avault, 1969).
5. In cyprinids, salinity tolerance value ranges roughly between 8.4 ppt (*Puntius conchonicus*, Nazneen and Begum, 1981) and 17.2 ppt (*Barbus callensis*, Kraiem and Pattee, 1988).
6. In catfish, the upper salinity mainly varies from 9.0 ppt (*Heterobranchus longifilis*, Fastina-Bombata and Busari, 2003) to 15 ppt (*Mystus vittatus*, Zullah and Ud-Din, 1982).

Table 5.2: Stenohaline Fishes (Salinity Tolerance)

Sl.No.	*Fish*	*Salinity Tolerance*	*Reference*	*Remarks*
1.	*Carassius auratus* (Goldfish)	15 ‰	Schofield *et al.* (2006)	Goldfish showed high levels of survival at salinities of 5 and 10 ‰, but significant mortality at salinities of 15 and 20 ‰.
2.	*Gasterosteus aculeatus* (Threespine stickleback)	50% SW	Armitage and Olund (1962)	Activity was normal in 10% and 20% SW and decreased progressively
3.	*Cyprinus carpio* (Common carp)	9 ‰	Azizi *et al.* (2010)	Common carp can survive successfully in brackish water with salinity of up to 9 ‰. However, it could tolerate 12 ‰ salinity by gradual acclimation. It has also been suggested that gradual acclimation was more effective than direct transfer to stimulate osmoregulatory mechanism.
		15‰	Abo Hegab and Hanke (1982)	
4.	*Pylodictis olivaris* (Flathead catfish)	14.5 ‰ direct transfer, gradual adaptation up to 15.8‰	Bringolf *et al.* (2005)	
5.	*Barbus callensis* (Barbel)	17.2‰	Kraiem and Pattee (1988)	Seasonal migration into Oued Sejnane and other tributaries in Tunisia
6.	*Melanotaenia splendida* (Rainbowfish)	29.8A ± 0.7 g/L (slow acclimation) 20.8 g/L (direct transfer)	Williams and Williams (1991)	(occurs in Murray-Darling river system)

Contd...

Table 5.2–Contd...

Sl.No.	*Fish*	*Salinity Tolerance*	*Reference*	*Remarks*
7.	*Mystus vittatus* (Catfish)	Exceeds 15.0 ‰	Zullah and Ud-Din (1982)	
8.	*Polyondon spatula* (Paddlefish)	14.0 ‰	Krayushkina *et al.* (1996)	
9.	*Colisia fasciata* (Giant gourami)	18.0 ‰	Das and Srivastava (1979)	
10.	*Ictalurus punctatus* (Channel catfish)	12 ‰ 15.5‰	Allen and Avault (1969) Clemens and Jones (1955)	3- day old channel catfish eggs are able to tolerate salinity up to 15.5 ‰. The post-larvae were able to tolerate salinities up to 10 ‰. Channel catfish 6-12 month old were able to survive 12 ‰ salinity.
11.	*Esox lucius* (Northern pike)	9-14 ‰ (fry)	Jacobsen *et al.* (2007)	*Exos* fry was able to tolerate 9-14 ‰ salinity in combination with temperature of 10,14 and 18°C
12.	*Pseudophoxinus stymphalicus* (Daska)	Up to 12-13 ‰ with gradual acclimation	Bianco and Nordlie (2008)	Tolerance up to 12-13 ‰ with gradual acclimation of 6 ‰ intervals and 11 ‰ in direct transfer
13.	*Clarias batrachus* (Walking catfish)	12.0 ‰	Synudeen (2003) Parwez *et al.* (2001)	
14.	*Clarias lazera* (Catfish)	25% SW (9.75‰)	Chervinski (1984)	No survival in 30% SW. Pre-adaptation had no effect
15.	*Micropterus salmoides* (Largemouth bass)	8 ‰	Meador and Kelso (1990)	

Contd...

Table 5.2–Contd...

Sl.No.	*Fish*	*Salinity Tolerance*	*Reference*	*Remarks*
16.	*Puntius conchonicus* (Rosy barb)	8.4 ‰	Nazneen and Begum (1981)	
17.	*Heterobranchus longifilis* (Vandu catfish)	9.0 ‰	Fashina-Bombata and Busari (2003)	
18.	*Perca flavescens* (Yellow perch)	9.1 ‰	Victoria *et al.* (1992)	
19.	*Ameiurus catus* (White catfish)	14.0 ‰	Kendall and Schwartz (1968)	
20.	*Ameiurus melas* (Black bullhead)	10.0 ‰ 13.8 ‰	Chipman (1959) Clemens and Jones (1955)	
21.	*Clarias gariepinus* (African catfish)	Eggs hatched by optimum hatching salinity (0-5‰). No survival up to 8 ‰	Gbulubo and Erondu (1998)	Eggs and hatched by optimum hatching salinity (0-5‰) Above salinity decreased hatching and no hatching at 8‰. Fry also showed survival up to 8‰
22.	Non-native Asian Swamp eels (Symbranchidae)	One population (14 ‰), another population (16 ‰)	Schofield and Nico (2009)	Occupy wide range of shallow water habitat including inland and coastal environment

Contd...

Table 5.2–Contd...

Sl.No.	*Fish*	*Salinity Tolerance*	*Reference*	*Remarks*
23.	*Eucalia inconstans* (Brook stickleback)	Active upto 20% SW Sluggish in 30% SW	Armitage and Olund (1962)	
24.	*Catostomus commersonii* (White Sucker)	0.94% NaCl	Wilkes and McMahon (1986)	4-days exposure showed an increase in plasma Na and Cl.
25.	*Oreochromis niloticus* (Nile tilapia)	Direct transfer to 20‰ – all dies (field strain). Genetically improved Farmed Tilapia (GIFT) strain showed 100% SW survival of *O. niloticus* but with skin lesions.	Ridha (2008) Avella *et al.* (1993)	Fish does not tolerate salinities above 20 ‰ and might not be suitable for culture in full strength seawater (37 to 40 ‰). Strain-specific variations with respect to the possible effect on salinity.
26.	*Oreochromis aureus* (Blue tilapia)	Field strain – *O. aureus*– more tolerant *O. niloticus* – less tolerant None survived direct transfer to 20‰	Avella *et al.* (1993)	
27.	*Heteropneustes fossilis* (Stinging catfish)	35% SW	Parwcz *et al.* (1979)	

Euryhaline Fishes

Only very limited number of teleost fishes (5 per cent) fall under this category. However, they have been extensively studied largely due to their remarkable ability to tolerate wide range of environmental salinities inhabiting even some of the most inhospitable environment (Table 5.3). Some of their generalized features are described below:

1. It is interesting to note that different species even within the same genus show a wide ranging of salinity tolerance. For instance in Cichlidae, the salinity tolerance of various species of tilapia normally ranging 29 to 65 ppt (*O. niloticus* 20 ppt; *O. aureus* 30 ppt. *O. mossambicus* 64 ppt.) (Avella *et al.*, 1993) and may even go up to 124 ppt in *Sarotherodon melanotheron* (Lemarie *et al.*, 2004).
2. Among euryhaline fishes, Cyprinodontoid species show a much higher salinity tolerance range from 100 ppt to the highest 167 ppt in case of *C. variegatus* which by far is the highest range reported for any teleost.
3. The Salmonid group has *Salvelinus* as a primitive genus relative to *Salmo* and *Oncorhynchus* and displays restricted pattern of seaward migration. For example lake trout *Salvelinus namaycush* restricted to cold freshwater lakes is a non-anadromous species whereas brook trout *Salvelinus fontinalis* largely non-anadromous, but has some anadromous populations too and Atlantic salmon *Salmo salar* exhibited greater anadromous role. The upper salinity limit of these fishes also vary according to their migratory nature. Lake trout had survival rate of 80 per cent following both direct and gradual transfer to 30 ppt. Brook trout has still higher euryhalinity having 50 per cent and 100 per cent survival following direct and gradual transfer and Atlantic salmon exhibited highest euryhalinity by showing 100 per cent survival under both protocols.
4. Claridae and Cyprinidae are primary freshwater fishes and therefore are able to tolerate low salinity upto 25 per cent SW. Other families which are secondary freshwater fishes *e.g.* Cichlidae, Cyprinidontidae and Poecilidae are able to tolerate gradual salinity adaptation in concentration exceeding that of sea water (Chervinski, 1984)

Table 5.3: Euryhaline Fishes (Salinity Tolerance)

Sl.No.	*Fish*	*Salinity Tolerance*	*Reference*	*Remarks*
1.	*Gambusia affinis* (Mosquito fish)	Abrupt transfer: low mortality up to 50% SW Through a gradual adaptation, tolerance up to 39.0‰ to 58.8‰ (50% Mortality) Good survival in transfer from 100% SW to FW	Chervinski, (1983)	
2.	*Oreochromis mossambicus* (Tilapia)	FW 180% SW (64‰)	Uchida *et al.* (2000)	Fish can adapt to FW and SW
3.	*Poecilia latipinna* (Sailfin Molly)	Salinity range 35-95‰ SW adapted fish	Gonzalez *et al.* (2005)	Inhabitant in salt marshes along the gulf coast
4.	*Sparus auratus* (Gilthead sea bream)	6 ‰– 55 ‰ SW adapted fish	Sangiao-Alvarellos *et al.* (2005)	Fish can survive in FW up to hypersaline SW (55‰)
5.	*Etroplus maculatus* (Orange chromide)	100% SW	Virabhadrachari (1961)	FW fish can be adapted up to 100% SW by gradual transfer through intermediate salinities.
6.	*Salaria pavo* (Peacock blenny) (marine inhabitant)	Can tolerate up to 0, 40, 100% SW	Plaut (1998)	*S. Pavo* lives in SW but is able to tolerate FW environment
7.	*S. fluviatilis* (Freshwater blenny)	Survive up to 100% SW	Plaut (1998)	*S. fluviatilis* is able to osmoregulate both in freshwater and seawater

Contd...

Table 5.3–Contd...

Sl.No.	Fish	Salinity Tolerance	Reference	Remarks
8.	*Fundulus zebrinus* (Plains killifish) *F. diaphanu* (Banded killifish) *F. waccamensis* (Waccamaw killifish)	74 – 114 ‰	Griffith (1974)	
	F. heteroclitus (killifish)	106-120 ‰ (avg: 113 ‰)		
9.	*Anguilla anguilla* (Yellow European eel)	200% SW FW to SW	Skadhauge (1969)	
10.	*Salvelinus namaycush* (Lake trout)	80% Survival up to 30‰ by direct or gradual transfer	Hiroi and McCormick (2007)	Lake trout survives high levels in 30 ‰ of both direct and gradual transfer
	Salvelinus fontinalis (brook trout)	50% and 100% survival rate by direct and gradual transfer		
11.	*Salmo salar* (Atlantic salmon)	100% survival in 30 ‰ by direct and gradual transfer	Hiroi and McCormick (2007)	
12.	*Chanos chanos* (Milkfish)	48‰ (juvenile)	Chen *et al.* (2004) Ferraris *et al.* (1988)	Survived more than 95% in 0, 16, 32, and 48 ‰, adapted well to abrupt changes of salinity.
13.	*Valencia letourneuxi* (Corfu toothcarp)	Upper limit 46 ‰ FW to SW	Bianco and Nordlie (2008)	

Contd...

Table 5.3–Contd...

Sl.No.	Fish	Salinity Tolerance	Reference	Remarks
14.	*Cyprinodon variegatus* (sheepshead minnow)	167 ‰	Gilmore *et al.* (1982)	Highest recorded salinity tolerance
15.	*Cyprinodon rubrofluviatilis* (Red River pupfish)	150 ‰	Echelle *et al.* (1972)	
16.	*Aphanius dispar*	145 ‰	Lotan (1971)	
17.	*Fundulus parvipinnis* (California killifish)	128 ‰	Rao (1975)	
18.	*Cyprinodon milleri* (Death valley pupfish)	105 ‰	Naiman *et al.* (1976)	
19.	*Mugil cephalus* (Flathead mullet)	126 ‰	Hotos and Vlahos (1998)	Marine species. The Mullet normally occupies fresh, brackish and marine habitats.
20.	*Salmo gairdneri* (Rainbow trout)	FW – SW (32 ‰) (960 mOsm)	Gordon (1963)	Upper salinity tolerance not noted.

Conventional Experimental Protocol to Determine the Stenohaline or Euryhaline Status of the Fish

For any comprehensive study on the mechanism of osmoregulation in fishes, the first and the foremost requirement is to determine whether the fish under investigation is a stenohaline or euryhaline. It requires the preparation of various dilutions of artificial seawater from full-strength (100 per cent SW). The ionic composition of various salts in full-strength SW is detailed in Table 5.4. Generally, SW is prepared by mixing these salts in the required quantity and further dilutions are made by mixing it with dechlorinated tap water. To check the veracity of this composition, the osmolarity of full strength SW is measured by Osmometer (Vapour pressure or Freezing point depression type). The value of this full-strength SW comes to approximately 1000 mOsm.

Normally, several dilution of SW (10 per cent, 20 per cent, 25 per cent, 30 per cent, 35 per cent, 40 per cent, 45 per cent, 50 per cent, 60 per cent, 70 per cent, 80 per cent, 90 per cent and 100 per cent SW) are made and approximately twenty well-acclimatized fishes are transferred directly to each salinity and daily mortality record is maintained. By the end of fifteen days of transfer, total mortality record is assessed and LC_{50} value (seawater concentration in which half the population survives/dies in a given period) is calculated which is regarded as upper salinity tolerance limit (USTL) of the fish. Similarly, in another set of experiment, USTL is determined following pre-adaptation in sub-lethal salinities for 3 days and subsequent transfer of the same group to next higher salinities progressively after every 3-day acclimation in the respective salinity. Hence, following the above protocol, USTL following direct transfer and pre-adaption in lower salinities can be easily determined. In some fishes, USTL in both conditions have been found to be either the same or shows enhancement following pre-adaptation in lower salinities.

Under the present nomenclature the FW-endemic fish which can survive full-strength SW or the SW-endemic fish which can survive in FW are termed euryhaline whereas those with limited salinity tolerance (the range may vary, see Table 5.2) are called stenohaline. For more details, the interested readers are advised to consult the references of various workers enlisted in Tables 5.2 and 5.3.

Table 5.4: Sea Water (SW) Composition and Osmotic Pressure of Various SW Dilutions

Seawater (SW) composition (mM)							
Salts	NaCl	KCl	$CaCl_2$	$MgCl_2$	Na_2SO_4	$NaHCO_3$	NaBr
Conc. (mM)	400.8	9.8	10.1	52.7	27.0	2.5	0.6

Osmotic Pressure of various SW dilutions								
Dilutions (SW)	100 per cent	60 per cent	50 per cent	40 per cent	35 per cent	30 per cent	20 per cent	10 per cent
Osmotic pressure (mOsm)	985	592	487	388	338	292	194	98

Osmoregulatory Mechanism in Higher Salinities

Teleost fishes in higher salinities face the twin problem of diffusional influx of salts and osmotic loss of water and classical model proposed by Smith (1932) and Krogh (1939) to explain osmoregulatory mechanisms operating in freshwater and marine teleost fishes is still essentially valid. Teleost fishes in higher salinities maintain osmo-ionic balance by coordinated function of gastrointestinal tract, renal complex and branchial apparatus. Any detailed study dealing with unraveling the above mechanism, apart from other parameters, it also requires the collection of urine from the fish which often become a daunting task. One has to keep the minimal mechanical intervention during urine collection to avoid laboratory induced diuresis caused due to procedural stress. Hence urine collection has been reported only in limited number of teleost fishes such as *Salmo gairdneri, Fundulus heteroclitus, Carassius auratus, Ictalurus punctatus* and *Anguilla anguilla*. In the catfish *H. fossilis*, of the various methods tested for urine collection, that of the'retention catheter' consisting of an assembly of 5-cm long polyethylene tubing, impermeable rubber balloon and 2.5 cm long thick-walled glass tubing proved to be the most satisfactory. It has also been conclusively proved that the catfish is not susceptible to stress by routine laboratory handling (Sherwani and Parwez, 2000).

In catfish, *H. fossilis* adaptation in higher salinities is evident from the drastic reduction in urine output upto 81 per cent facilitated by reduction in glomerular filtration rate(GFR) and free water clearance as a means of water conservation (Goswami *et al.*, 1983) which corresponds well with the similar data obtained in several euryhaline and stenohaline teleost fishes. Excess body salt elimination, a necessity of the catfish *H. fossilis* as also other teleost fish in higher salinities, is being achieved by enormous increase in urine osmolarity. What, then, limits the survival of the catfish only upto 35 per cent SW ? The absences of loop of Henle in fish kidney restrict the ability of these fishes to produce the urine which can at best be iso-osmotic to its body fluid. Hence, euryhaline fishes circumvent this limitation by adopting an excellent division of labour regarding salt excretion where majority of the monovalent ions are eliminated by branchial mechanism and the major divalent ions through renal route. Our studies on catfish suggest that the branchial apparatus possibly does not excrete the monovalent ions efficiently hence the elimination of even monovalent ions is being performed by the renal pathway as is evident by an enormous increase in urine osmolarity when the catfish is placed in NaCl solutions. Thus the inability of catfish to produce hyperosmotic urine coupled with the inability of the gills to efficiently excrete ions account for its limited survival up to 35 per cent SW or 1.1 per cent NaCl (Goswami *et al.*, 1983). Further, gut examination reveal no evidence of catfish drinking water in higher salinities which deprives it of its osmotically unobligated water. This together with the inability of renal tubules to increase reabsorption of water, unchanged osmolar clearance and reduction in free water clearance account for its inability to eliminate increased salt load hence limiting the salinity tolerance in this fish. On the contrary, the urinary sodium loss is virtually unaffected following injection of sodium chloride in goldfish suggesting a relatively more efficient branchial mechanism (Bourguet *et al.*, 1964). Based on the above, it is tempting to suggest that progression towards euryhalinity, among other factors, is intimately linked with the efficient functional reversal of branchial system from ion-uptake in FW to ion exertion in higher salinities. While the catfish seems totally unable to accomplish this reversibility, the goldfish does show considerable efficiency but not to the extent of a euryhaline fish.

Effect of Pre-adaptation in Sub-lethal Salinity on Upper Salinity Tolerance Limit of Fish

The data on *H. fossilis* and *C. batrachus* show that these fishes are able to survive up to 35 per cent SW and 30 per cent SW respectively by direct transfer and the pre-adaptation in lower salinities showed no improvement in survival rate of *H. fossilis* and only a marginal effect on *C. batrachus* (Parwez *et al.*, 1979, 2001). Similar absence of effect on prior acclimation has also been reported in channel catfish (Norton and Davis, 1977). However, the contrast in seen in flathead catfish in which upper salinity limit increases from a 14.5 ppt following direct transfer to about 15.5 ppt following pre-adaptation in lower salinities (Bringolf *et al.*, 2005).

Active Osmoregulation versus Passive Tissue Tolerance

Mere data on upper salinity tolerance limit may, however, not present the exact physiological state of the fish. Osmoregulatory adjustment is a bimodal process. The first phase called adaptive phase may last from few hours to few days and is characterized by abrupt increase in plasma osmotic pressure and ionic contents. This is followed by chronic regulative phase which marks the restoration of normalcy in all the elevated parameters. Studies on *H. fossilis* and *C. batrachus* clearly demonstrate the absence of regulative phase (Goswami *et al.*, 1983; Parwez *et al.*, 2001) and the same results were reported in barred surfperch *Amphistichus argenteus*, a marine stenohaline teleost (Holmes and Lockwood, 1970) but the exception is provided by stenohaline *I. punctatus* (Norton and Davis, 1977). Generally euryhaline fishes do show the existence of this bimodal phase as is evident in flounder, salmon and eel (Bentley, 1971).

Interestingly, in *H. fossilis* and *C. batrachus* following transfer to higher salinities, osmoregulatory parameters do not show any appreciable increase up to 10 per cent 15 per cent respectively and the fishes are said to be actively osmoregulating upto this level and survival beyond this up to their upper salinity tolerance limit is by mere tissue tolerance to increased ionic concentration in body fluid. Channel catfish *I. punctatus* and common carp, *C. carpio*, however, actively osmoregulate up to their upper salinity tolerance (Norton and Davis, 1977; Abo Hegab and Hanke, 1982) though the latter shows a marginal increase in plasma osmolarity in 45 per cent SW.

Osmoregulatory Target Organs

Gill

Teleost gill assumes considerable significance as an important osmoregulatory target organ largely because it offers up to 60 times more surface area compared to integument and opercular epithelial surface. Moreover, it, like integument, forms a direct contact point with external environment and hence directly experiences the osmotic fluctuation of the ambient medium. Hence, extensive studies have been carried out on its morphology and anatomy to elucidate its functional role. Interested readers may refer to comprehensive reviews of fish gill by Hughes (1984), Laurent (1984, 1989) and Wilson and Laurent (2002). Generally, gill consists of gill arch, gill lamellae, gill filament and four major types of epithelial cells which line two distinct types of surfaces-filament and lamellar epithelia also called primary and secondary epithelia.

Gill Cell types: The four major ubiquitously occurring cell types include the most abundantly occurring pavement cells (PVC) also termed respiratory cells constituting about 90 per cent of surface area, squamous or cuboid shaped with conflicting evidence for the presence of PVC gap junction communicating with mitochondrial rich cells (MRC).

The second cell type – Mucous or goblet cells contain mucopolysaccharides and are mostly associated with defense and protective role. Hence these cells are not implicated to any reasonable degree in osmoregulatory mechanism. The pillar cells basically provide structural support to gill. The other major type of branchial cells are MRCs also called Chloride cells which have been shown to be the site of ionic transport. Most studies of gills with reference to osmoregulation have been focused on the localization, distribution and functional attributes of these cells in osmoregulatory adjustment of teleost fishes.

Gastrointestinal Tract

Of all the osmoregulatory target organs, GI tract plays a more significant role in marine teleosts which drink SW as a part of strategy to compensate for osmotic water loss in hyperosmotic media (SW). Oesophagus is the first site of desaltation of SW specially NaCl which is absorbed by passive and active component reducing the osmolarity of the intestinal fluid. The main osmolytes in the intestinal fluid are Mg^{2+}, SO_4^{2-} and HCO_3^- which finally get excreted through rectal fluid. The GI tract role in FW teleost is not clearly defined. However, the ingested food does contain considerable electrolytes which make up for, partly though, the diffusional salt loss in hypoosmotic environment of FW. However, very little is known about the interaction between osmoregulation and feeding.

Renal Complex

It has been extensively documented that the process of osmoionic regulation does not remain confined to only kidney but extends even to the urinary bladder which also plays significant role. Hence, it is appropriate to use the nomenclature 'renal complex' rather than just the kidney to encompass the salt and water fluxes in this entire organ system. The renal complex of teleost is unable to produce urine that is hyperosmotic to blood because it lacks the loop of Henle which is present in other vertebrates. The renal complex of marine teleost is essentially the same as in FW teleost with the exception that distal segment is usually missing and the glomeruli are mostly reduced or are totally absent as in 23 marine teleosts notably goosefish (*Lophius*) and toadfish (*Opsanus*).

In FW teleost, glomerular filtration rate (GFR) is rapid and consequently the urine flow rate (UFR) is high, urine is highly hypotonic and output is copious to minimize the salt loss. On the contrary, in marine teleost, GFR is considerably reduced either due to reduced number of glomeruli or variations in the perfused glomeruli called 'glomeular intermittancy'. In aglomerular fishes, small volume of urine is produced by secretion. The urine in these fishes is isotonic with considerable concentration of divalent ions such as Mg^{2+}, SO_4^{2-} and Ca^{2+}. The urinary parameters of a few representative FW and SW teleost is given in Table 5.5.

Osmoregulatory Hormones

Hormonal control of osmoregulatory adjustment in teleost fishes first became apparent from the studies of Pickford (1953) and Burden (1956). They observed that killifish *Fundulus heteroclitus* failed to survive in freshwater following hypophysectomy and its mortality could be avoided if the fish was kept in dilute seawater. Similar observations were made in many other teleosts such as *Sarotherodon mossambicus*, *Gambusia affinis*, *Poecilia latipinna*, *Xiphophorus*, *Pleuronectes platessa* (Johnson, 1973). There is, however, another category of teleost fishes which survive for prolonged period following hypophysectomy but with deranged osmoregulatory parameters. Such category is examplified by *Anguilla anguilla*, *Carassius auratus*, *Salmo gairdneri*, *Platichthys flesus*, *Fundulus kansae* and *Channa punctatus* (Parwez *et al.*, 1984).

Massive literature on endocrine control of osmoregulation in teleost fishes seems to implicate, to varying extent, almost all conceivable endocrine glands. However, overwhelming body of evidence generated until 1980s points to the role of prolactin (PRL) as a dominant hormonal factor regulating hydromineral balance in FW while cortisol (F) may play the critical role in SW adaptation. It was also believed that F may primarily act at the ion pump level and PRL on osmotic permeability. However, subsequent years witnessed the emergence of new hormone candidates and their axis strongly suggestive of their role as osmoregulatory hormones. This included, among others, growth hormone (GH) and insulin like growth factor I (IGF-I) axis and thyroid hormones (T_3 and T_4), all favoring SW-adaptation. Interestingly, contrary to earlier classical concept of cortisol as "SW-adapting hormone", it was later shown to play a dual role both in hypo and hyperosmotic environments. A large

Table 5.5: Renal Parameters of a Few Representative Stenohaline and Euryhaline Teleosts

Sl.No.	Fish	GFR ml/hr/kg	UFR ml/hr/kg	Osmolarity mOsm	Reference
			Stenohaline Fishes		
1.	*Salvelinus namaycush* (Lake trout)	3.73	2.44	Plasma: 328 Urine: 36.2	Hammond (1969)
2.	*Ameiurus nebulosus* (Brown bullhead)	9.4	6.4		Lavoie *et al.* (1959) Haywood and Clapp (1942) Marshall (1934)
3.	*Carassius auratus* (Goldfish)	14.4	10.7	Plasma: 258 Urine: 35.9	Bourguet *et al.* (1964) Maetz (1963)
4.	*Cyprinus carpio* (Common carp)		1.1-10.8 at temp. between 6-28° C		Pora and Prekup (1960)
5.	*Esox lucius* (Northen Pike)	4.0	2.8	Plasma: 264 Urine: 37.7	Ginetsinkii *et al.* (1961) Hickman (1965)
6.	*Catostomus commersonii* (Lacepede)	2.2	1.15	Plasma: 233 Urine: 33.5	Hickman (1965) Mackay (1967)

Contd...

Table 5.5–Contd...

Sl.No.	Fish	GFR ml/hr/kg	UFR ml/hr/kg	Osmolarity mOsm	Reference
			Euryhaline Fishes		
1.	*Salmo gairdneri* (Rainbow trout)	Fw: 7.3 ± 0.1	Fw: 3.8	Urine: 32–48	Holmes and Stainer (1966)
2.	*Anguilla anguilla* (European eel)	Fw: 4.6 Sw: 1.03	Fw: 3.5 Sw: 0.63	Plasma: 323	Sharratt *et al.* (1964) Chester Jones *et al.* (1969) Kenyon *et al.* (1984)
3.	*Platichthys flesus* (Flounder)	Fw: 4.91 Sw: 2.4	Fw: 1.78 Sw: 0.68		Lahlou (1967)
4.	*Fundulus kansae* (Plains Killifish)	Fw: 25 Sw: 1.35	Fw: 8.33 Sw: 0.52	Plasma: 305 ± 4.4 Urine: 82.3 ± 8.4	Fleming and Stanley (1965) Stanley and Fleming (1967)
5.	*Paralichthys lethostigma* (Southern flounder)	Fw: 3.88 Sw: 1.69	Fw: 2.9 Sw: 0.22		Hickman (1965)
6.	*Anguilla japonica* (Japanese eel)	Fw: 2.80 Sw: 3.13	Fw: 2.26 Sw: 0.38		Oide and Utida (1968)
7.	*Salmo salar* (Atlantic salmon)		Sw: 0.72 Fw: 4.55 Fw: 1.2 Sw: 0.2		Talbot *et al.* (1989) Talbot *et al.* (1992)

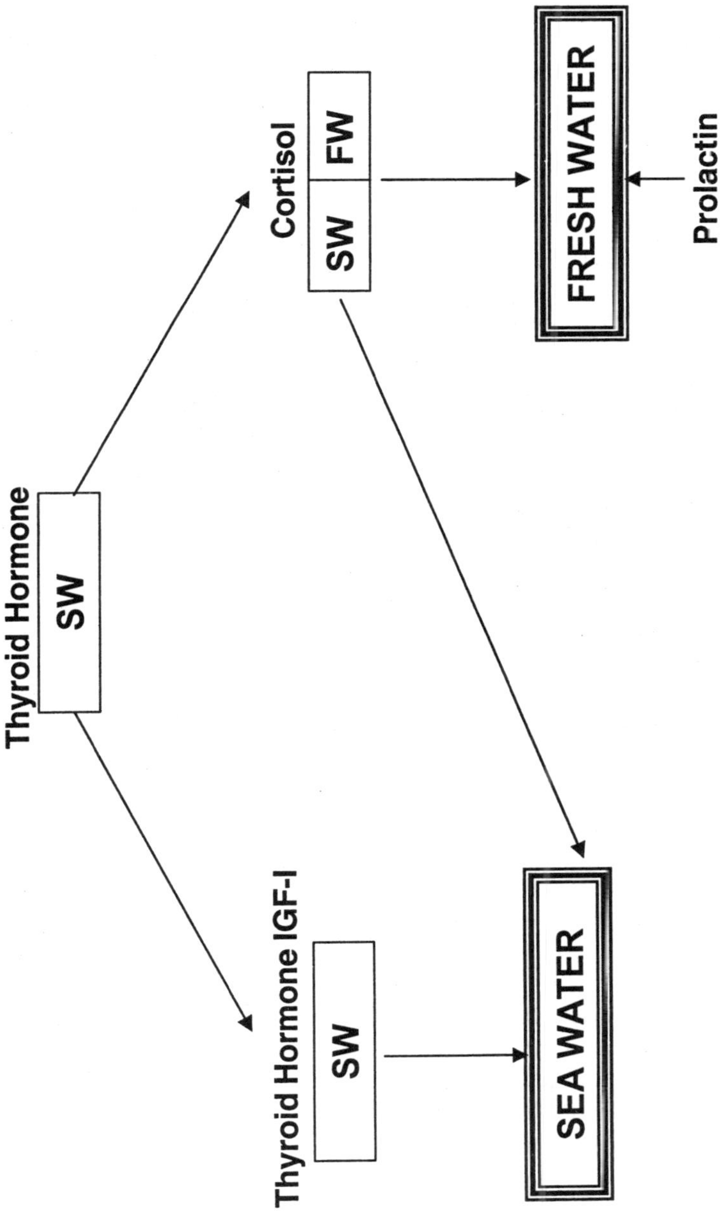

Figure 5.1: Major Hormones and their Role in Regulation in FW and SW

number of studies have also brought out a clear cut synergistic action among various hormones, notably GH/IGF-I, GH and F, T_4/GH potentiating the physiological response at various effector organs (Figure 5.1). Recently, a comprehensive list of rapid acting osmoregulatory hormones/factors emanating from different tissues have been added. Inhibition of chloride secretion has been demonstrated by epinephrine, urotensin II, acetylcholine and prostaglandin E_2. Other hormones which may be involved in stimulating chloride uptake through increased second messenger are glucagon, vasoactive intestinal peptide (VIP), leukotrienes and urotensin I. There is increasing evidence to show that atrial natriuretic peptide (ANP) plays an important role in ion transport particularly in SW-acclimated mummichog, flounder and toadfish. It must, however, be mentioned that most of the above studies on rapid regulatory hormones are limited to SW-adapted teleost and under *in vitro* system. There is also a need to examine FW-acclimated fish under *in vivo* condition to have a more realistic and complete picture. The above narrative presents a very brief account of the osmoregulatory hormones. For more detailed view, excellent reviews by McCormick (2001), McCormick and Bradshaw (2006) and Mancera and McCormick (2007) are suggested.

Future Prospectives

While catfish *H. fossilis* of the Indian subcontinent remains the most extensively studied fish on osmoregulatory mechanism in divergent media, certain very important aspects are uncovered and should be taken up as prospective studies. This includes the role of GH on the changes in branchial, renal and gut target organs, α and β chloride cells, changes in Na^+/K^+-ATPase, receptor dynamics and GH and PRL gene expression in different target organs. The last aspect relating to GH gene expression should now be easily possible since GH gene in the *H. fossilis* has already been sequenced (Anathy *et al.*, 2001). In addition to GH, the role of other hormones such as cortisol, prolactin, arginine vasotocin, thyroid hormones on the above mentioned osmoregulatory parameters have also not been studied. It must be conceded that the quantum of work proposed above on the catfish, *H. fossilis* is simply enormous but the availability of such data on these aspects will make catfish, *H. fossilis* as one of the most comprehensively studied fish on the osmoregulation and will serve as a model to understand the ion regulatory mechanism in a tropical stenohaline fish.

However, the above narration is not an advocacy in favour of studies on one single species. As already mentioned in the beginning of this review, Indian subcontinent abounds with a rich piscine biodiversity. This will provide an excellent opportunity to extend such studies on large number of fish species inhabiting divergent ionic environment to take the measure of species-specific variations in different teleost group.

References

Abo Hegab, S. and Hanke, W., 1982. Electrolyte changes and volume regulatory processes in the carp (*Cyprinus carpio*) during osmotic stress. *Comp. Biochem. Physiol.*, 71: 157-164.

Allen, K.O. and Avault, J.W., 1969. Effects of salinity on growth and survival of channel catfish, *Ictalurus punctatus*. *Proc. S.E. Assoc. Game Fish Comm.*, 23: 319-331.

Anathy, V., Venugopal, T, Koteeswaran, R., Pandian, T. J. and Mathavan, S., 2001. Cloning, sequencing and expression of cDNA encoding growth hormone from Indian catfish (*Heteropneustes fossilis*). *J. Biosci.*, 26(3): 315-324.

Armitage, K. B. and Olund, L. J., 1962. Salt Tolerance of the Brook Stickleback. *American Midland Naturalist*, 68(2): 274-277.

Avella, M., Berhaut, J. and Bornancin, M., 1993. Salinity tolerance of two tropical fishes, *Oreochromis aureus* and *O. niloticus*. I. Biochemical and morphological changes in the gill epithelium. *J. Fish Biol.*, 42(2): 243 – 254.

Azizi, S., Kochanian, P., Peyghan, R., Khansari, A., Bastami, K. D., 2010. Chloride cell morphometrics of common carp, *Cyprinus carpio*, in response in different salinities. *Comp. Clin. Pathol.*, DOI: 10.1007/s00580-010-1003-8

Bently, P. J., 1971. Endocrines and Osmoregulation. A comparative account of the regulation of water and salt in vertebrates, Vol. Berlin, Heidelberg, New York: Springer- Verlag.

Bianco, P. G. and Nordlie, F., 2008. The salinity tolerance of *Pseudophoxinus stymphalicus* (Cyprinidae) and *Valencia letourneuxi* (Valenciidae) from western Greece suggests a revision of the ecological categories of freshwater fishes. *Italian Journal of Zoology*, 75 (3): 285- 293.

Bourguet, J., Lahlou, B., and Maetz, J., 1964. Modifications experimentales de I'equilibre hydromineral et osmoregulation chez *Carassius auratus*. *Gen. Comp. Endocrinol.*, 4: 563-576.

Burden, C. E., 1956. The failure of hypophysectomized *Fundulus heteroclitus* to survive in freshwater. *Biol. Bull.*, 110: 8-28.

Bringolf, R. B., Kwak, T.J., Gregory, C. W. and Lorimore, M. S., 2005. Salinity tolerance of Flathead catfish: implications for dispersal of introduced population. *Transactions of the American Fish Society*, 134: 927-936.

Chen, C., Lin, L. and Lee, T., 2004. Ionocyte Distribution in Gills of the Euryhaline Milkfish, *Chanos chanos* (Forsskal, 1775). *Zool. Stud.*, 43(4): 772-777.

Chervinski, J., 1983. Salinity tolerance of the mosquito fish, *Gambusia affinis* (Baird and Girard). *J. Fish Biol.*, 22: 9-11.

Chervinski, J., 1984. Salinity tolerance of the young catfish, *Clarias lazera* (Burchell). *J. Fish Biol.*, 25: 147-149.

Chester Jones, I., Chan, D.K.O. and Rankin, J.C., 1969. Renal function in European eel (*Anguilla Anguilla* L.): Changes in blood pressure and renal function of freshwater eel transferred to sea-water. *J. Endocrinol.*, 43: 9-19.

Chipman, R. K., 1959. Studies of tolerance of certain freshwater fishes to brine water from oil wells. *Ecology*, 40: 299-302.

Clemens, H. P. and Jones, W. H., 1955. Toxicity of brine water from oil wells. *Transaction of the American Fisheries Society*, 84: 97-109.

Das, S., Srivastava, G. J. I., 1979. Salinity tolerance of giant *Colisa fasciatus* (Bl. and Schn.). *Bonner Zoologische Beitrages*, 25: 391–402.

Echelle, A.A., Echelle, A.F., Hill, L.G., 1972. Interspecific interactions and limiting factors of abundance and distribution in the Red River pupfish *Cyprinodon rubrofluviatilis*. *American Midland Naturalist*, 88: 109–130.

Fashina-Bombata, H. A., Busari, A. N., 2003. Influence of salinity on the developmental stages of African catfish *Heterobranchus longifilis* (Valenciennes, 1840). *Aquaculture*, 224: 213–222.

Ferraris, R. P., Almendras, J. M. and Jazul, A. P., 1988. Changes in plasma osmolality and chloride concentration during abrupt transfer of milkfish (*Chanos chanos*) from seawater to different test salinities. *Aquaculture*, 70: 145-157.

Fleming, W. R., and Stanley, J. G., 1965. Effects of rapid changes in salinity on the renal function of a euryhaline teleost. *Am. J. Physiol.*, 209: 1025-1030.

Gbulubo, A. J. and Erondu, E. S., 1998. Salinity influence on the early stages of the African catfish. *Aquaculture Int.*, p. 369- 379.

Gilmore, R.G., Cooke, D.W., Donohue, C.J., 1982. A comparison of the fish populations and habitat in open and closed salt marsh impoundments in east-central Florida. *Northeast Gulf Science*, 5: 25–37.

Ginetsinkii, A. G., Vasileva, V. F., and Natochin, Yu, V., 1961. Reaktsiya ryb na izmenenie solenosti sredy, (The reaction of fishes to a change in the salinity of the water). In "Problemy Evolyutsii Funksii I Enzimochimi Protsessov Voz-buzhdehiya" (Problems of the evolution of function and of enzyme chemistry of the processes of stimulation.), pp. 89-102. Akad. Nauk, S.S.S.R., Moscow.

Gonzalez, R. Z., Cooper, J., Head, D., 2005. Physiological responses to hyper-saline waters in sailfin mollies (*Poecilia latipinna*). *Comp. Biochem. Physiol. A Mol. Integr. Physiol.*, 142(4): 397-403.

Gordon, M.S., 1963. Water and salt balance in fish and amphibians. *Handbook of Physiology.*

Goswami, S.V., Parwez, I. And Sundararaj, B.I., 1983. Some aspects of osmoregulation in a stenohaline freshwater catfish, *Heteropneustes fossilis* (Bloch), in different salinities. *J. Fish Biol.*, 23: 475-487.

Griffith, R. W., 1974. Environment and salinity tolerance in the genus *Fundulus. American Society of Ichthyologists and Herpetologists*, 1974(2): 319-331.

Hammond, B. R., 1969. Renal function and the effects of arginine vasotocin in lake trout, *Salvelinus namaycush* (Walbaum). Doctoral thesis, Cornell Univ.

Haywood, C., and Clapp, M. J., 1942. A note on the freezing points of the urines of two freshwater fishes: The catfish (*Ameiurus nebulosus*) and the sucker (*Catostomus commersonii*). *Biol. Bull.*, 83: 363-366.

Hickman, C.P., Jr., 1965. Studies on the renal function in freshwater teleost fish. *Tran. Roy. Soc. Can. Sect.*, III [4] 3: 213-236.

Hiroi, J., McCormick, S.D., 2007. Variation in salinity tolerance, gill Na^+/K^+-ATPase, $Na^+/K^+/2Cl^-$ cotransporter and mitochondria-rich cell distribution in three salmonids *Salvelinus namaycush, Salvelinus fontinalis* and *Salmo salar. J. Exp. Biol.*, 210(6): 1015-24.

Holmes, W. N. and Lockwood L. N., 1970. Some aspects of osmoregulation in the barred surf perch (*Amphistichus argenteus. J. Zool. Lond.*, 161: 1-14.

Holmes, W. N., and Stainer, I. M., 1966. Studies on the renal excretion of electrolytes by the trout (*Salmo gairdneri*). *J. Exptl. Biol.*, 44: 33-46.

Hotos, G.N., Vlahos, N., 1998. Salinity tolerance of *Mugil cephalus* and *Chelon labrosus* (Pisces, Mugilidae) fry in experimental conditions. *Aquaculture*, 167: 329–338.

Hughes, G. M., 1984. General anatomy of the gills. In: *Fish Physiology* Eds: Hoar, W. S., Randall, D. J., Vol 10A. New York: Academic Press. 1-72.

Jacobsen, L., Skov, C., Koed, A., Berg, S., 2007. Short-term salinity tolerance of northern pike, *Esox lucius*, fry, related to temperature and size. *Fisheries Management and Ecology*, 14(5): 303-308.

Johnson, D. W., 1973. Endocrine control of hydromineral balance in teleost. *Amer. Zool.*, 13: 799-818.

Kendall, A.W. Jr. and Schwartz, F.L., 1968. Lethal temperature and salinity tolerance for white catfish, *Ictalurus catus*, from the Patuxent river, Maryland. Chesapeake *Science*, 9: 103 -108.

Kenyon, C. J., McKeever, A., Oliver, J. A. and Henderson, I. W., 1984. Control of renal and adrenocortical function by the rennin-angiotensin system in two euryhaline teleost fishes. *Gen. Comp. Endocrinol.*, 58: 93-100

Kraiem, M. M. and Pattee, E.(1988. Salinity tolerance of the barbel, *Barbus callensis* Valenciennes, 1842 (Pisces, Cyprinidae) and its ecological significance. *Hydrobiologia*,166 (3): 263-267.

Krayushkina, L. S., Semenova, O. G., Panov, A. A., Gerasimov, A. A., 1996. Functional traits of juvenile paddlefish *Polyodon spathula* (Polyodontidae). *Journal of Ichthyology*, 36: 787–793.

Krogh, A., 1939. *Osmotic Regulation in Aquatic Animals*. Cambridge Univ. Press.

Lahlou, B., 1967. Mise en evidence d,un "recrutement glomerulaire" dans le rein des Teleosteens d,après la mesure du Tm glucose. *Comp. Biochem. Physiol.*, 20: 925-938.

Lavoie, M. E., Chidsey, J. L., and Forster, R. P., 1959. Glomerular filtration rate and renal plasma flow in the freshwater brown bullhead or horned pout, *Ameiurus nebulosus*. *Bull. Mt. Desert Isl. Biol. Lab.*, 50-51

Laurent, P., 1984. Gill internal Morphology. In: *Fish Physiology*. Eds: Hoar, W. S., Randall, D. J., Vol 10A. New York: Academic Press. 73-183.

Laurent, P., 1989. Gill structure and function. In: *Comparative Pulmonary Physiology*. Eds. Wood, S. C. New York: Marcel Dekker. 69-120.

Lemarie, G., Baroiller, J. F., Clota, F., Lazard, J., Dosdat, A., 2004. A simple test to estimate the salinity resistance of fish with specific application to *O. niloticus* and *S. melanotheron*. *Aquaculture*, 240: 575-587.

Lotan, R., 1971. Osmotic adjustment in the euryhaline teleost, *Aphanius dispar* (Cyprinodontidae). *Zeitschrift für vergleichende Physiologie*, 75: 383–387.

Mackay, W. C., 1967. Plasma glucose levels in the northern pike, *Esox lucius* and the white sucker, *Catostomus commersonii*, and renal glucose reabsorption in the white sucker. Master's thesis, University of Alberta.

Maetz, J., 1963. Physiological aspects of neurohypophysial function in fishes with some reference to the amphibian. *Symp. Zool. Soc. London*, 9: 107-140.

Mancera, J. M. and McCormick, S. D., 2007. Role of Prolactin, Growth hormone, Insulin-like growth factor I and Cortisol in teleost osmoregulation. *In: Fish osmoregulation*. Eds. Baldisserotto, B., Mancera, J. M. and Kapoor, B. G. Science Publisher. 498-515.

Marshall, E. K., Jr., 1934. The comparative physiology of the kidney in relation to theories of renal secretion. *Physiol. Rev.*, 14: 133-159.

McCormick, S. D., 2001. Endocrine Control of Osmoregulation in Teleost Fish. *Amer. Zool.*, 41: 781-794.

McCormick, S. D. and Bradshaw, 2006. Hormonal control of salt and water balance in vertebrates. *Gen. Comp. Endocrinol.*, 147: 3-8.

Meador, M.R. and Kelso, W.E., 1990. Behaviour and movements of largemouth bass in response to salinity. *Trans. Am. Fish. Soc.*, 118: 409-415.

Naiman, R.J., Gerking, S.D. and Stuart, R.E., 1976. Osmoregulation in the Death Valley pupfish *Cyprinodon milleri* (Pisces: Cyprinodontidae). *Copeia*, 1976: 807–810.

Nazneen, S. and Begum, F., 1981. Salinity tolerance in some freshwater fishes. *Biologia*, 27: 33–38.

Norton, V. M. and Davis, K. B., 1977. Effect of abrupt change in the salinity of the environment on plasma electrolytes, urine volume, and electrolyte excretion in channel catfish, *Ictalurus punctatus*. *Comp. Biochem. Physiol.*, 56: 392-444.

Oide, H. and Utida, S., 1968. Changes in intestinal absorption and renal excretion of water during adaptation to sea-water in the Japanese eel. *Marine Biol.*, 1: 172-177.

Parwez, I. and Goswami, S.V., 1985. Effect of prolactin, adrenocorticotrophin, Neurohypophysial peptides, cortisol, and androgens on some osmoregulatory parameters of the hypophysectomized catfish, *Heteropneustes fossilis* (Bloch). *Gen. Comp. Endocrinol.*, 58: 51-68.

Parwez, I., Goswami, S.V. and Sundararaj, B.I., 1979. Salinity tolerance of the freshwater catfish, *Heteropneustes fossilis* (Bloch). *Indian J. Exp. Biol.*, 17: 810-811.

Parwez, I., Goswami, S.V. and Sundararaj, B.I., 1984. Effect of hypophysectomy on some osmoregulatory parameters of the catfish, *Heteropneustes fossilis* (Bloch). *J. Exp. Zool.*,23: 475-487.

Parwez, I., Nayyar, M., Sherwani, F.A. and Parwez, H., 2001. Salinity tolerance and the role of cortisol during osmotic adjustments of an air-breathing catfish, *Clarias batrachus*. *Journal of Aquaculture*, 9: 9-17.

Parwez, I., Sherwani, F.A. and Goswami, S. V., 1994. Osmoregulation in the stenohaline freshwater catfish, *Heteropneustes fossilis* (Bloch) in deionized water. *Fish Physiol. Biochem.*, 13: 173-181.

Pickford, G. E., 1953. A study of the hypophysectomozed male killifish, *Fundulus heteroclitus* (Linn.) *Bull. Bingham. Oceanogr. Coll.*, 14: 5-41.

Plaut, I., 1998. Comparison of salinity tolerance and osmoregulation in two closely related species of blennies from different habitats. *Fish Physiol. Biochem.*, 19(2): 181-188.

Pora, A. E., and Prekup, O., 1960. A study of the excretory processes of freshwater fish. Part II. Influence of environmental temperature on the excretory processes of the carp and Cruscian carp. *Vopr. Ikhtiol.* 15: 138-147; *Biol. Abstr.*, 37(4): 13391 (1962).

Rao, T.P., 1975. Salinity tolerance of laboratory-reared larvae of the California killfish, *Fundulus parvipinnis* Girard. *J. Fish Biol.*, 7: 783–790.

Ridha M. T.(2008. Preliminary Observation on salinity tolerance of three sizes of the GIFT and non-improved strains of the nile tilapia *Oreochromis niloticus*. *European Journal of Scientific Research*, 24(3): 374-377.

Sangiao-Alvarellos, S., Arjona, F. J., Martin del Rio, M.P., Miguez, J. M., Mancera, J. M. and Soengas, J. L., 2005. Time course of osmoregulatory metabolic changes during osmotic acclimation in *Sparus auratus*. *J. Exp. Biol.*, 288(22): 4291-4304.

Schofield, P. J., Brown, M. E. and Fuller, P. F., 2006. Salinity tolerance of goldfish *Carassius auratus*, a non-native fish in the United States. *Florida Scientist*, 69(4): 258-268.

Schofield, P. J. and Nico L. G., 2009. Salinity tolerance of non-native Asian swamp eels (Teleostei: Synbranchidae) in Florida, USA: comparisons of three populations and implications for dispersal. *Environ. Biol. Fish.*, 85: 51-59.

Sharratt, B. M., Chester Jones, I., and Bellamy, D., 1964. Water and electrolyte composition of the body and renal function of the eel (*Anguilla anguilla* L.). *Comp. Biochem. Physiol.*, 11: 9-18.

Sherwani, F.A. and Parwez, I., 2000. Effects of stress and food deprivation on the catfish, *Heteropneustes fossilis* (Bloch). *Indian J. Exp. Biol.*, 38: 379-384.

Sherwani, F.A. and Parwez, I., 2008. Changes in plasma thyroxine and cortisol profiles and gill and kidney Na^+/K^+-ATPase and SDH activities during acclimation of the catfish, *Heteropneustes fossilis* (Bloch) to higher salinities, with special reference to the effects of exogenous cortisol on hypo-osmoregulatory ability of the catfish. *Zool. Scie.*, 25: 164-171.

Skadhauge, E., 1969).The mechanism of salt and water absorption in the intestine of the eel (*Anguilla anguilla*) adapted to waters of various salinities. *J. Physiol.* 204: 135-158.

Smith, H.W., 1932. Water regulation and its evolution in the fishes. *Quart.Rev.Biol.*, 7: 1-26.

Stanley, J.G. and Fleming, W.R., 1967. The effect of hypophysectomy on the electrolyte content of *Fundulus kansae* held in freshwater and sea water. *Comp. Biochem. Physiol.*, 20: 489-497.

Synudeen, S. S., 2003. Salinity tolerance of *Clarias batrachus*. *Journal of Ecotoxicology and Environmental Monitoring*, 13: 319–320.

Talbot, C., Eddy, F.B., Potts, W.T.W. and Primmett, D.R.N., 1989. Renal function in migrating adult Atlantic Salmon, *Salmo salar* (L.). *Comp. Biochem. Physiol. Part A: Physiology*, Vol. 92, Issue 2, 241-245.

Talbot, C., Stagg, R. M. and Eddy, F.B., 1992. Renal, respiratory and ionic regulation in Atlantic salmon (*Salmo salar* L.) Kelt following transfer from freshwater to seawater. *J. Comp. Physiol.*, 162(4): 358-364.

Uchida, K., Kaneko, T., Miyazaki, H., Hasegawa, S. and Hirano, T., 2000. Excellent salinity tolerance of Mazambique tilapia (*Oreochromis mossambicus*): Elevated chloride cell activity in the branchial and opercular epithelia of the fish adapted to concentrated seawater. *Zool. Sci.*, 17: 149-160.

Victoria, C. J., Wilkerson, B. S., Klauda, R. J., Perry, E. S., 1992. Salinity tolerance of yellow perch eggs and larvae from coastal plain stream populations in Maryland, with comparison to a Pennsylvania lake population. *Copeia*, 1992: 859–865.

Virbhadrachari, V., 1961. Structural changes in the gills, intestine and kidney of *Etroplus maculatus* (Teleostei) adapted to different salinities. *Quarterly Journal of Microscopical Science*, 102 (3): 361-369.

Wilkes, P. R. H. and McMahon, B. R., 1986. Responses of a stenohaline freshwater teleost (*Catostomus commersoni*) to hypersaline exposure. *J. Exp. Biol.*, 121: 77–94.

Williams, M. D. and Williams, W. D., 1991. Salinity tolerances of four species of fish from the Murray-Darling River system. *Hydrobiologia,* 210: 145–160.

Wilson, J. M. and Laurent, P., 2002. Fish gill Morphology: Inside out. *J. Exp. Zool.*, 293: 192-213.

Zullah, A., Ud-Din, S., 1982. Salinity tolerance of *Mystus vittatus* (Bloch). *Biologia,* 28: 263–268.

Chapter 6

Ecotoxicological Risk Assessment of Pharmaceutical Effluent on Blood Chemistry Profiles of an Indian Major Carp, *Labeo rohita*

Chokkalingam Kavitha, Mathan Ramesh, Annamalai Malarvizhi and Jayanthi Prabhu Naveena*

Unit of Toxicology, Department of Zoology, School of Life Sciences, Bharathiar University, Coimbatore – 641 046, Tamil Nadu, India

ABSTRACT

The objective of the present study is to assess the toxicity of pharmaceutical effluent on certain hematological and biochemical parameters of an Indian major carp *Labeo rohita* for 96 h. Fish were exposed to different concentrations (100 per cent, 75 per cent, 50 per cent, 25 per cent, 10 per cent, 5 per cent, 1 per cent 0.5 per cent, 0.1 per cent) of the pharmaceutical effluent and based on the survival/mortality ratio 0.5 per cent concentration of the effluent was taken to assess the toxicity. Fish were exposed to above concentration and the alterations in haematological and biochemical parameters were observed at every 24 h interval for a period of 96 h. During the above treatment period, hemoglobin, hematocrit, erythrocytes,

* Corresponding author: E-mail: mathanramesh@yahoo.com

leucocytes, MCHC, plasma glucose and plasma protein levels were decreased, whereas MCV and MCH contents were increased in effluent treated fish. The alterations of the above said parameters can be effectively used to assess the health status of the aquatic organisms.

Keywords: *Pharmaceutical effluent, Hematology, Plasma glucose and protein, Labeo rohita.*

Introduction

Pharmaceuticals are an important group of potential endocrine disrupting chemicals (EDCs) which has attracted much attention of the internationals scientific community. They are promising environmental contaminants, widely and increasingly being used in human and veterinary medicine (Nikolaou *et al.*, 2007). Due to their high production level and pharmacokinetical behaviour during normal therapeutic use (*e.g.* half-life, urinary and fecal excretion, and metabolism) the presences of these compounds and their metabolites have been detected in wastewaters; sewage treatment plants (STPs) were pointed out as the major source of discharge of these compounds to the environment (Daughton and Ternes, 1999). Discharged pharmaceuticals in variable quantities can reach surface waters, ground waters (Farre *et al.*, 2001), and sediments (Zuccato *et al.*, 2000).

To date, over 80 compounds have been found in sewage effluent, surface waters, and even in ground waters (Heberer, 2002). Drugs are frequently detected in effluents at levels from below 1 ng/L up to a few μ/L (Halling-Sorensen *et al.*, 1998). Buchberger (2007) reported that the concentrations of pharmaceuticals found in surface water downstream from sewage treatment plant effluents are generally in the ng L^{-1} range and do not inevitably represent a serious threat to drinking water quality. They have been detected in low concentrations in many countries in many environmental samples, for example sewage plant effluents, surface water, seawater, and groundwater (Fent *et al.*, 2006).

Potential risks associated with releases of pharmaceuticals into the environment have become an increasingly important issue for environmental regulators and the pharmaceuticals industry (Jorgensen and Halling-Sorensen, 2000). Fent *et al.* (2006) pointed out that a wide range of human pharmaceuticals, including analgesics, antibiotics, steroids, cardiovascular drugs etc., are present in sewage treatment work (STW) effluents and enter rivers. As a result many aquatic organisms are exposed to these ill-defined mixtures of pharmaceuticals at low concentrations (usually nanograms per litre) (Runnalls *et al.*, 2007). These hot spot pollutants are designed to have a specific mode of action, and many are persistent in the body. Although many pharmaceuticals have relatively short environmental half-lives, they assume the qualities of highly persistent pollutants because they are continually introduced into the environment (Daughton and Ternes, 1999; Brain *et al.*, 2004). It is well known that industrial wastes in aquatic environments have a toxic effect on organisms, especially on fish (Sjobeck *et al.*, 1984). The responses of aquatic ecosystems and aquatic organisms to pharmaceuticals and their metabolites are largely unknown. Unlike non-point aquatic pesticide exposures that may occur over short periods of time following rainfall events, potentially resulting in acute toxicity to aquatic organisms, lower-level pharmaceutical releases to effluent-dominated streams over longer time periods may subtly modulate and alter normal biochemical, physiological, reproductive, and ecological processes (Daughton and Ternes, 1999; Wilson *et al.*, 2003).

For most of these compounds, the ecotoxicological characteristics are unknown. Like mammalian system, biomarkers of exposure and effect that are specific to the mechanism of action for individual pharmaceutical classes should be developed for aquatic organisms. Many studies have demonstrated changes in blood variables as a result of environmental conditions and presence of contaminants (Houston and Murad, 1992; Zbanyszek and Smith, 1984; Houston and Schrapp, 1994; Houston and Gingras-Bedard, 1994). In addition to the hematological parameters, biochemical variables are of fundamental importance in the physiopathological evaluation of animals (Ranzani-Paiva *et al.*, 1999; Osman *et al.*, 2010). Hence in the present study it was aimed to study the effect of pharmaceutical effluent on blood chemistry profiles of an Indian major carp, *Labeo rohita*.

Materials and Methods

Specimens of *Labeo rohita*, a freshwater fish belonging to the family cyprinidae (Hamilton) were procured from Tamil Nadu

Fisheries Development Corporation Limited, Aliyar Fish Farm, Aliyar, Tamil Nadu, India. It is the most important group among the 3 Indian major carp species used in carp polyculture systems. The collected fish were safely brought to the laboratory and acclimatized for a month in a large cement tank (1000 L capacity). During the acclimatization period, the fish were fed *ad libitum* with rice bran and groundnut oil cake. The feeding was done once in a day. The water was renewed daily to avoid accumulation and contamination of excretory materials and feeding was withheld 24 h before the commencement of the experiment. After acclimatization, fish with an average length of 8.0 ± 0.2 cm and weight 10.2 ± 1 g were selected and transferred in the clean glass aquaria (75 × 35 × 37 cm). Fish of both sexes were used. To maintain a healthy environment for the fish, during both acclimatization and experimental period the water was replaced every 24 hours after feeding. This ensures sufficient oxygen supply for the fish and the environment is devoid of any accumulated metabolic state.

The pharmaceutical effluent used in the present study was collected from Salem (Salem district, Tamil Nadu). The effluent was collected to the point of discharge in plastic cans and brought to the laboratory and kept immediately in refrigerator to avoid any microbial decomposition. For the assessment of pharmaceutical effluent toxicity, 9 circular plastic tubs with 50 litres of water were taken. Then to each tub, different concentrations of effluent (*i.e.* 100 per cent, 75 per cent, 50 per cent, 25 per cent, 10 per cent, 5 per cent, 1 per cent 0.5 per cent, 0.1 per cent) were added. A control tub with 10 litres of water was also taken. Ten healthy fish were selected and introduced into each plastic tub.

The manifestation and survival time of fish was observed in each concentration according to the method of Wuhman (1950) and graphically expressed as survival curve. The manifestation time, the time at which fish loose their sense of balance and float on their sides were determined and presented as manifestation curve (Warren, 1990). Based on the method of Powers (1971), the relationship between the reciprocal of survival time and percent effluent concentration was determined and graphically expressed as fatality curve.

Based on survival time, fish exposed to 0.5 per cent effluent concentration were taken for acute studies. Three tubs with 50 litres of water were taken for acute concentration. 0.5 per cent of effluent was added to each tub. Then, 10 fishes were introduced into each tub. A common control was also maintained. At the end of 24, 48, 72 and 96 h, alive fish from control and experimental fish were taken and sacrificed for blood chemistry profiles.

Blood samples were collected from heart by puncturing it by using plastic disposable syringe fitted with 26 gauge needle. The syringe and needle were prechilled and moistured with heparin (Beparine R heparin sodium, IP 1000 IU/ml derived from beef intestinal mucosa containing 0.15 per cent w/v chlorocresol IP preservative), an anticoagulant manufactured by Biological E Limited, Hyderabad, India. It was transferred into small vials, which is previously rinsed with heparin. The whole blood was used for the estimation of hemoglobin, erythrocytes and leucocytes count. The remainder of the blood sample was centrifuged at 10,000 rpm for 20 minutes to separate the plasma, which was used for plasma glucose and protein estimation.

The hematocrit value was estimated by the method of Nelson and Morris (1989), Total erythrocytes and leucocytes were counted by the method of Rusia and Sood (1992), Hemoglobin was estimated by the method of Drabkin (1946), plasma glucose by the method of Cooper and McDaniel (1970) and plasma protein by the method of Lowry *et al.* (1951). The significance of sample mean between control and effluent treated fish was tested using Student's t-test (Campbell, 1981).

Results

Changes in hematological and biochemical profiles of the freshwater fish *Labeo rohita* during acute treatment of pharmaceutical effluent for 96 hours at 24 h interval were presented in Figures 6.1 and 6.2. Hematological profiles like hemoglobin (Figure 6.1a) and hematocrit (Figure 6.1b) levels were decreased in the experimental fish throughout the study period showing a minimum percent decrease of 6.61 and 3.24 at the end of 24 h and a maximum percent decrease of 53.46 and 50.02 at the end of 72 h, respectively. Similarly, erythrocyte (Figure 6.1c) and leucocyte (Figure 6.1d) counts were also decreased throughout the treatment period showing a minimum percent decrease of 37.29 and 17.56 at the end of 24 h and a maximum percent decrease of 66.40 and 43.26 at the end of 96 h, respectively.

Figure 6.1: Hematological Changes

6.1a: Hemoglobin; 6.1b: Hematocrit; 6.1c: Erythrocytes; 6.1d: Leucocytes; 6.1e: MCV, 6.1f: MCH; 6.1g: MCHC) in an Indian Major Carp, *Labeo rohita* Exposed to Pharmaceutical Effluent for 96 h at 24 h Interval

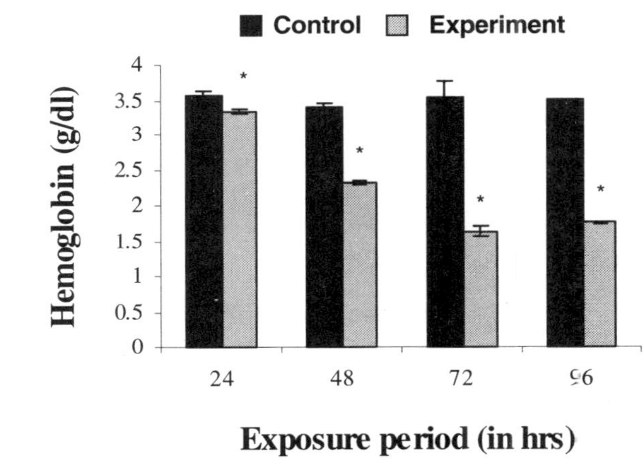

6.1a

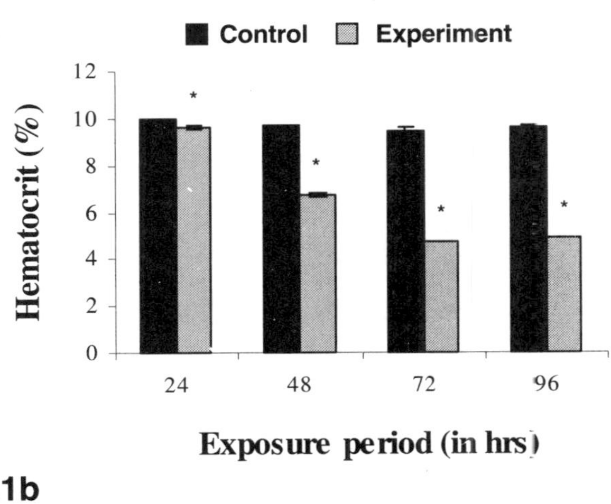

6.1b

Contd...

Figure 6.1–Contd...

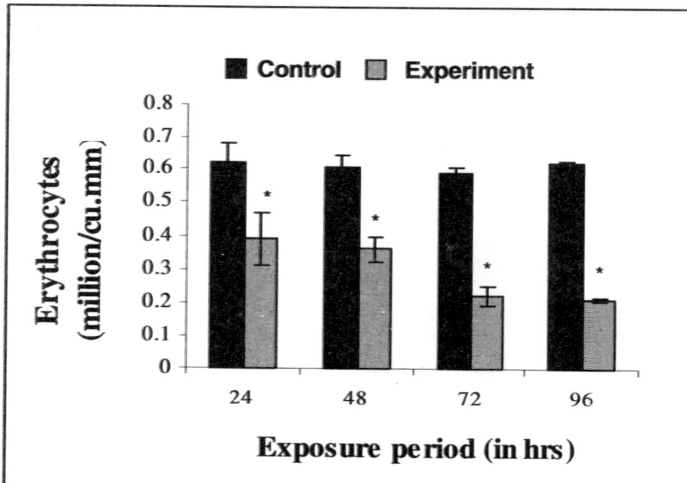

6.1c

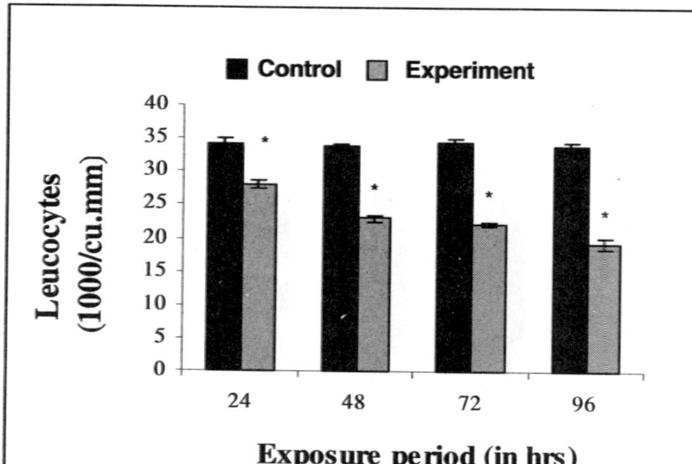

6.1d

Contd...

Figure 6.1–Contd...

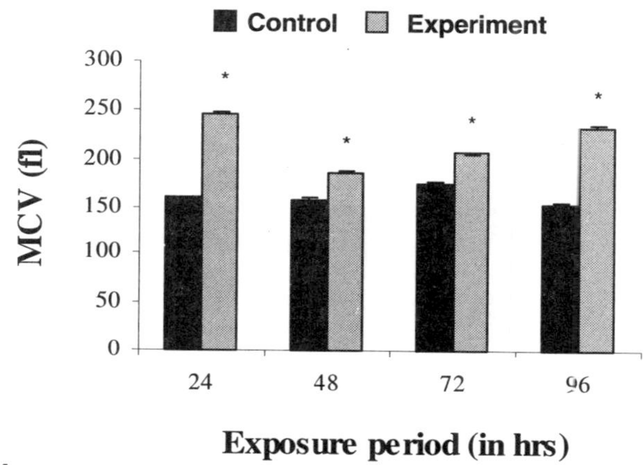

6.1e

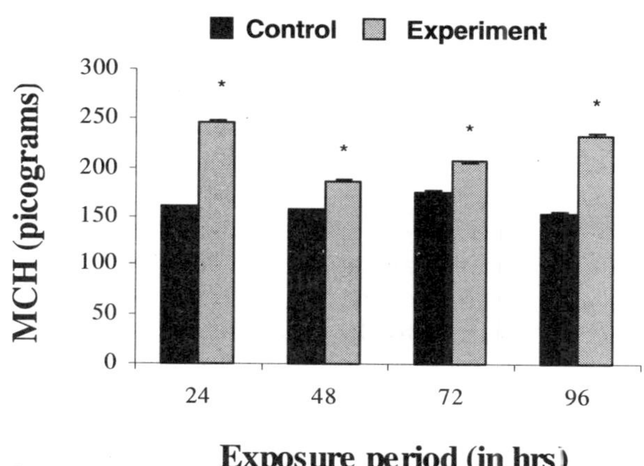

6.1f

Contd...

Figure 6.1–Contd...

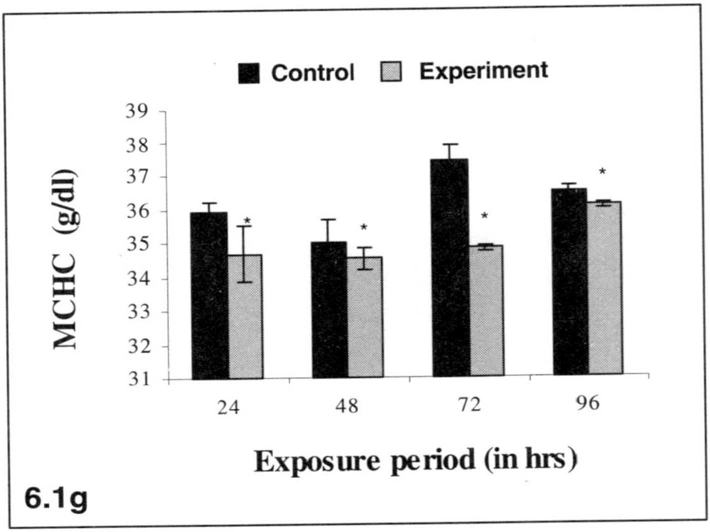

Hematological indices like MCV (Figure 6.1e) and MCH (Figure 6.1f) were increased in the experimental fish throughout the treatment period while decreasing of MCHC (Figure 6.1g) content.

Biochemical profiles such as plasma glucose (Figure 6.2a) and protein (Figure 6.1b) levels were decreased throughout the exposure period showing a minimum percent decrease of 18.50 and 10.66 at the end of 24 h and a maximum percent decrease of 42.15 and 72.03 at the end of 96 h, respectively.

Discussion

Effluents are important sources of direct input of pollutants into the aquatic environment. Thereby posing significant environmental hazards to the receiving biota and ecosystems, Adverse ecotoxicological effects induced by effluent exposure may be acute or chronic, and can occur at all levels of biological organization, from the molecular to the ecosystem level (Adams *et al.*, 2000; Porter and Janz, 2003), Among them are changes in cellular energy budgets (Smolders *et al.*, 2004), physiological alterations related to stress induction (Linton *et al.*, 2005), impairment of reproduction (Sepulveda *et al.*, 2003) and ultimately effects on fish

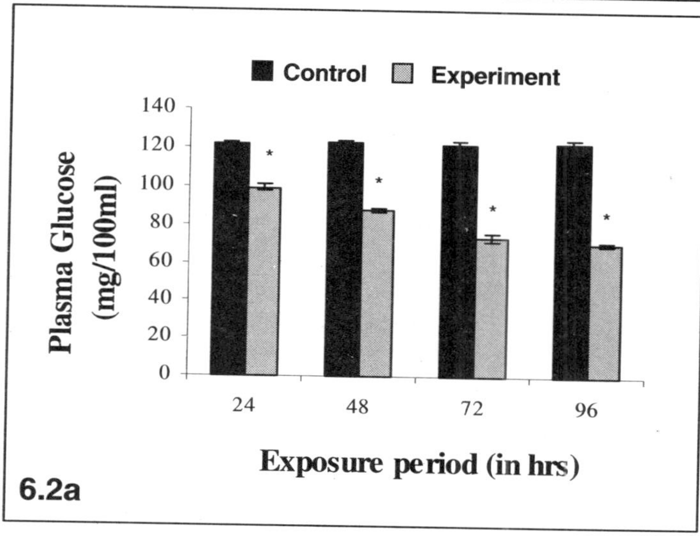

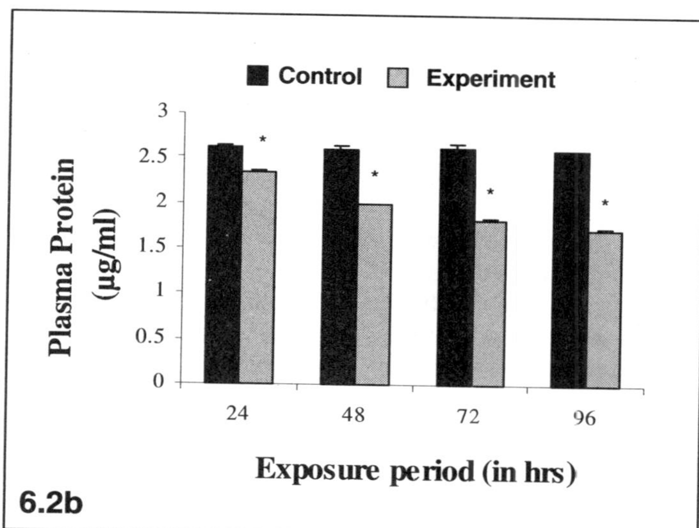

Figure 6.2: Biochemical Changes (2a: Plasma glucose; 2b: Plasma protein) in an Indian Major Carp, *Labeo rohita* Exposed to Pharmaceutical Effluent for 96 h at 24 h Interval

populations and communities (Adams *et al.*, 1992; Porter and Janz, 2003).

A common strategy to investigate potential adverse effects and toxicological modes of action following effluent exposure, and/or to assess contamination to certain classes of chemicals (*e.g.* heavy metals or estrogenic compounds), is the use of biomarkers. Over the past decade, a variety of biomarkers, covering a range of molecular, biochemical and cellular alterations, have been used to evaluate effects of contaminant exposure in aquatic environments. These proved to be very valuable in providing measures of the molecular mechanisms that underlie toxicity (Hinton *et al.*, 2005).

Behavioural toxicology is a tool for hazard assessment of water pollution. In the present study, the behavioural pattern of fish was dependent upon the effluent concentration. In 100, 75, 50 and 25 per cent effluent concentration, the fish exhibited hyper excitability, enhanced operator movements, erratic and jerky movements and vigorous activity before they become lethargic. In 10 per cent, 5 per cent, 1 per cent 0.5 per cent and 0.1 per cent fish were found at the bottom of the tank at the initial stage, and subsequently they come upto the surface and remained in the surface thereafter.

Hematological parameters are closely related to the response of the animal to the environment, an indication that the environment where fishes live could exert some influence on the hematological characteristics (Gabriel *et al.*, 2004). These indices have been employed in effectively monitoring the responses of fishes to the stressors and thus their health status under such adverse conditions. They can provide substantial diagnostic information once reference values are established under standardized conditions. It is well known that blood sampling, laboratory techniques, seasonal variations, size, genetic properties, sex, population density, lack of food supply, environmental stress and transportation could affect hematological data (Van Vuren and Hattingh, 1978; Hardig and Hoglung, 1984; Wilhem *et al.*, 1992; Orun and Erdemli, 2002).

Erythrocytes are the dominant cell type in the blood of the vast majority of fish species. Ueda *et al.* (2001) reported that erythroblast abundance as a result of the acceleration of erythropoiesis in different physiological conditions, while Shaperclaus (1979) reported abnormal forms of erythrocytes caused by haemolysis for intoxication which is accompanied by observation of triangular erythrocytes.

Erythrocyte level was found to be depressed in fishes subjected to stressful conditions. The reduction in RBC may be caused either by the inhibition of erythropoiesis or by the destruction of red cells (Sakthivel, 1988). Iwama *et al.* (1986) reported that the destruction of hematopoietic tissue in kidney and spleen could result in decreased blood cell production and a subsequent reduction in RBC counts. In the present study, the decrease in RBC count in effluent exposed fish up to 96 h may be due to severe anemic state or hemolysing power of the drug present in the effluent particularly on the red cell membrane.

Natarajan (1981) was of the view that reduction in RBC counts, haemoglobin concentration and haematocrit values resulting in hypo-chronic anaemia could be attributed utilization of haemoglobin synthesis. The decreased utilization levels of hematological parameters like hemoglobin and hematocrit in the present study might have been caused due to the destruction of mature erythrocytes resulting in reduced RBC levels. In addition to alterations of blood cell volume regulation, treatment plant effluents also probably lead to impaired membrane structure. Subramanian *et al.* (1988) reported decreased level of hemoglobin in *Macrones keletius* exported to tannery effluent and suggested that the low level of haemoglobin may be due to disruptive action of the tannery efficient on the erythropoietin tissues. In the present study also, the loss of erythrocytes may be the reason for anemia which reflects decreased level of hemoglobin.

It is widely accepted that fishes, like most other vertebrates, have a common leucocyte pattern consisting of granulocytes, monocytes, lymphocytes and thrombocytes (Vazquez and Guerrero, 2007). Variation in leucocytes count provide more sensitive index of stress than do changes in erythrocyte abundance (Mcleay and Gordon, 1977). Jezierka and Witeska (2001) showed that poisoning of fish with pollutant might cause not only alteration in count or share of particular white blood cell types, but it might also result impairment of their function causing suppression of non-specific and specific immune response. The gradual decrease in white blood cell count indicates possible impairment of immune mechanisms in the intoxicated fish. The decrease in total WBC count in the present investigation may be due to a response to an increased ACTH level in a reaction to stress produced by the presence of the drugs. Another cause can be inhibition of white blood cell maturation and the release from tissue reservoirs.

The fluctuation in the MCH clearly indicates that the concentration of haemoglobin in the red blood cells were much lower in the exposed fish than in the control fish, thereby, depicting an anaemic condition (Adeyemo, 2005). The lower values measured for MCHC coupled with high MCV in fish are indicative of adrenalin mediated cell swelling (Nikinmaa, 1992). In the present study the significant increase of MCV and MCH indicates the swelling of red blood cells or increase in the erythrocyte volume due to toxic stress of drugs in the effluent. In the present study the decrease in MCHC value may be due to red blood cell swelling or release of young erythrocytes containing less hemoglobin into the circulation.

It was shown that serum glucose levels in fish were affected by many stress factors. The changes in the blood glucose level may be attributed to the changes in the respiration and activity of the animals, as pointed out by Ghosh (1989). Bhattacharya *et al.* (1987) observed hypoglycemia with persistent depletion of hepatic glycogen content. *In vitro* exposure of hepatocytes to epinephrine and norepinepohrine has shown the catacholamines (CAs) promote glycogenolysis through stimulation of glycogen phosphorylase, a β_2-receptor-mediated process. In the present study the decreased level of plasma glucose during effluent treatment may be due to hypoxic condition caused by drugs present in the pharmaceutical effluent.

Direct utilization of proteins as immediate source of energy demands also cannot be ruled out. Decrease in the plasma protein level may be due to the excretion of proteins by kidney due to kidney disorder (albuminuria) or impaired protein synthesis as a result of liver disorders (Dalela *et al.*, 1981). Similarly Lynch *et al.* (1969) suggested that reduced level of serum protein may be due to nephrosis or liver cirrhosis. In the present study, the reduction of plasma protein of fish during pharmaceutical effluent exposure may be due to inhibition of protein synthesis or direct utilization of protein in gluconeogenesis to produce energy during stress or either cirrhosis or nephrosis or increased activity by proteolytic enzymes.

From the present study, it is concluded that, pharmaceutical effluent has a profound influence on the hematological and biochemical profiles of fish. These parameters could be effectively used as potential biomarkers of pharmaceutical toxicity to the freshwater fish in the field of environmental biomonitoring.

References

Adams, S.M., Crumby, W.D., Greeley Jr, M.S., Shugart, L.R., Saylor, C.F., 1992. Responses of fish populations and communities to pulp mill effluents: a holistic assessment. *Ecotoxicol. Environ. Saf.*, 24: 347-360.

Adams, M.S., Greeley, M.S., Ryon, M.G., 2000. Evaluating effects of contaminants on fish health at multiple levels of biological organization: extrapolating from lower to higher levels. *Hum. Ecol. Risk Assess.*, 6: 15-27.

Adeyemo, O.K., 2005. Haematological and histopathological effects of Cassava Mill Effluent in *Clarias gariepinus*. *Afr. J. Biomedi. Res.*, 8: 179 -183.

Brain, R.A., Johnson, D.J., Richards, S.M., Sanderson, H., Sibley, P.K., Solomon, K.R., 2004. Effects of 25 pharmaceutical compounds to *Lemna gibba* using a seven-day static- renewal test. Environ. *Toxicol. Chem.*, 23: 371-382.

Buchberger, W.W., 2007. Novel analytical procedures for screening of drug residues in water, wastewater, sediment and sludge. *Analytica Chimica Acta.*, 593: 129-139.

Campbell, R.C., 1981. Statistics for biologists. 2nd ed. Cambridge, London. 66.

Cooper, G.R. and Mc Daniel, V., 1970. The determination of glucose by the O-toluidine method. *Stand. Meth. Clin. Chem.*, 159.

Dalela, R.C., Rani, S., Kumar, V., Verma, S.R., 1981. *In vivo* haematological alterations in a freshwater teleost, *Mystus vittatus* following subacute exposure to pesticides and their combinations. *J. Environ. Biol.*, 2: 79-86.

Daughton, C.G., Ternes, T.A., 1999. Pharmaceuticals and personal care products in the environment: agents of subtle change? *Environ. Health Perspect.*, 107 (6): 907-938.

Drabkin, D.L., 1946. Spectrometric studies, XIV- The crystallographic and optimal properties of the hemoglobin of man in comparison with those of other species. *J. Biol. Chem.*, 164: 703-723.

Farre, M., Ferrer, I., Ginebreda, A., Figueras, M., Olivella, L., Tirapu, L., Vilanova, M., Barcelo, D., 2001. Determination of drugs in surface water and wastewater samples by liquid chromatography–mass spectrometry: Methods and preliminary results including toxicity studies with *Vibrio fischeri*. *J. Chromatogr. A.*, 938: 187-197.

Fent, K., Weston, A.A., Caminada, D., 2006. Ecotoxicology of human pharmaceuticals. *Aquat. Toxicol.*, 76: 122-159.

Gabriel, U.U., Ezeri, G.N.O., Opabunmi, O.O., 2004. Influence of sex, source, health status and acclimation on the haematology of *Clarias gariepinus* (Burch, 1822). *Afr. J. Biotechnol.*, 3: 463-467.

Ghosh, T.K., 1989. Toxic impact of three organophosphates on carbohydrate metabolism in a freshwater Indian catfish (*Clarias batrachus*). Proceedings of Indian Natural Sciences Congress, IEEE Explore, London, pp.142-135.

Halling-Sorensen, B., Nielsen, S.N., Lanzky, P. F., Ingerslev, F., Holten Lutzhoft, H.C., Jorgensen, S.E., 1998. Occurrence, fate, and effects of pharmaceutical substances in the environment- A review. *Chemosphere*, 36: 357-393.

Hardig, J., Hoglung, L.B., 1984. Seasonal variation in blood components of reared Baltic Salmon, *Salmo salar*. *J. Fish Biol.*, 24: 565-579.

Heberer, T., 2002. Occurrence, fate, and removal of pharmaceutical residues in the aquatic environment: a review of recent research data. *Toxicol. Lett.*, 131: 5-17.

Hinton, D.E., Kullman, S.W., Hardman, R.C., Volz, D.C., Chen, P.J., Carney, M., Bencic, D.C., 2005. Resolving mechanisms of toxicity while pursuing ecotoxicological relevance? *Mar. Pollut. Bull.*, 51: . 635-648.

Houston, A., Gingras-Bedard, J., 1994. Variable versus constant temperature acclimation regimes: effects on hemoglobin isomorph profile in goldfish, *Carassius auratus*. *Fish Physiol. Biochem.*, 13: 445–450.

Houston, A., Murad, A., 1992. Erythrodynamics in goldfish, *Carassius auratus* L. temperature effects. *Physiol. Zool.*, 65: 55–76.

Houston, A., Schrapp, M., 1994. Thermoacclimatory hematological response: have we been using appropriate conditions and assessment methods? *Can J. Zool.*, 72: 1238–1242.

Iwama, G.K., Greer, G.C., Randall, D.J., 1986. Changes in selected haematological parameters in juvenile chiriook salmon subjected to bacterial challenge and a toxicant. *J. Fish. Biol.*, 28: 563- 572.

Jezierska, B., Witeska, M., 2001. Metal toxicity to fish. *Wyclawnictwo Akademi Podlaskiej*, Siedlce.

Jorgensen, S.E., Halling-Sorensen B., 2000. Drugs in the environment. *Chemosphere*, 40: 691-699.

Linton, E.D., Scuton, D.A., McKinley, R.S., 2005. Physiological effects of thermo mechanical newsprint mill effluent on Atlantic salmon *Salmo salar* L. *Ecotoxicol. Environ. Saf.*, 62: 317-330.

Lowry, O.H., Rosebrough, N.J., Farr, A.L., Randall, R.I., 1951. Protein measurement with folin phenol reagent. *J. Biol. Chem.*, 193: 265-275.

Lynch, M.J., Raphelss, Mellor, L.D., Spare, P.D., Inwood, M.J.H., 1969. *In*: 'Medical technology and clinical pathology'. 2nd ed. (Eds.), *W. B. Saunders Company*, London, UK.

Mcleay, D.J., Gorden, M.R., 1977. Leucocrit: A simple hematological technique for measuring acute stress in salmonoid fish, including stressful concentrations of pulp mill effluents. *J. Fish. Res. Bel. Can.*, 34: 2164-2175.

Natarajan, G. M., 1981. Changes in the bimodal exchange and some blood parameters in the air breathing fish, *Channa striatus* following lethal exposure to *Meta systox* (Demeton). *Curr. Sci.*, 50: 40-41.

Nelson, D.A., Morris, M.W., 1989. Basic methodology. Chap. 27. Hematology and coagulation, part IV. In: Clinical diagnosis and management by laboratory methods. (Eds.,) Nelson, D.A., Henry, J.B. 17th ed. (Ed.) Henry, J. B. *W.B. Saunder Company*, Philadelphia, U.S.A. 578 – 625.

Nikinmaa, M., 1992. Membrane transport and control of hemoglobin–oxygen affinity in nucleated erythrocytes. *Physiol. Rev.*, 72: 301-321.

Nikolaou, A., Meric, S., Fatta, D., 2007. Occurrence patterns of pharmaceuticals in waterand wastewater environments. *Anal. Bioanal. Chem.*, 387: 1225-1234.

Orun, I. and Erdemli, A. U. 2002. A study on blood parameters of *Capoeta trutta* (Heckel, 1843). *J. Biol. Sci.*, 2 (8): 508-511.

Osman, A.G.M., Koutb, M., Sayed, E-D.H., 2010. Use of hematological parameters to assess the efficiency of quince (*Cydonia oblonga* Miller) leaf extract in alleviation of the effect of ultraviolet – A radiation on African catfish *Clarias gariepinus* (Burchell, 1822). *J. Photochem. Photobiol. B. Biol.*, 99: 1–8.

Porter, C.M., Janz, D.M., 2003. Treated municipal sewage discharge affects multiple levels of biological organization in fish. *Ecotoxicol. Environ. Saf.*, 54: 199-206.

Powers, E.B., 1971. The gold fish, *Carassius carassius* as a test animal in the study of toxicity. *Illions Biol. Monoger.*, 4: 127-193.

Ranzani-Paiva, M., Salles, F., Eiras, J., Ishikawa, C., Alexandrino, A., 1999. Análise hematológica de curimbatá (*Prochilodus scrofa*), pacu (*Piractus mesopotamicus*) e tambaqui (*Colossoma macropomum*) das estações de piscicultura do instituto de pesca. *Boletim do Instituto de Pesca.*, 25: 77–83.

Runnalls, T.J., Hala, D.N., Sumpter, J.P., 2007. Preliminary studies into the effects of the human pharmaceutical clofibric acid on sperm parameters in adult fathead minnow. *Aquat. Toxicol.*, 84: 111-118.

Rusia, V., Sood, S.K., 1992. Routine hematological tests. *In*: 'Medical *Laboratory Technology*' Kanai, L. Mukerjee. (Ed.), Vol.1. Fifth reprint. Tata McGraw Hill Publishing Company Limited, New Delhi, p. 252-258.

Sakthivel, M. 1988. Effects of varying dietary protein level on blood parameters of *Cyprinus carpio*. *Proc. Ind. Acad. Sci.* (*Anim. Sci*)., 97: 363-366.

Sepulveda, M.S., Quinn, B.P., Denslow, N.D., Holm, S.E., Gross, T.S., 2003. Effects of pulp and paper mill effluents on reproductive success of largemouth bass. *Environ. Toxicol. Chem.*, 22: 205-213.

Shaperclaus, W., 1979. Fish Diseases, Akademie Verlag, Berlin. 570.

Sjöbeck, M.L., Haux, C., Larsson, A., Lithner, G., 1984. Biochemical and haematological studies on perch, *Perca fluviatilis*, from the cadmium-contaminated river. *Ecotoxicol. Environ. Saf.*, 8: 303-312.

Smolders, R., Bervoets, L., De Coen, W., Blust, R., 2004. Cellular energy allocation in zebra mussels exposed along a pollution gradient: linking cellular effects to higher levels of biological organization. *Environ. Pollut.*, 129: 99-112.

Subramanian, M.A., Hameed, M.S., Varadaraj, G., 1988. Haematological changes in the fish *Macrones keletinus* (Gunther) after exposure to the tannery effluent. *Indian Zool.*, 71- 74.

Ueda, I.K., Egami, M.I., Sasso, W.S., Maushima, E.R., 2001. Cytochemical aspects of the peripheral blood cells of *Oreochromis* (tilapia) *niloticus*. Linnaeus, 1758 (Cichlidae, Teleostei): Part II. *Braz. J. Vet. Res. Anim. Sci.*, 38: 273-277.

Van Vuren, J.H.J., Hattingh, J., 1978. A seasonal study of haematology of wild freshwater fish. *J. Fish Biol.*, 13: 305-313.

Vazquez, G.R., Guerrero, G.A., 2007. Characterization of blood cells and hematological parameters in *Cichlasoma dimerus* (Teleostei, Perciformes). *Tissue Cell.*, 39: 151-160.

Warren, E., 1990. On the reaction of *Daphnia magna* (Stratus) to certain changes in its environment. *Quast. J. Micer. Sci.*, 43: 199-204.

Wilhem, D.F., Eble, G.J., Kassner, F.X., Dafre, A.L., Ohira, M., 1992. Comparative hematology in marine fish. *Comp. Biochem. Physiol.*, 102: 311-321.

Wilson, B.A., Smith, V.A., Denoylles, F., Jr, Larive, C.K., 2003. Effects of three pharmaceutical and personal care products on natural freshwater algal assemblages. *Environ. Sci. Technol.*, 37: 1713-1719.

Wurhman, E., 1952. Sur quelgues principles dela toxicologiedes poisen. *Bull. Centre. Belge. Et Document. Eaux.*, 15: 49–60.

Zbanyszek, R., Smith, L., 1984. The effect of water soluble aromatic hydrocarbon on some hematological parameters of rain bow trout *Salmo gairdneri* Richardson, during acute exposure. *J. Fish Biol.*, 24: 245–252.

Zuccato, E., Calamari, D., Natangelo, M., Fanelli, R., 2000. Presence of therapeutic drugs in the environment. *Lancet*, 355: 1789-1790.

Chapter 7

Behavioural Alterations of Freshwater Airbreathing Teleost, *Channa punctatus* (Bloch) in Response to Heavy Metal Exposure

Mohit Tiwari[1], N.S. Nagpure[1], D.N. Saksena[2] and W.S. Lakra[1]*

[1]*Molecular Biology and Biotechnology Division, National Bureau of Fish Genetic Resources, Lucknow – 226 002, U.P., India*

[2]*Aquatic Biology and Aquaculture Unit, School of Studies in Zoology, Jiwaji University, Gwalior – 474 011, M.P., India*

ABSTRACT

In recent times, the occurrence of metal contaminants, especially the heavy metals in excess of natural loads has become a problem of increasing concern. This situation has arisen as a result of the rapid growth of population, increased urbanization and expansion of industrial activities, exploration and exploitation of natural resources, extension of irrigation and other modern agricultural practices as well as the lack of environmental regulations. Present study deciphers the ethological responses of a freshwater airbreathing teleost,

* Corresponding author: E-mail: mohittiwari2002@yahoo.com

Channa punctatus due to waterborne exposure of heavy metal, cadmium at various concentrations in a time span of 96 hrs. At lower concentrations fish tried to adopt themselves, but at higher ones they could not cope up with the surroundings and ultimately showed death.

Keywords: *Cadmium, Channa punctatus, Ethological responses, Freshwater teleost, Heavy metal.*

Introduction

Metals are non-biodegradable materials and once they enter into the environment, bio-concentration may occur in fish tissue by means of metabolic and bio-absorption processes. From the surrounding water, fish may absorb dissolved heavy metals that may accumulate in various tissues and organs and even biomagnified in the food-chain or web. In the absorption process there are four possible routes for metals to enter a fish *viz.*, the food ingested; simple diffusion of the metallic ions through gill pores; through respiration; and by skin absorption (Abdullah and Javed, 2006).

Heavy metal, cadmium present in nature, is a relatively rare element which is not essential for any biological process in plants or animals. It occurs mainly as a component of minerals in the earth's crust at an average concentration of 0.18 mg L^{-1} (Babich and Stotzky, 1978). In natural freshwaters, cadmium sometimes occurs at concentrations of less than 0.01 µg L^{-1}, but in environments influenced by man, concentrations can be several micrograms per litre or greater (U.S. EPA, 2000). Cadmium (Cd) is an odourless, white, crystalline powder and is used in the manufacture of fungicides, dyeing, and printing textiles, and in metal finishing baths. Cadmium is released into the environment through mining and metal processing operations, burning fuels, making and using phosphate fertilizers, and disposing of metal products. One of the reasons that cadmium has been listed as a PBT (persistent, bioaccumulative and toxic) is that inhaling cadmium fumes at high exposures can cause heart and lung irritation, including shortness of breath, chest pain, coughing, and a build-up of fluid in the lungs. Cadmium is considered to be toxic, and is a probable cancer-causing agent in humans. It is believed that cadmium can have toxic effects on the prostate, kidney, lung and testes, and may also affect the female reproductive cycle. Cadmium has long been known to be toxic and itai-itai disease which was originated in Japan, is the most severe form of chronic cadmium poisoning caused by prolonged oral cadmium ingestion (Takaki *et al.*, 2004) and the World Health Organization has fixed the provisional tolerable weekly intake of cadmium to 7 mg kg^{-1} of cadmium per person.

In freshwater, the presence or absence of fish has been widely used as a biological indicator of the degree of pollution. Data obtained on the concentration of selected individual pollutants which are lethal to fish provide very necessary information, apart from identifying a boundary limit above which fish are likely to be killed. The contamination of aquatic ecosystem by heavy metals has gained increasing attention in recent decades. Discharge of industrial wastewater, causing serious consequence for fisheries resulting in impairment of important function such as respiration and osmoregulation (Kumaraguru, 1995). The ethological changes in fishes have been considered to be sensitive indicator of toxicity and among aquatic fauna, fishes are more sensitive to pollutants. Aquatic pollution is significant to fisheries and aquaculture industries. The changes of physical, chemical, and biological parameters of water alter the behaviour of fishes besides causing mortality (Yadav *et al.*, 2007).

Therefore, present study was conducted to evaluate the effect of heavy metal salt, cadmium chloride on behavioural responses to common edible murrel, *Channa punctatus* (Bloch). This species was selected for ethological study because it is fulfilling most of the requirements of a model test species *viz.*, availability throughout the year, raised easily under laboratory conditions and easy handling etc.

Materials and Methods

Experimental Animals

Healthy specimens of freshwater teleost, *Channa punctatus* were procured from local sources. The specimens had an average wet weight and length of 20.15 ± 1.88 g and 13.11 ± 0.62 cm (mean ± SE) respectively. The fishes were acclimatized for 15 days under laboratory conditions prior to metal exposure. The fishes were fed, *ad libitum*, with boiled chicken eggs, goat liver and poultry waste material. The faecal matter and other waste were siphoned off daily to reduce ammonia content in water. Every effort was made to maintain optimal conditions during acclimatization and no mortality occurred during this period.

Test Chemical

For the present study, analytical-grade cadmium chloride ($CdCl_2.H_2O$) (98 per cent), manufactured by Himedia Laboratories Pvt. Limited, Mumbai, India was used as the test compound.

Behavioural Responses

The acclimatized specimens were randomly transferred to eight test concentrations of cadmium chloride *i.e.*, 20, 22, 24, 26, 28, 30, 32 and 34 mg L^{-1} in 40 L aquaria. During the experiment conducted for 96 hrs in semi static system of cadmium exposure, behavioural responses of animals of exposed as well as control group were examined. For this various parameters *viz.*, convulsions, equilibrium status, fin movement, hyperactivity, somersaulting activity and swimming rate were observed in the test fish as suggested by Rand (1985).

Observations

Physico-chemical Properties of the Test Water

During the experiment the temperature of the test water ranged from 18.9 to 23.1 (20.3 ± 0.25) °C, dissolved oxygen from 7.11 to 8.25 (7.94 ± 0.27) mg L^{-1}, and pH from 7.25 to 7.99 (7.33 ± 0.11) respectively. The total hardness and total alkalinity of the test water varied from 157 to 188 (171.6 ± 1.99) and 245 to 281 (259.8 ± 3.24) mg L^{-1} as $CaCO_3$ respectively, during the experiment.

Ethological Observations

All the parameters of behavioural study, such as convulsions, equilibrium status, fin movement, hyperactivity, somersaulting activity and swimming rate were found to be altered in the test fish depending on dose and duration of metal exposure. At the start of the exposure, the fish exposed with the cadmium became restless. With the progression of the experiment, the fish stopped swimming and remained static in position in response to the sudden changes in the surrounding environment. There were no behavioural changes observed in the control group.

The magnitude and duration of behavioural changes increased with increased metal concentration. On initial exposure at higher concentration (28 mg L^{-1} and onwards), the fish exhibited characteristic avoidance behaviour by rapid and erratic swimming with jerky movements and hyper-excitability, stretching half of their body out of water surface and trying to jump out. Faster opercular activity was observed as surfacing and in gulping of air increased. The drastic subsequent increase and decrease in surface activities such as linear movement, distance travelling, and movement of fins were also observed. Their fins became hard and stretched due to stretching of body muscles. They secreted copious amounts of mucus from whole body continuously, and soon a thick layer of mucus was deposited on body, buccal cavity and gills. Ultimately, fish lost their balance, became exhausted, lost consciousness, and became lethargic. Lastly fish sank down to the bottom and became motionless; after some time their bellies turned upward and the fish died finally.

Discussion

The alterations in the behavioural pattern are the most sensitive indication of potential toxic effects (Sardo and Soares, 2010). The behavioural changes observed in fish were: swimming in imbalanced manner, difficulty in breathing and slowness in surfacing motion, capsizing and sinking down to bottom. These toxic effects increased with the dose and duration. In the present experiment conducted with *C. punctatus*, the fish exposed at 20 to 34 mg L^{-1} cadmium chloride concentrations exhibited abnormal behaviour in the form of erratic swimming, loss of equilibrium and enhanced surfacing behaviour. They become lethargic and mucous was secreted from the whole body. These observed behavioural alterations in the fish are consistent with the previous reports on cadmium (Yilmaz *et al.*, 2004) and other heavy metals like chromium (Begum *et al.*, 2006; Mishra and Mohanty, 2008), mercury (Pandey *et al.*, 2005) and lead (Olojo *et al.*, 2005).

At initial exposure they tried to avoid the toxic water with fast swimming and jumping. Such abnormal behaviour and altered movements are considered to be the result of excessive elimination of skeletal minerals, thus, causing skeletal deformities (Pragatheeswaran *et al.*, 1987), while heavy exudation of mucus over the body and dispigmentation is attributed to dysfunction of the endocrine (pituitary) gland under toxic stress and causes reduction in number and size of chromatophores (Pandey *et al.*, 1990). Fish secrete copious amount of mucus, as a defence mechanism to neutralize the effect of metal, from whole body continuously, and soon a thick layer of mucus was deposited in the buccal cavity and gills. In their study, Bisht and Agarwal (2007) observed hypertrophy and hyperplasia of mucous cells in copper sulphate ($CuSO_4$) exposed fish, and suggested that this phenomenon is an adaptive and defence mechanism to prevent cutaneous entry of toxicant by coagulation through increased mucus production.

The behavioural alterations of fish and subsequent death imply that the toxic effect is mediated through the disturbed coordinating systems, which are involved in control of almost all vital activities. In earlier studies, heavy metals have been shown to affect Na^{2+}-K^{2-}-ATPase in the brain and Ca^{2+}-ATPase in the gills (Verma *et al.*, 1983; Bansal *et al.*, 1985) of fish. Heavy metals are known to have a neurotoxic action on the 'calcium pump' in fish brain as confirmed by the study of Reddy *et al.* (1988) in freshwater catfish, *Ictalurus punctatus*.

Inactivation of acetylcholinesterase causes, accumulation of acetylcholine at synaptic junctions due to which fish shows hyperactivity, swimming in imbalanced manner and becomes lethargic (Fulton and Key, 2001; Yilmaz *et al.*, 2004), and stimulation of peripheral nervous system which results in to increased metabolic activities. The higher metabolic rate leads to more oxygen utilization. Previous studies have shown that erratic and jerky swimming may be caused due to inhibition of the acetylcholinesterase in the brain and neuromuscular junctions (Rao *et al.*, 2005; Agrahari *et al.*, 2006). Likewise, the faster opercular movement in fish has been reported to increase considerably following the exposure of toxicants (Omitoyin *et al.*, 2006; Yadav *et al.*, 2007). The deficiency of oxygen causes hypoxic condition in fish resulting increase in the breathing rate and to cope with the condition fish gulp air by frequent surfacing.

Changes in behaviour were indicative of stress in the toxicant exposed fish. These alterations indicate that the toxicant is present in the environment and is bioavailable to the organism and, thus, causing deleterious effects to the organism.

Acknowledgements

The authors express their gratitude to Director, National Bureau of Fish Genetic Resources (ICAR), Lucknow, U.P., India, for providing necessary facilities for carrying out this work.

References

Abdullah, S. and Javed, M., 2006. Studies on acute toxicity of metals to the fish, *Catla catla*. *Pak. J. Biol. Sci.*, 9(9): 1807-1811.

Agrahari, S., Gopal, K. and Pandey, K.C., 2006. Biomarkers of monocrotophos in a freshwater fish *Channa punctatus* (Bloch). *J. Environ. Biol.*, 27: 453-457.

Babich, H. and Stotzky, G., 1978. Effects of cadmium on the biota: influence of environmental factors. *Adv. Appl. Microbiol.*, 23: 55-117.

Bansal, S.K., Murthy, R.C. and Chandra, S.V., 1985. The effect of some divalent metals on cardiac and branchial Ca^{2+}-ATPase in a freshwater fish *Saccobranchus fossilis*. *Ecotoxicol. Environ. Saf.*, 9: 373-377.

Begum, G., Venkateswara, R.J. and Srikanth, K., 2006. Oxidative stress and changes in locomotor behaviour and gill morphology of *Gambusia affinis* exposed to chromium. *Toxicol. Environ. Chem.*, 88: 355-365.

Bisht, I. and Agarwal, S.K., 2007. Cytomorphological and histomorphological changes in mucous cells of general body epidermis of *Barilius vagra* (Cyprinidae, Pisces) following exposure to herbicide-BLUE VITROL ($CuSO_4$): A statistical analysis. *J. Exp. Zool. India*, 10: 27-36.

Fulton, M.H. and Key, P.B., 2001. Acetylcholinesterase inhibition in estuarine fish and invertebrates as an indicator of organophosphorus insecticide exposure and effects. *Environ. Toxicol. Chem.*, 20: 37-45.

Kumaraguru, A.K., 1995. Water pollution and fisheries. *Ecol. Environ. Cons.*, 1: 143-150.

Mishra, A.K. and Mohanty, B., 2008. Acute toxicity impacts of hexavalent chromium on behaviour and histopathology of gill, kidney and liver of the freshwater fish, *Channa punctatus* (Bloch). *Environ. Toxicol. Pharmacol.*, 26: 136-141.

Olojo, E.A.A., Olurin, K.B., Mbaka, G. and Oluwemimo, A.D., 2005. Histopathology of the gill and liver tissues of the African catfish, *Clarias gariepinus* exposed to lead. *Afr. J. Biotechnol.*, 4(1): 117-122.

Omitoyin, B.O., Ajani, E.K., Adesina, B.T. and Okuagu, C.N.F., 2006. Toxicity of Lindane (Gamma Hexachloro-CycloHexane) to *Clarias gariepinus* (Burchell, 1822). *World J. Zool.*, 1(1): 57-63.

Pandey, A., Kumar, G.K. and Munshi, J.S.D., 1990. Integumentary chromatophores and mucus glands of fish as indicator of heavy metal pollution. *J. Freshwater Biol.*, 2: 117-121.

Pandey, S., Kumar, R., Sharma, S., Nagpure, N.S., Srivastava, S.K. and Verma, M.S., 2005. Acute toxicity bioassays of mercuric chloride and malathion on air-breathing fish, *Channa punctatus* (Bloch). *Eco. Toxicol. Environ. Saf.*, 61: 114-120.

Pragatheeswaran, V., Loganathan, P., Natarajan, R. and Venugopalan, V. K., 1987. Cadmium induced vertebral deformities in an esturine fish, *Ambassis commersoni. Proc. Indian Acad. Sci. (Anim. Sci.)*, 94: 389-394.

Rand, G.M., 1985. Behaviour. In: *Fundamentals of Aquatic Toxicology Methods and Applications*, (Eds.) G.M. Rand, S.R. Petrocelli. pp. 221-256. Hemisphere Publishing Corporation, Washington.

Rao, J.V., Begum, G., Pallela, R., Usman, P.K. and Rao, R.N., 2005. Changes in behaviour and brain acetylcholinesterase activity in mosquito fish, *Gambusia affinis* in reference to the sublethal exposure of chlorpyrifos. *Int. J. Environ. Res. Public Health*, 2: 478-483.

Reddy, R.S., Jinna, R.R., Ujodinma, J.E. and Desaiah D., 1988. *In vitro* effect of mercury and cadmium on brain Ca^{2+}-ATPase of the catfish *Ictalurus punctatus. Bull. Environ. Contam. Toxicol.*, 41: 324-328.

Sardo, A.M. and Soares, A.M.V.M. (2010. Can behavioural responses of *Lumbriculus variegatus* (Oligochaeta) assess sediment toxicity? A case study with sediments exposed to acid mine drainage. *Environ. Pollut.*, 158(2): 636-640.

Takaki, A., Jimi, S., Segawa, M., Hisano, S., Takebayashi, S. and Iwasaki, H., 2004. Long-term cadmium exposure accelerates age-related mitochondrial changes in renal epithelial cells. *Toxicology*, 203: 145-154.

U.S. EPA., 2000. 2000 Update of Ambient Water Quality Criteria for Cadmium. EPA-68-C-98-134. U.S. Environmental Protection Agency, Office of Water, Office of Science and Technology, Washington, DC.

Verma, S.R., Jain, M. and Tonk, I.P., 1983. *In vivo* effects of mercuric chloride on tissue ATPase of *Notopterus notopterus*. *Toxicol. Lett.*, 16: 305-309.

Yadav, A., Neraliya, S. and Gopesh, A., 2007. Acute toxicity levels and ethological responses of *Channa striatus* to fertilizer industrial wastewater. *J. Environ. Biol.*, 28(2): 159-162.

Yadav, A., Neraliya, S. and Gopesh, A., 2007. Acute toxicity levels and ethological responses of *Channa striatus* to fertilizer industrial wastewater. *J. Environ. Biol.*, 28(2): 159-162.

Yilmaz, M., Gul, A. and Karakose, E., 2004. Investigation of acute toxicity and the effect of cadmium chloride ($CdCl_2.H_2O$) metal salt on behaviour of the guppy (*Poecilia reticulata*). *Chemosphere*, 56: 375-380.

Chapter 8

Fisheries and Aquaculture in India–Dimension Towards Development: A Review

Meenakshi Jindal and Kavita Sharma*

Department of Zoology and Aquaculture, CCS Haryana Agricultural University, Hisar – 125 004, Haryana, India

ABSTRACT

Aquaculture has already assumed the status of fast expanding industry, not only in India, but also, in several Asiatic countries over the recent past. India is not only blessed with rich natural resources, but also, with a climate which is suitable for quick growth and maturity of finfish or shellfish. India also holds big potential in the fishery sector, as India has vast and varied fisheries resources both in marine and freshwater. Fisheries and aquaculture play a crucial role for food supply, food security and income generation. Million people work directly as fishers and fish farmers, with hundreds of millions more engaged in associated activities – the great majority in developing countries. Fish exports boost foreign currency earnings – particularly important in developing economies. In fact, aquatic foods are the most widely traded foodstuffs,

* Corresponding author: E-mail: meenjind@gmail.com

outpacing agricultural products. In India aquaculture has been in progress for the past 5 decades. India's aquaculture industry is highly dependent on exports. World demand exceeds production and per capita consumption is also steadily increasing. Therefore, India has great scope in expanding its aquaculture industry. There has been a remarkable improvement in the productivity level of aqua culture ponds. From the nutritional point of view as well, aquaculture has a special significance as fish is a rich source of protein for human being and also for other livestock populations. The abundance of fish is the solution to fight against malnutrition, in developing societies and countries, on account of the high content of essential amino acids and high digestibility. Nutritionally, fish is often presented as an important source of protein, especially where other sources of animal protein are scarce or expensive. The importance of fish as a crucial element in the diet of a population, therefore, is now widely recognized, especially in the diets of young children, infants and pregnant women. We should realise that aquaculture can produce significant quantities of food, income and employment and if planned and applied effectively can revitalise rural life and supply products of high nutritional value. It can assist in enhancement and maintaining wild aquatic stocks, thereby improving capture fisheries. It is an efficient means of recycling and upgrading low grade food materials and waste products into high grade protein rich food. With proper management and essential inputs, we can certainly develop aquaculture as a major avocation thereby opening up a new frontier for food and wealth for our country.

Keywords: *Aquaculture, Fisheries, Fish farming, Importance of fish, Nutritional value.*

Introduction

Fishery is the occupation or industry of catching, processing or selling fish or shell fish. However, Aquaculture is the cultivation of aquatic animals and plants, especially, fish shell fish and seaweed, in natural or controlled marine or freshwater environments. It is commonly known as 'Fish Farming' and since marine or freshwater animals and plants are grown on a commercial scale, it can be termed as 'Commercial Underwater Agriculture'. There has been a continuous increase worldwide, in the demand for both fin-fish and shell-fish.

As we know three-fourth of our planet's surface is hydrosphere and 97 per cent of the hydrosphere is oceans. Now a days, increasing urbanization reduced the available land for agriculture and agriculture alone, is not sufficient to meet the requirement of protein rich, balanced diet for the population, which is growing at an alarming rate. This demographic flame is likely to consume this planet, unless, the problem of food production is efficiently tackled in time. So aqua farming can also be a vocation to generate employment and income in the rural sector and also in earning foreign exchange for the nation. Aquaculture has become one of the most lucrative of the farming practices (Agarwal, 2006).

Aquaculture has already assumed the status of fast expanding industry, not only in India, but also, in several Asiatic countries over the recent past.

Fisheries and aquaculture play a crucial role for food supply, food security and income generation. Million people work directly as fishers and fish farmers, with hundreds of millions more engaged in associated activities – the great majority in developing countries. Fish exports boost foreign currency earnings – particularly important in developing economies. In fact, aquatic foods are the most widely traded foodstuffs, outpacing agricultural products.

There is an increasing global demand for food. It is predicted that in another fifteen years animal proteins alone will provide 40 per cent of the world's need. As the growing population needs more food, increased aquaculture production would reduce the pressure on natural population. Aquaculture helps to promote economic development in rural and under developed areas. The desirable fish being cultured in pond makes the process of harvesting easy and economical. Fishes are healthy sources for animal proteins and are easy to digest and such an animal protein can be harvested on demand.

World Aquaculture and Asian Countries

The aquaculture technology has advanced to such an extent that fish can be produced where there is light and water. Aquatic products are among the most widely traded foods. About 40 per cent of global production enters international trade. Asian countries dominate the scene and account for 60 per cent of the total production in which India and China take a sizeable share in the freshwater fish production. The world production of conventional fish varieties is nearing an almost saturation level and may even exceed the maximum sustainable yield by 2015 A.D. The aquaculture production has been steadily increasing over the last decade. Aquaculture production was 51.7 million tonnes in 2006. It continues to grow more rapidly than all other animal food producing sectors, with a average global growth rate of 8.8 per cent per year since 1970, compared to 2.8 per cent for terrestrial farmed meat production systems. If growth in aquaculture can be sustained, it is likely to fulfil the increasing demand for aquatic food supplies by supplying more than 50 per cent of the total aquatic food consumption by 2015. (FAO, 2008)

Marine fisheries constitute a source of valuable food and employment. Marine fish production comes from the coastal resources and progressively, increased by nearly six times, during the last 55 years. Technological progress in boat and gear design, use of new hull material, such as, steel engine and equipment, preservation and processing, acoustic fish detective and other navigational aids including the increasing use of hand help GPS in recent years has facilitated access to the whole range of marine fishery resource in the exclusive economic zone (EEZ). But, after decades of growth, the marine fishery in the country has shown the sign of stagnation, due to overfishing in coastal waters, destructive fishing practices and pollution (Yadava, 2006). Declination in marine fisheries, shifts the fish production, increasing towards inland fisheries, which constitutes about 8 per cent of the world's total fish production. Such growth has been possible due to impressive developments in aquaculture, such as, genetic improvement, induced breeding techniques, scientific management and commercial farming (Ayyappan, 2006).

The Indian Scenario

Indian fisheries has diverse resources both in aquatic habitats ranging from glaciers lakes to deep seas and a rich biodiversity of fish and shellfish of more than 10 per cent of global biodiversity. Our country has a vast potential for marine, brackish and freshwater fisheries development.

The country is endowed with 8,129 km of coastline and 2.02 million sq. km of perennially, clear and mercury free water, within the Exclusive Economic Zone (EEZ). In the inland sector, the country has 4, 5000 km of rivers, 1, 26,334km network of canals, reservoirs and lakes, covering 3.3 million hectares and freshwater ponds and tanks, which are nearly 2.4 million hectares. By virtue of its geographical situation in the monsoonal belt, India is blessed with good rainfall, which accounts for extensive fresh and brackish water bodies ideal for aquacultural operations. Lakes in the high altitudes provide suitable conditions for the culture of coldwater species such as trouts. Therefore, in Inland sector, the fish production increased comparatively much more than marine sector after 2000 as evident from Table 8. 1 and Figure 8.1.

Table 8.1: Fish Production (In lakh tonnes) in Marine and Inland Sector of Fisheries in India from 1991 to 2007

Year	*Marine*	*Inland*	*Total*
1991- 92	2447	1710	41.57
1992- 93	2576	1789	43.65
1993- 94	2649	1995	46.44
1994- 95	2692	2097	47.89
1995- 96	2707	2242	49.49
1996- 97	2967	2381	53.48
1997- 98	2950	2438	53.88
1998- 99	2696	2566	52.98
1999- 2000	2852	2823	56.75
2000- 01	2811	2845	56.56
2001- 02	2830	3126	59.56
2002- 03	2990	3210	62.00
2003- 04	2941	3458	63.99
2004- 05	2778	3526	63.04
2005- 06	2816	3755	65.71
2006- 07	3024	3845	68.69

Source: Annual report, 2007- 2008.

In India aquaculture has been in progress for the past 5 decades. India's aquaculture industry is highly dependent on exports. World

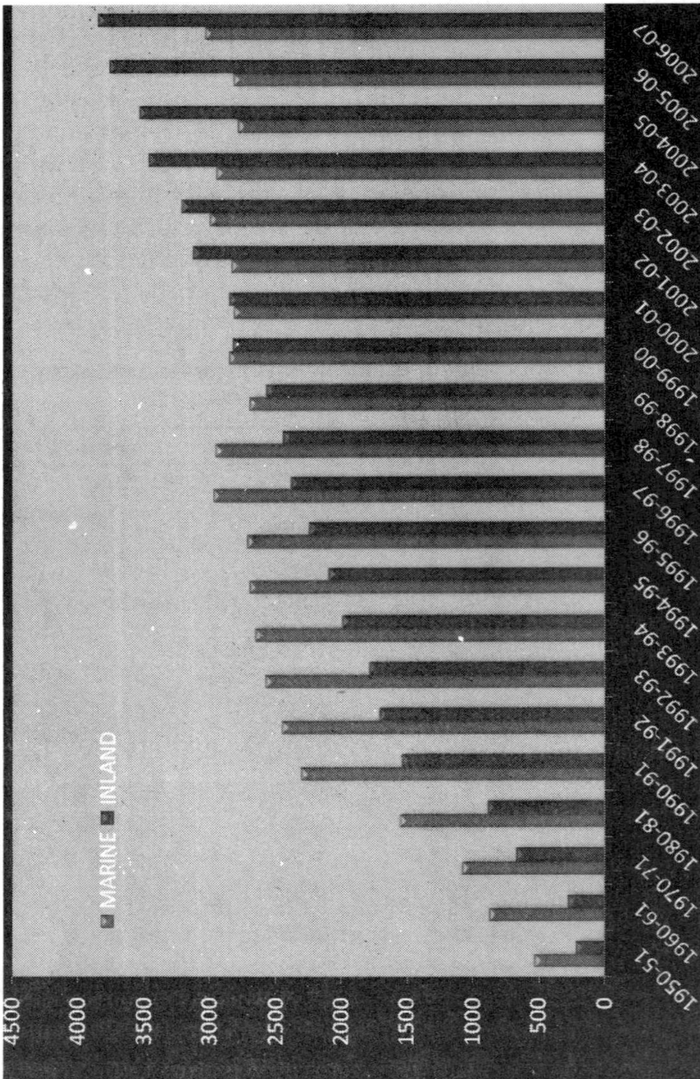

Figure 8.1: Fish Production in India in Marine and Inland Sector of Fisheries from 1950- 2007 (*Source:* Annual report, 2007- 2008)

demand exceeds production and per capita consumption is also steadily increasing. There has been a remarkable improvement in the productivity level of aqua culture ponds. Therefore, India has great scope in expanding its aquaculture industry.

The fish production of the country has increased from 0.75 million tonnes in 1950 to over 68.69 lakh tonnes at present (Figure 8.1). Therefore, an overall eight fold increase with production of over 30.24 lakh tonnes from the marine fisheries and 38.45 lakh tonnes from the inland sector (Table 8.1). With this production, the country has occupied the 2nd position in the world in terms of inland fish production and third position in overall fish production (Annual report, 2007-08).

Freshwater Aquaculture

Within the culture fisheries, the major contributors have been the freshwater aquaculture as evident from Table 8.1. India is being basically a carp country. Carp culture in India is believed to be as old as carp culture in China. Carp contributes more than 80 per cent of the total aquaculture production of the country. Carps mainly divided into two groups.

Indian Major Carps

- Catla (*Catla catla*)
- Rohu (*Labeo rohita*)
- Mrigal (*Cirrihinus mrigala*)

Exotic Carps

- Silver *carp* (*Hypophthalmichthys molitrix*)
- Grass carp (*Ctenopharyngodon idella*)
- Common carp (*Cyprinus carpio*)

The indigenous and the exotic carps account for the bulk of the production. The three Indian major carps (catla, rohu, mrigal), together, contribute a lion's share of two million tones with exotic carp (silver carp, grass carp, common carp), forming the next important group (Figure 8.2).

Composite Fish Culture

Culture of different species of fishes together is called composite

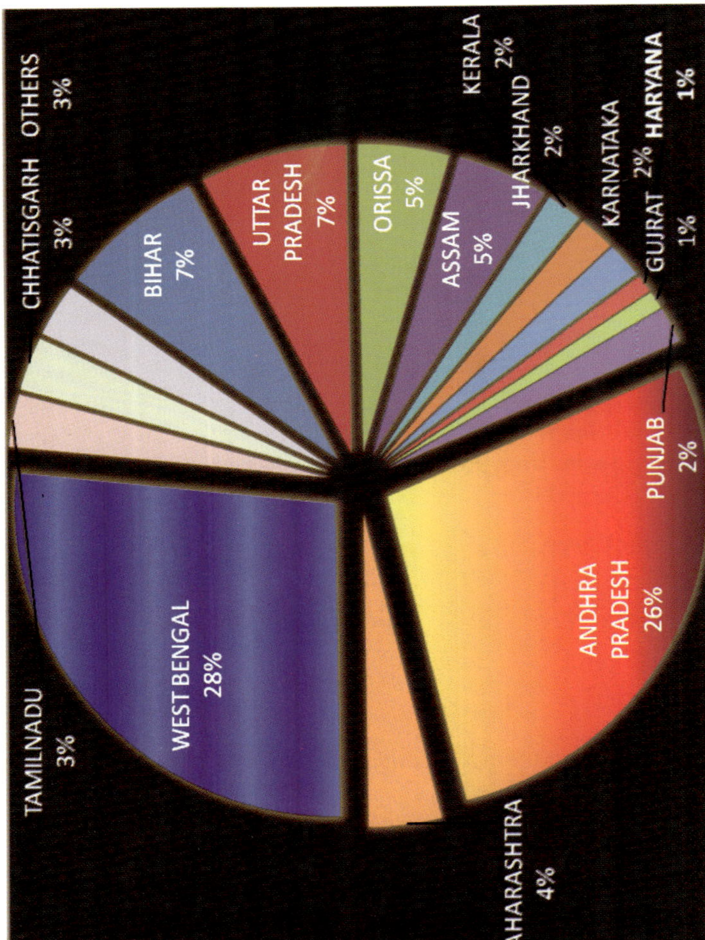

Figure 8.2: State-wise Inland Fish Production
(*Source:* Annual report, 2007- 2008)

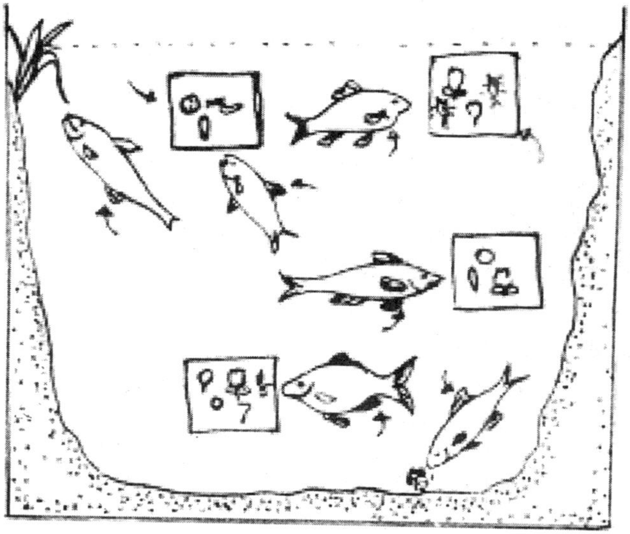

Figure 8.3: Composite Fish Culture

fish culture. It is also known as polyculture. The objective of this type of fish culture is to select and grow fishes of different feeding habits in order to exploit all types of food available in different regions of pond. In this type of fish culture, fast growing fishes namely Indian major carps *i.e.* catla, rohu, mrigal; silver carp, common carp and grass carp are usually cultured. This system is first developed in China. But now, this system is widely practiced with great success with different combinations of fishes in many countries.

Table 8.2 Some Combination of Fishes Used in Composite Fish Culture

(A)	Catla	:	Rohu	:	Mrigal		
	2	:	6	:	2.5		
(B)	Silver carp	:	Grass carp	:	Common carp		
	5	:	2	:	2.5		
(C)	Catla	:	Rohu	:	Mrigal	:	Common carp
	40%		30%		15%		15%

Integrated Fish Culture

Culture of fish along with agricultural crops such as paddy, banana and coconut and livestock such as poultry, duck, cattle and pigs is known as integrated fish farming. The integration of aquaculture with livestock and crop farming offers great efficiency in resource utilization, reduces risk by diversifying crop, and provides additional food and income. This system involves recycling of waste or by-products of one farming system as input for another system and efficient utilization of farming space for maximum production.

Culture of Catfishes

In recent years, culture of catfishes, has also received increased interest, due to their high market price and hardy nature. In all tropical regions of the world, oxygen depletion in shallow water is of common occurrence. The atmospheric temperature has a direct effect on the temperature of the water. There occur diurnal pulses of dissolved oxygen values, influenced by seasonal changes. Such water areas become unutilisable for the conventional human activities, pertaining to their commercial prospecting and are regarded as, derelict and swampy. Survival of carps in such inherently catastrophic environment is meagre but there are number of teleosts in tropical region which are able to thrive in the adverse ecological conditions. Air breathing carnivorous fishes such as murrels, koi, singhi and magur are suitable economically important catfishes for culture (Figures 8.4 and 8.5).

Brackish Water Aquaculture

Brackish water is saltier than freshwater, but not as salty as sea water. The culture of aquatic organisms in saline water having salinity range >0.5 – 30‰ is known as brackish water culture. In brackish water areas, milk fish, sea bass, mullet, mugil species and prawns are cultured by installing bamboo or nylon enclosures. These enclosures are called pens. In brackish water, mussels and oysters are also cultured by pole, rack, raft and rope culture methods.

Brackish water aquaculture in India is an important activity for increasing the fish production and to provide rural employment. Though brackish water aquaculture is traditionally practiced in the coastal areas technology improvements in this sector in recent years have motivated farming in new areas.

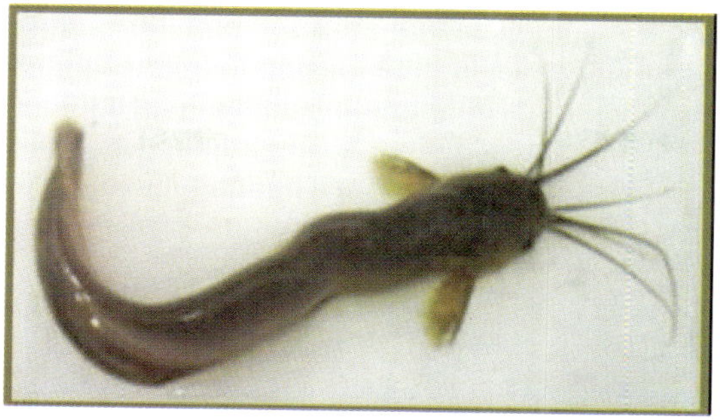

Figure 8.4: Singhi Fish

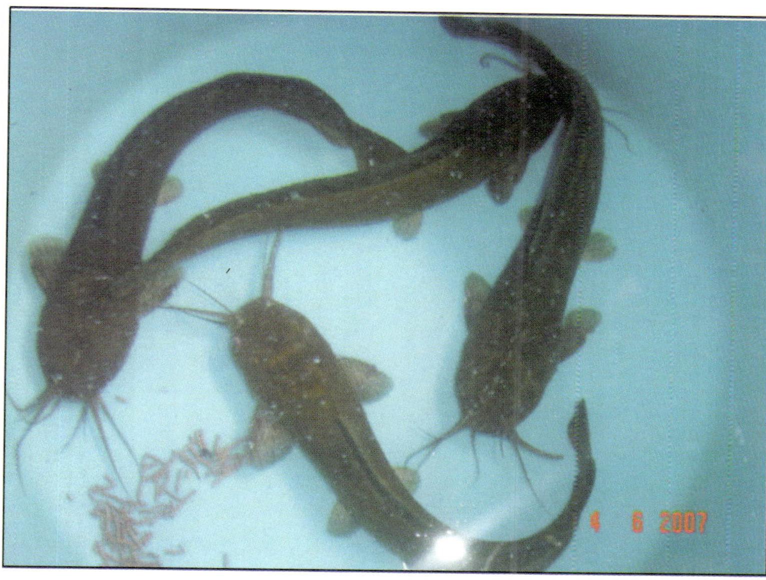

Figure 8.5: Magur Fish

Along the Indian coast line, the potential area of 1,909 million ha is amenable for brackish water. It has been estimated that we have 9 million ha salt affected land which are unfit or marginally fit for agriculture existence in the hot semi-arid and arid eco-region of northern plains in Haryana, Rajasthan, UP and Gujarat. the salinization is threatening the productivity of agricultural enterprises affecting the fragile ecosystem and damaging the infrastructure

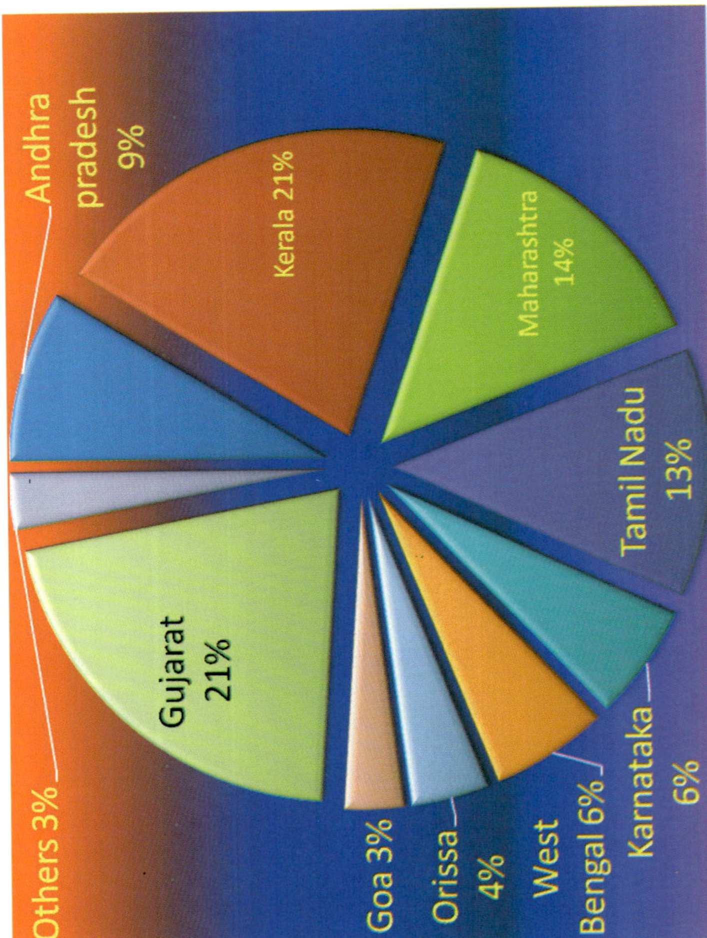

Figure 8.6: State-wise Marine Fish Production
(*Source*: Annual report, 2007- 2008)

facilities in these areas. The saline water resources, however can be used as a potential opportunity for the development of inland brackish water aquaculture adopting the technologies followed in the aquaculture practices of the coastal areas with site specific modifications.

Marine Fisheries

India is having a long coastline of 8,129 km with 10 million ha of land which is one of the greatest biodiversities in the world. It is delicately balanced with wetlands, mangroves, coral reefs and river basins sustaining 429 million rural people spread over 53 coastal districts and 10 maritime states. Major islands such as Andaman-Nicobar and Lakshadweep add to the biodiversity and bio wealth. These things offer high scope for the marine fisheries in India.

Among the Asian countries, India ranks second in culture and third in capture fisheries production and is one of the leading nations in marine products export. The present marine fisheries scenario is characterized by declining yields from the inshore waters and increasing conflicts among different stakeholders, whereas the demand for fish in domestic and export markets indicate good prospects for large scale sea farming and coastal mariculture.

Mariculture is the rearing of the aquatic organisms under control or semicontrolled conditions in the coastal and offshore waters where the salinity is maximal and not subject to significant daily or seasonal variations. Mariculture contributes to the production of protein rich food and has been the source of livelihood of millions of coastal villages.

The mariculture potential of India is vast as there is great scope for developing farming of shrimps, pearl oysters, mussels, crabs, lobsters, sea bass, groupers, mullets, milkfish, rabbitfish, sea cucumber, ornamental fishes, sea weeds etc. Although about 1.2 million ha is suitable for land based saline aquaculture in India, currently only 13 per cent is utilized. In India till date mariculture activities are confined only to coastal brackishwater aquaculture, chiefly shrimp farming.

Artisanal Mariculture

The other activities which can be categorized as artisanal mariculture include green mussel farming, lobster fattening, crab farming, edible oyster culture, clam farming and seaweed culture. A flourishing international trade of marine ornamental fishes is also in vogue which offers scope for the culture of marine ornamental fishes.

Marine Crustaceans Farming

- ☆ Shrimps
- ☆ Crabs
- ☆ Lobsters

Farming of Molluscs

- ☆ Oyster farming
- ☆ Clams farming
- ☆ Mussels farming
- ☆ Pearl farming

Marine Finfish Farming

Seaweed Farming

Oysters are most valued sea foods and are farmed extensively nearly 12 species of oysters which are commercially popular. *Crassostera madrasensis, C. gryphoides, C. rivularis* are most common oyster sp. available and preferred for farming.

Shrimp Farming

Shrimp is the most demanded product from coastal aquaculture and India is the 5th top most shrimp producer. Shrimp is major export earner (Over Rs. 3,500 crores every year).150,000 ha is under shrimp farming. *Penaeus monodon* alone accounts for more than 95 per cent of the production (Annual production of 1,15,000 tonnes shrimp). Shrimp seed production started in the experimental scale in Central Marine Fisheries Research Institute (CMFRI) in 1975 and till date country has 351 shrimp hatcheries with the total production capacity of 14 billion PL20/year wherein induced maturation technique have been standardized for the shrimp.

Fishery Trade

Fishery trade is particularly important as a source of foreign currency for developing countries. At present, their net earnings from aquatic products are greater than the combined earnings from the major agricultural commodities of rice, coffee, bananas, rubber, sugar and tea. In the last 50 years, the fish eaters of the world have doubled with a turnover. India's seafood industry is one of the biggest foreign exchange earners. Fishery trade plays an important role in the India.

The major marine products traded by India can be grouped into 9 categories:

Frozen Shrimp

Accelerated Freeze Dried (AFD) shrimp, block frozen shrimp, cooked salad shrimp, Individually Quick Frozen (IQF) and cultured shrimp.

Frozen Fish

Chinese pomfret, white and black pomfrets, fish lions/fish steaks, eels, fish fillets, fish roe, freshwater fish, mackerel, reef cod, ribbonfish, sardine, seabreams, seerfish, shark meat, snapper, big eye tuna, skipjack tuna, yellow fin tuna, gutted finless shark and shark tail.

Frozen Cuttlefish/Squid

Cuttlefish beak, cuttlefish blanched, cuttlefish bones, cuttlefish deskined, cuttlefish fillets, cuttlefish IQF, cuttlefish ink, cuttlefish meat trimmed, cuttlefish rings, cuttlefish roe, cuttlefish tentacles, cuttlefish tray packed, cuttlefish whole cleaned and cuttlefish wings.

Frozen Lobster

Rock lobster whole, sand lobster whole, IQF, deep sea lobster, rock lobster tail, sand/slipper tail, whole cooked lobster and lobster meat.

Live Items

Aquarium fish, crab, fish, lobster, shrimp, snail and whelk.

Chilled Items

Clam meat, fish, freshwater fish, lobster, pomfret and shrimp.

Dried Items

AFD shrimp powder, agar agar (seaweed), Beche-de-mer (sea cucumber), Bombay duck, chitin, chitosan, clam meat, cuttlefish, cuttlefish bones, fish maws, fish meal, fish nails, fish paste, isinglass, mussel meat, oyster shell powder, prawn feed, seahorse, shark fin rays, shark fins, shrimp powder, squid, fish skin, jellyfish salted, shark bones and shark tail.

Shells

Crab shell, seashell and turtle shells.

Others

Canned clams, chemeen chutney with and without coconut, fish pickles, fish vegetable barbeque, fish chutney, fish oil, fish powder, frozen mud crab, frozen crab meat, IQF whole crab, pasteurized crab, stuffed crab, freeze dried clam, fried fish and prawn, seafood vegetable mix, shark cooked and crushed, shrimp pickle, frozen snail meat, frozen surimi and frozen crab stick.

Seafood Export

The share of Indian seafood in the world market has shown an increasing trend over the years. During 2001-07 this increase has been 40 per cent in terms of value (Table 8.3). In the last decade the seafood trade doubled both in value and quantity. In 2006-07, India exported 6.12 lakh tonnes worth marine products valued at Rs. 8,363 crores.

Table 8.3: Seafood Export from India during 2001 to 2007

Year	*Exports*			
	Quantity (MT)	*% Variation*	*Value (Rs. Crore)*	*% Variation*
2001-02	424470	-3.63	5,957.05	-7.56
2002-03	467297	+10.09	6,881.31	+15.52
2003-04	412017	-11.83	6,091.95	-11.47
2004-05	461329	+11.97	6,646.69	+9.11
2005-06	512164	+11.02	7,245.30	+9.05
2006-07	612641	+19.62	8,363.53	+15.43

Source: MPEDA, 2007.

Major Items Exported

Frozen Shrimp continued to be the largest item exported in terms of value with 54 per cent of the total value of export as evident from

Table 8.4 and frozen Fish continued to be the major item exported in terms of quantity with 44 per cent of the total volume of marine products exported from the country. Cephalopods, squids and cuttlefish are other important commodities earning good market price.

It is worth noting that although frozen shrimp contributed to only 22 per cent in quantity of marine products exported, in terms of value realization it contributed nearly 54 per cent. In contrast frozen finfish, which contributed to 44 per cent in quantity, could only earn 17 per cent in terms of values as clearly shown in Table 8.4.

Table 8.4: Item-wise Exports of Marine Products During 2006-07

Items	*Exports*			
	Quantity (MT)	*% Share*	*Value (Rs. Crore)*	*% Share*
Frozen shrimp	137397	22.43	4,506.08	53.88
Frozen finfish	270751	44.19	1,452.88	17.37
Frozen cuttlefish	55701	9.09	797.37	9.53
Frozen squid	47252	7.71	568.32	6.80
Dried items	24293	3.97	183.16	2.19
Live items	2478	0.40	64.06	0.77
Chilled items	7200	1.18	117.30	1.40
Others	67571	11.03	674.35	8.06
Total	612641	100.00	8,363.53	100.00

Source: MPEDA, 2007.

Code of Conduct for Responsible Fisheries

The fisheries sector is an important source of life and livelihood for millions of people around the world. As the world's largest wild food harvest, fish provides a vital source of protein as well as cash income for many families in the developing world.

Fisheries (which includes the management, catching, processing, and marketing of fish stocks) and aquaculture (the farming of fish) provide an important source of food, employment, income and recreation for people throughout the world. Millions of people depend upon fish for their livelihood. If there is to be enough fish for future generations, everyone involved in fishing must help conserve and manage the world's fisheries.

According to the Food and Agricultural Organization (FAO) of the United Nations, about 36 million people worldwide a directly engaged in fishing and fish farming. Most are in the South and the majority are small-scale, artisanal fishers eking out a living from coastal and inshore resources. Worldwide, fish products provide 15 per cent or more of the protein consumed by nearly 3 billion people and support the livelihood of 520 million people, many of them women (FAO, 2009; World Fish Center, 2008).

The highest numbers of fishers and aquaculture workers are in Asia (85 per cent of the world total), followed by Africa (7 per cent), Europe, South America, North and Central America (about 2 per cent each) and Oceania (0.2 per cent).

With this situation in mind, more than 17O Members of the Food and Agriculture Organization of the United Nations (FAO) adopted the Code of Conduct for Responsible Fisheries in 1995. The Code is voluntary rather than mandatory, and aimed at everyone working in, and involved with, fisheries and aquaculture, irrespective of whether they are located in inland areas or in the oceans. Because the Code is voluntary, it is necessary to ensure that all people working in fisheries and aquaculture commit themselves to its principles and goals and take practical measures to implement them (FAO, 1995).

As a renewable natural resource, fish can be harvested year after year if countries have sound policies in place and if responsible fishing and utilization practices are followed. Similarly, with aquaculture, fish farming that does not harm the environment should be promoted because this type of culture will make important social and economic contributions to farming communities and the economies of their countries.

Role of Women in Fisheries

There are hardly any authentic statistics available on the number of women involved in fisheries-related work, though it is well known that women play important roles in the sector (ICSF, 2007).

Women are engaged in a wide range of activities, some of which have been enlisted below, in the fisheries and in fishing communities all around the world as:

- As workers (paid and unpaid) within the fisheries, in pre- and post-harvest activities, including liaison work with institutions and agencies. In many countries, it is mostly women who are engaged in inland fishing and aquaculture.
- As workers in seafood processing plants
- As caregivers of the family and in maintaining social networks and the culture of the community
- As workers in non-fisheries sectors to supplement the household income, and the often erratic returns from the fisher
- As members of fish worker movements and fishers' organizations

Nutritional Contribution of Aquaculture to Food Security

Fish are a major source of food protein for billions of people and their domesticated animals. Fish is a major source of protein in many poor people's diets, which are often dominated by starchy staples. Fish comprises about 20 per cent of animal protein in the diets of over 2.8 billion people – and can reach 50 per cent in the world's poorest regions, notably Africa and South Asia, and up to 90 per cent in small island developing states and coastal areas.

From the nutritional point of view as well, aquaculture has a special significance as fish is a rich source of protein for human being and also for other livestock populations. The diet of an average Indian is very low in calories, that's why, fish is considered as rich food for poor people, containing proteins and micronutrients such as iron, iodine, zinc, calcium, vitamin A and vitamin B. (Bene, 2005).The abundance of fish is the solution to fight against malnutrition, in developing societies and countries, on account of the high content of essential amino acids and high digestibility. Nutritionally, fish is often presented as an important source of protein, especially where other sources of animal protein are scarce or expensive. The share of fish in animal protein consumption can for instance exceed 25 per cent in many poor countries and reach 90 per cent in small-island states and isolated parts of coastal or inland areas.

Fish makes a minor contribution to calorie provision. Fish offers up to 180 calories per capita per day, but reaches such levels only in a few countries where there is a lack of alternative locally produced protein or where a preference for fish has been developed and maintained. More generally on a national basis, fish provides an average of 20 to 30 calories per day.

In low-income countries, staples such as rice, wheat, maize and cassava make up the bulk of the food consumed by people, supplying the majority of energy and nutrients. However there are some essential micro-nutrients which are not found in these staples or found only in small quantities–for example: iron, iodine, zinc, calcium, vitamin A and vitamin C. These nutrients must be supplied by other foods such as fish or vegetables. Fish is particularly rich in these micro-nutrients. Fish are also an important source of fatty acids that are necessary for the development of the brain and body. The importance of fish as a crucial element in the diet of a population, therefore, is now widely recognized, especially in the diets of young children, infants and pregnant women

Ornamental Fisheries: New Possibilities

Ornamental fish keeping is one of the most popular hobbies in the world today. This is a new and upcoming trade in India. It is an enjoyable hobby that brings relaxation and enlightment for persons of every age and interest. Through aquarium one can show the limitation of nature in a limited area and educate public for its conservation besides enhancing the beauty of place through living organisms.

Aquarium keeping has been rated as the second most popular hobby and the most popular type of pet (Olivier, 2001). The growing interest in aquarium fishes has resulted in steady increase in aquarium fish trade globally. The reason for the increasing popularity of aquarium fish trade is due to environmental awareness, the great variety of species and relative ease of care of fish.

Ornamental Fish Trade

Despite the huge potential offered by the rich diversity and environment, export of ornamental fish from India continues to remain negligible. Ornamental fish exports have increased from Rs. 3.2 crore in 2001-02 to Rs 5.6 crore in 2006-07, but it remains quite insignificant compared to the export of food fish, which is worth Rs. 8,000 crore per annum.

A study conducted by the School of Industrial Fisheries of the Cochin University of Science and Technology reports that India's share of the total global trade worth ($282 million) stands at 0.4 per cent. Experts say that India can emerge as a big supplier for ornamental fish with the rich biodiversity in the north eastern hills and Western Ghats. There are more than 300 species of freshwater fish in the Western Ghats alone, out of which 150 can be bred and promoted for trade.

The ornamental fish industry in the nation was scattered with low production volumes. Inadequate transport facility, high airfreight charges and lesser or non-availability of quality brood stock was hampering growth. The study also points out that 90 per cent of the ornamental fish export was based on wild collection. Unlike food fisheries, capture based export is not sustainable in ornamental fish trade and it is a matter of concern for the industry. In order to sustain the growth it is necessary to shift the focus from capture to culture based development. Organised trade in ornamental fish depends on assured and adequate supply of demand, which is possible only by mass breeding.

MPEDA is working towards the goal by developing captive breeding technology for indigenous varieties of ornamental fish. Other capacity building measures include developing strategies to network ornamental fish breeders in India, standardising methods for diagnosing viral diseases in ornamental fishes, cluster development and facilitating access to cheaper credit.

Need for Future Technology to be Developed

Despite the several new developments, India is still lagging behind many other countries in the use of modern aqua cultural technologies. We are not fully and effectively using vital information on technology already available, developed and successfully being practised with great advantage in many Asian countries. Water quality studies are important and have been taken up as a key subject in aquaculture. Innovative techniques are available with computer control, systems for continuous water quality monitoring and feeding. Since massive production of seed is basic for successful culture, a chain of hatcheries have to be established all over the coastal areas to boost production of seed. At the same time, collection and culture of larvae from natural sources be encouraged and expanded to save this precious resource being wasted or destroyed at present.

High energy feed has really boosted the production in aquaculture systems in many countries and we are yet to develop these items in India. Poly culture of freshwater prawn with major carps and other suitable species combinations in brackish water systems should be taken up. Other than above mentioned steps some more steps to be taken such as:

1. Emphasis on organic farming, integrated farming, utilization of hill stream resources, water log and saline soils etc.
2. Reducing pressure on wild fisheries
3. Raising productivity in aquaculture
4. Creation of infrastructure for facilities like icing, post harvest processing and value addition etc.

We should realise that aquaculture can produce significant quantities of food, income and employment and if planned and applied effectively can revitalise rural life and supply products of high nutritional value. It can assist in enhancement and maintaining wild aquatic stocks, thereby improving capture fisheries. It is an efficient means of recycling and upgrading low grade food materials and waste products into high grade protein rich food. With proper management and essential inputs, we can certainly develop aquaculture as a major avocation thereby opening up a new frontier for food and wealth for our country.

Threat to Fisheries: Global Warming

Global warming affects aquatic ecosystems and their fishery productivity. Fisheries and aquaculture are also threatened by the secondary effects of warming: changes in ocean currents, precipitation that affects lake levels and river flows, and increasing storminess and extreme floods and droughts. This makes living near water and catching or farming fish more hazardous than it is already. The physical, biological and ecological impacts of climate change in aquatic ecosystems are becoming increasingly apparent. Coral reefs are bleaching and their associated fisheries collapsing rapidly. Commercially exploited fishes are moving northward and into deeper waters at rapid rates, invading polar seas, and withdrawing from subpolar seas, semi-enclosed seas and the tropics. Climate change may affect fisheries, and their contribution to local livelihoods, national economies and global trade-flows, through both direct and indirect pathways. High-quality research that involves resource users, builds strong partnerships and harnesses political will is crucial for making fisheries and aquaculture systems more resilient to the challenge of global climate change and securing a bright future for the people that depend upon them (Allison, 2009).

References

Agarwal, V.P., 2006. *Aquaculture and Fisheries Science*. S. R. Scientific Publications, Agra, Delhi, p. 1-19.

Allison, E.H., A.L. Perry, M-C. Badjeck, W.N. Adger, N.L. Andrew, K. Brown, D. Conway, A. Halls, G.M Pilling, J.D. Reynolds and N.K. Dulvy. 2009. Vulnerability of national economies to potential impacts of climate change on fisheries. *Fish and Fisheries,* 10: 173-196.

Annual report 2007-2008, Department of Animal Husbandry, Dairying and Fisheries, Ministry of Agriculture, Government of India, New Delhi, p. 60-81.

Ayyappan, S., 2006. Showing signs of stagnation. In: *The Hindus Survey of Indian Agriculture 2006*. (Edited by N. Ram), p. 156-160.

Bene, C. and Heck, S., 2005. *Naga, World Fish center Quarterly*, 28(3): 8-9.

FAO, 2009. *The State of World Fisheries and Aquaculture, 2008*. FAO Fisheries and Aquaculture Department, Rome, 176 p.

ICAR, 2006. *Handbook of Fisheries and Aquaculture*. Directorate of Information and Publications of Agriculture, ICAR, New Delhi.

ICSF, 2007. *Gender Focus: Women in Fisheries: A Collection of Articles from Yemaya 2007*, ICSF, India.

Olivier, K., 2001. *FAO/Globefish Research Programme*, Vol. 67. United Nations Food and Agriculture Organisation, Rome, Italy.

World Bank and Food and Agriculture Organization, 2008. The sunken billions: the economic justification for fisheries reform. Agriculture and Rural Development Department. The World Bank: Washington DC.

Yadava, Y.S., 2006. Showing signs of stagnation. In: *The Hindus Survey of Indian Agriculture 2006*, (Edited) N. Ram, p. 139-142.

Chapter 9

A Critical Review on Certain Aspects of Anuran Integument

*Prahlad Dube**

Biodiversity Research Laboratory, Department of Zoology, Government College, Kota, Rajasthan, India

ABSTRACT

Integument is the exterior most covering of the body. It provides protection against the invasion of microorganisms, provides flexibility in motion, and seals in moisture. Anuran integument also gives rise to a variety of differentiated structures like various layers, glands, skin secretion, colour and pattern, but without the covering of protective derivatives like scales, feathers, hairs etc. Various glands are found on the layers of anuran integument like cutaneous glands which is belong to four main types- mucous, serous, lipid and mixed (sero-mucous) glands. Many specialized cells are developed from epidermal and dermal layers in the Anurans integument. The skin secretion of anurans is a rich source of biologically active compounds, including biogenic amines, alkaloids, steroids, peptides and proteins. The colors and patterns of anurans are determined by pigments produced by chromatophore cells in the skin. Therefore, anuran integument has remained preferred subject for research that attracted the

* Corresponding author: E-mail: dube_prahlad@rediffmail.com

researchers of various fields to work on it. The present chapter critically reviews available literature related to different aspects of anuran integument such as: Gross anatomy, histology and detailed structure, Histochemistry, Cellular details and Molecular biology.

Keywords: *Anuran integument, Layers, Cells, Glands, Skin secretion, Colour, Pattern, Morphology.*

Introduction

The skin is the largest organ of the integumentary system made up of multiple layers of ectodermal tissue, and guards the underlying muscles, bones, ligaments and organs. The skin is a soft outer covering of an animal, in particular a vertebrate. The epidermis of fish and of most amphibians consists entirely of live cells, with only minimal quantities of keratin in the cells of the superficial layer. It is generally permeable, and, in the case of many amphibians, may actually be a major respiratory organ. It is the exterior most covering of the body which provides protection against the invasion of microorganisms, provides flexibility in motion, and seals in moisture.

Anuran integument (Latin *integumentum,* from *integere* to cover, from *in-* + *tegere* to cover) having without the covering of protective derivatives like scales, feathers, hairs etc, but also gives rise to a variety of differentiated structures like various layers, glands, skin secretion, colour and pattern. Previous studies described that the integument of anuran amphibians is basically formed by an epidermal and a dermal layer. The epidermis is three cells thick. Epidermal layer is subdivided into the stratum cornium having keratinized cells, and the stratum germinativum having desmosomes and tonofilaments. The vast majority of the constituting cells are keratinocytes. Several types of cells have been recorded in the larval and adult anuran epidermis. The epidermal cell types that appear during early amphibian larval life include the ciliary cells, ordinary epidermal cells (keratinocytes), mucus-secreting (club) cells and mitochondria-rich cells (Fox, 1985). Other types of cells that appear at later larval stages include Merkel cells, Leydig cells and Flask cells (Warburg *et al.,* 1994). The dermal layer shows a classic structural morphology into the stratum spongiosum and the stratum compactum. Various glands are found on the layers of anuran integument like cutaneous glands which is belong to four main types- mucous, serous, lipid and mixed (sero-mucous) glands. Glands, specialized to secrete specific products are derived by an infolding of epidermal layer. In many cases, they retain a connection to the stratum corneum, whereby their secretions can be released at the skin surface. The skin secretion of anurans is a rich source of biologically active compounds, including biogenic amines, alkaloids, steroids, peptides and proteins. The colors and patterns of anurans are determined by pigments produced by chromatophore cells in the skin.

Although some 335 living species have been described in the world for the family Bufonidae (Duellman and Trueb, 1994), the integument has been studied in only a few of them. This chapter aims at obtaining a critical review on certain aspects of anuran integument biology.

Gross Anatomy and Histology

Detailed macroscopic and histological studies of the amphibian integument by Rabl (1931) and Elias and Shapiro (1957) have shown that the epidermis varies in thickness and may have projections or indentations, and that there are elevations and thickenings of various kinds in the dermis, especially in anurans. Elias and Shapiro (1957) provided definition and a terminology of the fine structure of the anuran integument. Fox (1972) described the structure of *R. temporaria* epidermis, Voute (1963), Parakkal and Matoltsy (1964) and Lavker (1974) studied *R. pipiens*. The epidermis of adult *Xenopus laevis* was studied by Farquahar and Palade (1965). The structural difference present in the skins of different species were observed and described by several workers (*e.g.* Verma *et al.*, 1969). Light and electron microscopical studies by Ernst (1973a, 1973b) and Green (1979) have shown that the epidermal cells in the toe-pads are structurally different from other epidermis on the body.

In *B. ictericus*, flask cells were visualized between the keratinocytes in both integument surfaces. Flask cells, also known as mitochondria-rich cells, constitute a specialized cell type of amphibian epidermis characterized by a 'flask-like' morphology and the existence of a high number of mitochondria in the cytoplasm (Villalba *et al.*, 1993). Willumsen *et al.* (2002) pointed out that flask cells represent a highly specialized pathway for passive transepithelial transport of chloride. Fox (1986a, b) reported that flask cells are involved in keratinization and sloughing. In *B. ictericus*, flask cell do not respond to PAF-staining, indicating the absence of cytokeratin filaments; then they do not participate, directly, in the keratinization process.

In adult anurans such *B. ictericus* (Azevedo *et al.*, 2005), *Bufo marinus* (Schwinger *et al.*, 2001) and *Xenopus laevis* (Greven *et al.*, 1995), the compact dermis is not a continuous layer, but is a series of alternating layers of bundles of collagenous fibers (arranged in a criss crossed manner) that join the hypodermis to the spongious dermis (Duellman and Trueb, 1994; Fox, 1988 a, b).

In the literature, reports of different epidermal elevations or projections have been reported. Quay (1972) and Duellman and Trueb (1994) reported to the largest elevation as 'warts' or 'verrucae'. Toledo and Jared (1993) named the roughened skin structures as 'verrucae hydrophilica'. Goniakowska-Witalinksa and Kubiczek (1998) relate regular 'ridges' to the elevations of ventral skin. The outermost epidermal layer of *B. ictericus* is covered with polygonal, usually pentagonal squamous cells, exhibiting elevation on the nuclear region and on the cell membrane border. Kaltenbach *et al.* (1980) described similar features in *Rana pipiens* epidermis. Warburg and Rosenberg (1997) cited that the ventral integument of the new *Tritturus vittatus* shows several 'tuberculi'. However, the authors do not suggest any morphological significance for these structures.

The anuran integument exhibit distinct structural morphology with respect to the dorsal and the ventral regions, as described for *Bufo ictericus* (Azevedo *et al.*, 2005; de Brito-Gitirana and Azevedo, 2005). De Brito-Gitirana and Azevedo (2005) reported that in *B. ictericus*, by using stereoscopic and low vaccum scanning electron images, three types of projections are observed on the dorsal surface: verrucae, tubercles and spines with distinct morphological features at light microscopy. Their macroscopical analysis revealed structural differences between the dorsal and ventral surfaces. The dorsal surface is rougher than the ventral, which is devoid of proturberances (verrucae). However, the ventral surface is the flattest. In the *Proceratophrys* genus, the tubercles showed neither an increase in the number of cellular layers nor an increase of keratin content, as observed for *B. ictericus*.

Felsemburgh *et al.* (2006) investigated the morphological characteristics of the leptodactylid integument of proceratophrys and odontophrynus genera using stereoscopic, low vaccum scanning electron and light microscopy. The integument morphology showed peculiar characteristics that may be helpful for to characterize and to differentiate anuran species. Their macroscopical observation revealed that all studied leptodactylids have a rougher integument. However, in *P. boiei, P. laticeps* and *P. appendiculata* the integument is rougher than O. americanus integument. This gross anatomical data has been confirmed by SM and SEM. In the Proceratophrys genus, the integument possesses several verrucae with numerous spine-like projections, and the dorsal surface has a heterogenous profile, while the ventral surface is more homogenous. In all leptodactylids, both integument surfaces have an anastomosed network of grooves between the verrucae. The grooves may contribute to spreading and retention of the glandular secretion on the integument, and could also be important for water distribution.

Bovbjerg (1963) indicated that the two types of glands and secretory cells develop independently without intermediate or transitional type in *Rana pipiens*. In studies of *Ambystoma mexicanum* and *Nectophrynoides occidentalis*, Le Quang Trong (1966, 1967) noted that some glands have granular cells basally and mucous cells in or below the neck region. In the literature, there are some different descriptions of these cutaneous elevations. For Lynch (1971), the cutaneous surfaces of *Proceratophrys* genus were covered with numerous tubercles, while on the *Odontophrynus* integument the tubercles were rarely observed. In both surfaces of *B. ictericus* integument there are several epidermal elongated orifices that correspond to the opening of glands, also visualized by light microscopy. Kaltenbach *et al.* (1980) reported that the openings of cutaneous glands are frequent, whereas Mills and Prum (1984) mentioned that the ductal cells are continuous with the lining epithelial cells, showing a gradual transition with the cornified layer reaching down into the two types of ducts, and ends up approximately in the middle third. Cutaneous glands of all living amphibians usually belong to four main types located in the spongious dermis: mucous, serous (granular or poison), lipid (or wax), and mixed (seromucous) glands (Duellman and Trueb, 1994; Brizzi *et al.*, 2002). Brizzi *et al.* (1999) described the granular cutaneous gland in the frog *Physalaemus biligonigeous* (Anura, leptodactylidae), comparison between ordinary serous and inguinal glands. In addition, there are various subtypes of serous glands indicating a high morphological variability (Warburgh *et al.*, 2000).

The cutaneous secretory products of bufonids have been characterized, and different compounds are described and divided into four main categories: biogenic amines, bufodienolides (bufogenins and bufotoxins), alkaloids, peptides and proteins (Daly *et al.*, 1987; Toledo and Jared, 1995; Erspamer, 1994).

In the spongious dermis of the anuran integument, two exocrine glands occur: mucous gland and granular (venom) gland (Porter, 1972; Delfino *et al.*, 1987; Duellman and Trueb, 1994; de Brito-Gitirana and Azevedo, 2005; Felsemburgh *et al.*, 2006). Experiments by Emerson and Diehl (1980) and Green (1981) provided evidence that surface tension (capillarity) enhanced by mucous secretions is the principal means by which anurans adhere to smooth surfaces. Many antimicrobial compounds have been isolated from mucous secretions of different tissues/organs (Brogden, 2005).

Mixed glands are constituted by mucous and serous cells. According to the established histology which uses histo-chemical and structural parameters (Weiss and Greep, 1977; Kierszenbaum, 2002), mixed secretory units are made up of mucous cells and serous cells; they produce a seromucous secretion delivered into the same lumen. The cytoplasm of mucous cells is basophilic provided that they contain neutral glycoproteins and acid mucosubstances. The nucleus is flattened, and appears at the basal portion of the cell (Kierszenbaum, 2002). The serous cells have a round nucleus centrally placed and its cytoplasm is acidophilic.

Bufonids have peculiar glandular structures symmetrically disposed in a post-orbital position, known as the parotoid glands (Young, 1985; Pough *et al.*, 2003). Although toads do not have a venom inoculation system, they are considered poisonous animals due to their cutaneous glandular secretions that contain a variety of compounds such as proteins, peptides, steroids, alkaloids, and biogenic amines (Sakate and Lucas de Oliveira, 2000; Maciel *et al.*, 2003). These glands are composed of large aggregations of granular glands responsible for the production and storage of a thick and creamy secretion which may contribute to the anuran protection against predators and parasites (Porter, 1972; Croce *et al.*, 1973; Duellman and Trueb, 1994; Clarke, 1997; Sakate and Lucas de Oliveira, 2000). Hutchinson and Savitzky (2004) commented that the large vessels provide the precursor molecules necessary to formation of toxins contained in the secretion of the parotoid gland. In *B.ictericus*, large vessels occur in the hypodermis of the parotoid gland region. A remarkable glandular type, different from the mucous, serous, and seromucous glands in anuran integument, was described in *Odontophrynus americanus* (Felsemburgh *et al.*, 2006). These glands have an acidophilic secretion constituted by a granular intake scattered by a homogeneous secretion. The homogeneous secretion showed continuity to glandular cell cytoplasm, and this continuity characterizes a glandular type with an apocrine mechanism of secretion, which was not previously described for the amphibian cutaneous glands. De Almeida *et al.* (2007) studied the re-evaluation of the morphology of the Bufo ictericus parotoid glands. They showed that the parotoid gland is a specialized region of the integument, in which three gland types occur: the mixed, the smaller granular, and the larger granular glands. The parotoid gland integument of the medial surface showed rounded depressions with small pores that connect with the duct openings of the larger granular glands. The larger granular glands are the main glandular component, and are responsible for the macroscopic protuberances known as parotoid gland. Under light microscopic evaluation the integument is constituted by typical epidermis, supported by dermis subdivided into a spongious dermis, a reticular dermis, and a compact dermis. The Eberth-Kateschenko layer is identified as a basophilic material scattered throughout the superficial spongious dermis. Thus, the end product released by the parotoid glands, known as venom, represents a mix of secretions which are elaborated by these three glandular types. In addition, the histochemical methods revealed that the end product of the mixed gland is enriched with proteins produced by serous cells and neutral glycoproteins as well as sulfated and carboxylated acid mucosubstances produced by mucous cells.

Toledo *et al.* (1992) described rounded depressions on the parotoid gland surface as pores. They pointed out that the secretion of granular glands is PAS-negative and AB-positive. The granular glands produce an alcianophilic secretory product. In this work, Almeida *et al.* (2007) showed that the pores are located at the bottom of the rounded depressions. De Brito-Gitirana and Azevedo (2005) described rounded orifices on the dorsal and ventral integument, which corresponded to the openings of the glandular ducts. Thus, the pores in the bottom of the depressions are the excretory duct openings through which the milky venom is extruded.

Breeding glands in the skin of the chest region of the microhylid Gastrophryne carolinensis were described by Conaway and Metter (1967); similar glands have been noted in other microhylids. The breeding glands are about the same size as the granular glands. The secretion is released by the fragmentation of the superficial part of the gland, and the sticky secretion adhere the male to the dorsum of the female. Histochemically, the secretion is similar to that of the mucous glands, but it lacks the sulfate group's characteristic of mucous (Holloway and Dapson, 1971).

Amphibian chromatophores are located in either the epidermis or dermis. Melanophores are the predominant type of epidermal chromatophores, although erythrophores have been observed in the epidermis of some amphibians (*e.g. Notophthalmus viridescens*, Forbes *et al.*, 1973). Epidermal melanophores are thin, elongate cells with long dendritic processes that extend between surrounding cells. For example, in tadpoles of *Bombina orientalis*, epidermal melanophores form an elaborate orthogonal network composed of melanophores each with four dendritic processes radiating symmetrically from a central cell body (Ellinger, 1980). In addition to the presumably genetically based colour dimorphism observed in many species of amphibians, there are occasional examples in nature of melanism and albinism (Dyrkacz, 1981). Richards (1982) determined that chromatophore pigments change ontogenetically with the development of sex hormones in the African tree frog *Hyperolius viridiflavus*. During and subsequent to metamorphosis, the majority of pterinosomes in xanthophores are replaced by carotenoid vesicles in the dorsal skin of Bombina orientalis (Frost and Robinson, 1984) and *Notophthalmus viridescens* (Forbes *et al.*, 1973). Thus, the chromatophores and pigment compositions of the amphibian integument represent a highly dynamic system. The colors and patterns of anurans are determined by pigments produced by chromatophore cells in the skin. According to Frost *et al.* (1984), there are three major factors contributing to green colour in frog skin: 1. Kind of yellow pigment: carotenoids (pteridines in xanthophores, 2. quantity of yellow pigment in xanthophores and, 3. the arrangement of pigment organelles in iridophores below the xanthophores.

The occurrence of morphological colour change in the absence of the physiological change was noted by Taylor (1969) for *Hyla cinerea*; when the frogs were treated with MSH (melanocyte-stimulating hormone; intermedin) there was dimunition of purines in the iridophores, but the organelles remained aggregated. Nielsen's (1978a) ultrastructural studies of colour change in *Hyla arborea* also demonstrated that during the change from a pale to dark colour phase. Anurans may be brightly coloured or completely cryptic. Toledo and Haddad (2009) reported the use of colours and some morphological traits as defensive mechanisms in anurans. They reviewed this subject, added new data, and provided information about the evolution of colour usage in anurans, with special reference to Neotropical species. They divided the use of colours into three major categories: mimicry, deceptive coloration, and aposematism. All amphibian scientific names follow Frost (2008), and the species nomenclature for colouration was adapted from Pasteur (1982).

Cellular Details

Conspicuous thread-like structures in the epidermal cells of middle and late tadpoles of the frog were discovered by Rudneff (1865). These same structures were described by Eberth, apparently independently, in 1866. Subsequent investigators have chosen to call the structures "mitochondrial threads" (Saguchi, 1913; Speidel, 1926), "figures of Eberth" (Weed, 1934), or "bodies of Eberth" (Cameron, 1936). Thus, Saguchi (1913) considered the structures to arise from the fusion of mitochondria and to penetrate the basal cell membranes to bind the dermis and epidermis together. Weed (1934) believed the structures to be fine fibrillar continuations of the connective tissue of the corium which supported the basal epidermal cells and strengthened the connection of the epidermal layer to the corium. Cameron (1936) regarded the bodies as reserve accumulations of secreted material which were used up in the formation of the dermal connective tissue. Chapman and Dawson (1961) reported the fine structure of the larval anuran (*Rana clamitans*) epidermis, with special reference to the figures of Eberth. They pointed out the relationship between the aggregation of fibrillar material seen with the electron microscope in the epidermal cells of the tadpole and the classical figures of Eberth. They showed that aggregates of fibrous material in the cells of the inner layer of epidermal cells are identical in disposition and size with the classical figures of Eberth. These figures do not arise from an aggregation of mitochondrial filaments. Numerous mitochondria are located in the distal region of the cells of the outer layer of epidermis in association with the secretory vacuoles. Microvilli are seen occasionally on the free surface of the skin. Cisternae are found only in the cells of the outer epidermal layer, while vesicular endoplasmic reticulum is found in the cells of both epidermal layers.

Almeida *et al.* (2007) showed that the parotoid gland is a specialized region of the integument, in which three gland types occur: the mixed, the smaller granular and the largest granular glands. They reported the EK layer in the parotoid gland integument region.

The several types of cells have been recorded in the larval and adult anuran epidermis. The epidermal cell types that appear during early amphibian larval life include the ciliary cells, ordinary epidermal cells (keratinocytes), mucus-secreting (club) cells and mitochondria-rich cells (Fox, 1985). Other types of cells that appear at later larval stages include Merkel cells, Leydig cells and Flask cells (Warburg *et al.*, 1994).

In a previous work, Qar and Al-Adhami (2003) described the flank skin of the green toad, *Bufo viridis viridis*, in which a new type of cell was described. Then Al-Adhami *et al.* (2005) extends the description of another type of rare cell, the dark cells, in the pre-metamorphic larval epidermis of the green toad, *Bufo viridis viridis*, by the help of electron microscopy. It is a ramified cell with a number of cytoplasmic processes intervening in between the keratinocytes. Cells of this type partially rest on the basal lamina but do not attach to it through hemidesmosomes or inter-digitations as do ordinary basal keratinocytes omit (Fox, 1986). It is worth mentioning that the non-epidermal cells reported previously (Qar and Al-Adhami, 2003) did not contain hemidesmosomes, even though they rest on the basal lamina as do the dark cells of their study. Further investigation is needed to test this hypothesis and to determine the origin of this type of cell. Other types of cells were observed include surface mucous cells and mitochondria-rich cells. This general histological description of the pre-metamorphic skin of the green toad is in general accordance with descriptions of the larval skin in other amphibians, particularly anurans, previously studied (Billet and Gould, 1971; Rosenberg and Warburg, 1992; 1995).

Azevedo *et al.* (2005) had studied the dermal collagen organization in *Bufo ictericus* and in *Rana catesbeiana* integument (anuran, amphibian) under the evaluation of laser confocal microscopy, and statistical analyzed collagenous elements of the dermis. Their study provide evidence that *B. ictericus* and *R. catesbeiana* integument has well-organized compact dermis, constituted by collagenous lamellae in a plywood manner. In both animals, the thick collagenous columns are formed by association of alternating lamellae, and have a perpendicular trajectory, jointing the hypodermis to the spongious dermis without interfere in the compact dermis integrity. Then, the dermal arrangement is essential to the biochemical property of both anuran integuments.

Burton (1980) had studied the two cutaneous muscle, the *M. rectus abdominis pars anteroflecta* and the *M. cutaneous dorsalis*, that may help in the adoption of a defensive posture and in the secretion of fluids from integumentary glands in some microhylids. In some anurans, the mucous glands lack a distinct myoepithelium, but a distinct myoepithelium is present in caecilians (Fox, 1983).

Schwartz *et al.* (2003) investigated the effect of skin secretion of the amphibian *Siphonops paulensis* by monitoring the changes in conductance of an artificial planer lipid bilayer. They reported that the skin secretion of *Siphonops paulensis* (Gymnophiona, Amphibia) is able to form voltage-dependent ionic channels in lipid membranes.

The dermis contains many unmyelinated nerve fibers, and some of these axons extend into the epidermis. Investigations of these receptors were summarized by Catton *et al.* (1976).

Biochemistry

Cutaneous glands of amphibians usually belong to four main types: mucous, serous (or granular glands or poison glands), lipid (or wax) and mixed or seromucous gland (Brizzi *et al.*, 2002).

The mucous secretion released onto the anuran integument exerts both mechanical and chemical functions. This secretory product maintains the integument moist and contributes to cutaneous respiration (cutaneous gas exchange). Muhse (1909) believed that only one kind of integumentary gland was present in amphibians even in toads. It is now known that all amphibians have both mucus and granular (poison or serous) glands. The mucus glands secrete muco-polysaccharides (mucus) that keep the skin moist and facilitate oxygen transport. Granular glands secrete a variety of substance (*e.g.* peptides and alkaloids) that commonly are noxious and sometimes highly toxic, and therefore are important defense mechanisms. In amphibians, the cutaneous mucous is produced by intra-dermal multicellular glands (Duellman and Trueb, 1994).

Le Quang Trong (1974) demonstrated the presence of neutral glycoprotein in mucous glands of the anurans integument using the PAS method. Park (1974) also detected acidic carboxylated and acidic sulphated mucopolysaccharides in the *Rana nigromaculata* mucous glands using the AB method, at pH 2.5 and 1.0 respectively. Faszewski and Kaltenbach (1995) observed the presence of fucose residues in the epidermis of *Ceratophrys ornate* and they assumed that it may act as a partial barrier to water loss. Since amphibians occupy a wide spectrum of different habitats, histochemical properties of the cutaneous glands possibly fit changes in environmental conditions (Choi *et al.*, 1997). Choi *et al.* (1997) employing the AB method in the *Rana rugosa* integument, did not observe any positive reaction in the extra cellular matrix, but not only in the mucous gland.

Mucous consist of complex molecules containing proteoglycans and glycoproteins produced by specific glandular cells (Kierszenbaum, 2004). De Brito-Gitirana *et al.* (2007) reported the expression pattern of glycoconjugates in the integument of *Bufo ictericus* (Anuran, Bufonidae): biochemical and histochemical (lectin) profiles. In anurans, the cutaneous mucous is produced by intra-dermal glands and displays both mechanical and chemical protection function. In this work, the carbohydrate moiety distribution was investigated in the integument of *Bufo icterícus* using conventional and lectin histochemistry to describe the pattern of cutaneous glycoconjugate expression, including both secretory and structural proteoglycans. The paper chromatography identified galactose, fucose and mannose as characteristic sugar residues. They suggested that the different glycoconjugate location reflects in two glycoconjugates categories: the secretory which participate in the water flow regulation, and the structural which is involved in the dermal maintenance. The integument carbohydrate content in the *B. ictericus* mucous gland is demonstrated by the positive reactions in AB and PAS methods, revealing neutral glycoprotein and acidic carboxylated and/or sulphated mucopolysaccharides as prevailing components. According to Gitirana *et al.* (2007), the spongious dermis extra-cellular matrix is rich in acid mucopolysaccharides. Once detected through the histochemical techniques, the biochemical method of chromatography in Whatmann paper characterized fucose, mannose and galactose as the sugar residues in the Brazilian toad integument.

Danguy and Genten (1989) detected binding sites for LCA, PSA and Con A in the epidermis and in the mucous glands of *Bufo bufo* and *Xenopus laevis*. Lectins which exhibit biochemically identical carbohydrate affinities may differ in their histochemical binding patterns. Villalba *et al.* (1993) applied the lectin histochemistry in *Rana perezi* and detected strong positive reaction for UEA in the flask cells. However, in the *B. ictericus* integument these cells do not have binding site for UEA. In fact, flask cells show negative reaction for all lectins used in the study of Gitirana *et al.* (2007).

The mannose sugar residues observed in the dermis should play a structural role since it participates in the collagen synthesis, influencing the collagen type synthesized by the fibroblasts (Kossi *et al.*, 2004).

Azevedo *et al.* (2006) was suggested that hyaluronan (HA) was localized in the pericellular epidermal matrix and in the spongious dermis of anuran integument; it plays an important role in hydric balance, and is essential for integument integrity and functionality.

Cutaneous lipids are present in the serous gland of phyllomedusine anurans (Blaylock *et al.*, 1976), and in hylids (Warburgh *et al.*, 2000) and the rhacophorid frog (Lilly White *et al.*, 1997).

Delfino *et al.* (1998) described two types of syncytial granular glands occurring in the *M. stelzneri* integument, and each gland line plays a peculiar role in the production of specific active molecules.

Some groups of anurans (*e.g. Phyllomedusine hylids*) contain large amount of unique polypeptides, and each species has its own characteristic polypeptide spectrum (Cei, 1963). Cei *et al.* (1972) demonstrate the analyses of biogenic amines and, Low, 1972 demonstrate the secretion of the parotoid gland of *Bufo* from throughout the world that trends in these biochemical traits corresponded to morphological groups of toads presumable representing different evolutionary lineages. The dendrobatids are well known for their strong toxins; phyllobates produce mainly batrachotoxins, which are extraordinarily toxic steroidal alkaloids, whereas Dendrobates secretes a variety of less toxic and chemically simpler piperidine alkaloids (Myers *et al.*, 1978). Serotonin was identified in the secretion of parotoid glands of *Bufo alvarius*, but not compound was absent in secretions from the macrogland on the hind limb (Cannon *et al.*, 1978).

Simmaco *et al.* (1997) suggested that amphibian skin is a promising resource for antimicrobial peptides that are assumed to have diverse physiological and defense functions. They isolated the natural antimicrobial peptides from amphibian skin could provide lead structures for either the chemical, or rDNA synthesis of novel antimicrobials. The skin plays key roles in the everyday survival of amphibians and their ability to exploit a wide range of habitats and ecological conditions. The biology and natural history of amphibian skin, its glands, their secretions, their normal functioning and potential medical applications are briefly reviewed by Clarke (1997). They suggested that the four categories of compounds are found in the granular or poison glands, these are: biogenic amines, bufodienolids (bufogenins), alkaloids and steroids, peptides and proteins.

Matutte *et al.* (2000) reported that extensive studies have been conducted on amphibian antimicrobial peptides of frogs belonging to the genus Rana. Members of the Rana genus comprise more than 250 species and are distributed worldwide, except for the Polar Regions, Southern South America and most of Australia. About 160 antimicrobial peptides have been identified from more than 20 Ranid amphibians.

Mangoni *et al.* (2001) demonstrated that the expression of antimicrobial peptides in *Rana esculenta* is induced by the exposure to microorganisms and this induction is mediated through the NF-kB cascade.

Granular glands in the skin of anuran amphibians, particularly those belonging to the families Pipidae, Hylidae, Hyperolidae, Pseudidae, and Ranidae, synthesize and secrete a remarkably diverse array of antimicrobial peptides, 10-15 residues in length, that are released onto the outer layer of the skin to provide an effective and fast-acting defense against harmful microorganisms (Duda *et al.*, 2002; Conlon *et al.*, 2004).

Vanhoye Damien *et al.* (2003) reported that the dermal glands of hylid and ranin frogs produce antimicrobial peptides originated from a 150-million years old ancestral precursor with a conserved signal peptide but a hypermutable antimicrobial domain. These antimicrobial peptides protect the skin against noxious microorganisms and assist in wound repair.

Macfoy *et al.* (2005) suggested that certain of the skin alkaloids of poison frogs, in addition to being noxious to predators, may also benefit the frog through protection against skin infections. More recently a large number of peptides exhibiting hemolytic and/or antimicrobial activities have been isolated from numerous species of anurans (frogs and toads), included mainly in the genera *Phyllomedusa, Rana, Litoria* and *Bombina*. Rollins Smith *et al.* (2005) suggested that a 25b amino-acid residue, C-terminally alpha-amidated peptide with antimicrobial activity, which has been termed fallaxin, was isolated in high yield from the norepinephrine-stimulated skin secretions of the mountain chicken frog *Leptodactylus fallax*. Fallaxin inhibited the growth of reference strains of Gram-negative bacteria (*E. coli, Pseudomonas aeruginosa, Enterobacter cloacae, Klebsiella pneumoniae*) but with relatively low potency and was inactive against the Gram-positive bacteria (*Staphylococcus aureus*) and the yeast *Candida albicans*. Castro *et al.* (2005) reported the purification and structural characterization of two novel hemolytic peptides isolated from the skin secretion of the Brazilian tree frog (Hylidae frog) *Hyla biobeba,* using reversed-phase chromatographic procedures. These peptides could be included in the bombinin H-antimicrobial peptide group because of some common structural features, including amino acid sequences, high hydrophobic profile, amidated C-termini, as well as, hemolytic properties. These two novel peptides are the first examples of bombinins H- like peptides isolated from anurans species not related to *bombina* species. They also observed a mass difference between the experimental and theoretical molecular masses of each peptide, indicating the presence of post-translational modification, possibly an amidated C-terminus.

Conlon *et al.* (2007) isolated two peptides (Dermaseptin-L1 and Phylloseptin-L1) with differential cytolytic activity against bacteria, a fungus pathogenic to amphibians, and mammalian cells from norepinephrine-stimulated skin secretions of the Lemur leaf frog *Hylomantis lemur* Boulenger, 1882 (Hylidae: Phyllomedusinae).

Dermaseptin-L1 was active against the Gram-negative bacterium *E. coli* (MIC=8 μM) but inactive against the Gram-positive bacterium *Staphylococcus aureus*. Phylloseptin-L1 was active against *S. aureus* (MIC=8 μM) but was inactive against *E. coli*. Dermaseptine-L1 showed selective cytolytic activity against HepG2 human hepatoma-derived cells (LC_5 = 45 μM) compared with human erythrocytes (LC_{50} = 35 μM) and erythrocytes (LC_{50} = 40 μM). The potential anti-cancer and anti-bacterial functions of the peptides demonstrate the importance of this species and biodiversity in general to human medicine and the urgency of the need for conservation of rapidly disappearing amphibians. The dermaseptins are an extensive family of peptides whose members have been isolated from the skins of a range of species belonging to the Phyllomedusinae–*Phyllomedusa sauvagei* (Mor and Nicholas, 1994; Chen *et al.*, 2003), *Phyllomedusa bicolor* (Charpentier *et al.*, 1998), *Phyllomedusa oreades* (Brand *et al.*, 2002), *Phyllomedusa distincta* (Brand *et al.*, 2002), *Phyllomedusa hypochondrialis* (Brand *et al.*, 2006), *Pachymedusa docnicolor* (Wechselberger, 1998), *Agalychnis annae* (Wechselberger, 1998), and *Agalychnis callidryas* (Vanhoye *et al.*, 2003). The primary structure of dermaseptin-L1 from H. lemur is compared with the structures of the eight members of the dermaseptin family identified in *P. sauvagei*. The phylloseptins are a family of structurally related peptides identified in the skin secretions of the Brazilian tree frogs, *P. hypochondrialis* (Leite *et al.*, 2005; Conceicao *et al.*, 2006) and *P. oreades* (Leite *et al.*, 2005). Their primary structures are compared with that of Phylloseptin-L1.

Cytolytic peptides are synthesized in granular glands present in the skins of a wide range of anuran species (frogs and toads) and constitute an important component of the animal's system of innate immunity (Hancock, 2001). The peptides are released into skin secretions, often in very high concentrations, in response to infection or stress (Davidson *et al.*, 2007).

The Phyllomedusinae sub-family of the Hylidae family comprises 56 species and has proved to be a rich source of peptides may be grouped together on the basis of limited structural similarity and the following families have been identified: (a) dermaseptins, (b) dermatoxins, (c) phylloxins, (d) phylloseptins, and (e) Gly-Leu-rich peptides (reviewed in Nicolas and Amiche, 2006). The members of the different families differ appreciably in both primary structures and biological activities, but strong conservation of the amino acid sequences of the signal peptide and N-terminal pro-regions of the biosynthetic precursors of the peptides demonstrated that they are related evolutionarily (*Vanhoye et al.*, 2003).

Skin secretions from a single species frequently contain several members of a particular peptide family with varying degrees of antimicrobial potency and selectivity that are presumed to have arisen from multiple duplications of an ancestral gene (Tennessen and Blouin, 2007). It is speculated that the molecular diversity may provide a broader spectrum of defence against pathogenic microoraganisms although firm evidence to support this hypothesis is lacking.

Conlon *et al.* (2009) described the purification and characterization of two families of structurally related C-terminally α-amidated antimicrobial peptides (alyteserin-1, alyteserin-2a) in norepinephrine-stimulated skin secretions of the midwife toad *Alytes obstericans* (Alytidae). The alyteserin-1 peptides show selective growth inhibitory activity against the Gram-negative bacteria *E. coli* (MIC = 25 μM) whereas alyteserin-2a is more potent against the Gram-positive bacteria *Staphylococcus aureus* (MIC = 50 μM). The data demonstrated that the frogs belonging to the family Alytidae are among those producing dermal antimicrobial peptides that may represent a component of the animal's system of innate immunity. The alyteserin-1 papetides show limited structural similarity (between 37 and 39 per cent) to the C-terminally α-amidated antimicrobial peptides ascaphin-1 and ascaphin-8, previously isolated from *Ascaphus truei* (Conlon *et al.*, 2004) and *Ascaphus montanus* (Conlon *et al.*, 2007) belonging to the family Leiopelmatidae. Similarly, the alyteserin-2 peptides show limited structural similarity (between 41 and 65 per cent) to bombinin H-6, previously identified in the skin secretions of the toad *Bombina bombina, B. orientalis,* and *B. variegate* belonging to the family Bombinatoridae (Mangoni *et al.*, 2007). Bombinin H6 is unusual in that isoforms have been found to contain either Δ-leusine or Δ-alloisoleusine instead of Λ-leusine at position 2 in the molecule (Mignogna *et al.*, 1993) and the enzyme responsible for effecting this transformation has been isolated from frog skin (Jilek *et al.*, 2005).

Myers *et al.* (1978) noted a decline in the toxicity of secretions produced by *Phyllobates terribilis* maintained in captivity. There even may be differences in the presence of a substance in secretions from glands on different parts of the body in the same species. Lima *et al.* (1991) reported the utilization of o-phthalaldehyde-sulphuric acid as a spray reagent in thin-layer chromatographic detection of some indole alkylamines and application to cutaneous secretion extracts of toad species (*Bufo ictericus* and *Odontophrynus cultripes*).

Erspamer (1971) noted the presence of three groups of aromatic amines and five groups of polypeptides. The amines are indolealkylamine (found in pipids, leptodactylids, Bufonids, hylids, ranids), imidazolealkylamines (*e.g.* Leptodactylus, Taudactylus and Litoria), and hydroxyl phenylalkylamines (found in leptodactylids, bufo).

Martenson *et al.* (1974) demonstrated that the frog myelin basic protein, unlike those of all other species hitherto examined, contains a single cysteinyl residue in its polypeptide chain. The skin of the frog, *Rana temporaria,* has similar physiological properties to this mammalian kidney tissue.

In this study, an immuno-histological method involving an antibody to human Tamm-Horsfall protein was used to investigate the distribution of this distinctive protein in frog kidney and skin, and to compare its distribution with that found in the kidney tubules of rat and rabbit. It is suggested that its presence in amphibian skin is consistent with the hypothesis that THP is an important component of tissue that absorb sodium and chloride ions but remain impermeable to water (Alexander *et al.,* 1990).

Bv8, a small protein from skin secretions of frog *Bombina variegate* and *Bombina bombina* and its homologue from snake venom induce hyperalgesia in rats. Bv8 is related to protein A, a component of the venom of the lack mamba (Mollay *et al.,* 1998). Alibardi (2001) had studied the keratinization in the epidermis of amphibians and the lungfish by electron microscopy, autoradiography and immuno-cytochemistry to determine whether histidine rich protein, filaggrin and loricin are present and compare with amniote keratinization. Baptiste *et al.* (2006), reported the first analysis of the frog cutaneous mucus proteome (in search for protein chemoattractants), leading to the identification, purification, and characterization of two new protein candidate ligands for the vomeronasal organ (VNO).

Simon Pitman (2008) believed that the frog skin adds to growing list of animal-based anti-aging solutions (first snail slime, then snake venom, now it is frog skin), scientists in South Korea are claiming that a new study has shown the skin of bullfrogs produces antioxidants that can help fight human skin aging.

In India, Garg *et al.* (2007), reported the antimicrobial activity of skin secretion isolated from Indian toad, *Bufo melanostictus* Schneider 1799. Amphibians like toads secrete such antimicrobial secretion both inside their body like other organisms as well as outside their body into the environment, through skin pores and parotid glands. Toad skin-secretions contain four types of compounds namely, biogenic amines, bufadienolides, alkaloids and steroids, and peptides and proteins.

Histochemistry

Elkan (1968) had studied more than 100 anuran species (except *Bufo ictericus*), described that an additional layer is absent in tadpole stages, which is known as ground substance or the Eberth-Kateschenko layer. According to Elkan (1968) in most species, but not all, the intermediate layer is located between the stratum spongiosum and stratum compactum, with thickness varying from 5 to 30 μm depending on the species. The EK layer has no cellular structure, and is basically composed of gycosaminoglycans (GAGs) in association with calcium salts (Elkan 1976). Toledo and Jared (1993) suggested that the calcium located in the EK layer participates in hydric balance, affecting the hydric absorption and retention.

Elkan (1968) mentioned that the EK layer is weakly stained with haematoxilin, faintly PAS but strongly alcianophilic, besides exhibiting a metachromatic staining with Toluidine and Thionine blue. Elkan also described the loss of metachromasia by pre-treatment with commercial hyaluronidase. This finding is in contrast with the results of Imamura *et al.* (1965), who believed that other mucopolysaccharides, instead of chondroitin sulfate or hyaluronic acid, could be responsible for metachromatic staining.

In *P. nattereri*, the EK layer occurs in the body integument (Lenzi-Mattos *et al.*, 1995), but lacks in the inguinal gland of *Cycloramphus dubius* (de-Lucas *et al.*, 1996). In *Triturus phyrrogaster*, the EK layer was not detected (Kikuyama *et al.*, 1975) as well as in the integument of *Melanophryniscus stelzneri* (Delfino *et al.*, 1998) and in the inguinal gland region (Lenzi-Mattos *et al.*, 1995). For Elkan (1968), the EK layer should have significant intra- and inter-specific variations.

Elkan used animals fixed with formaldehyde, Bouin's liquid and alcohol, and some of them were collection animals; however he commented that the type of fixative does not seem to affect the EK layer detection. The results of Elkan (1968) were based on a personal communication from Prof. Mathews, who has performed biochemical analysis in the Brazilian toad (*B. bufo*) integument, and identified two types of chondroitin sulfate.

On the other hand, Azevedo *et al.* (2005) observed that integument strips, removed from the same animal and fixed in Bouin's liquid, did not usually show the EK layer while in the formaldehyde fixed material the EK layer was preserved. They concluded that the fixative type might affect the EK layer preservation in paraffinized tissues. Azevedo *et al.* (2005) reported the structural aspects of the Eberth-Katschenko layer of the ventral and dorsal integument of a Brazilian toad *Bufo ictericus* with the aid of light microscopy using histochemical techniques in combination with biochemical analysis of the cutaneous calcium (Amphibian, Bufonidae). Anuran such as Brazilian toad *Bufo ictericus* spix, 1824, possess a calcified dermal layer called the Eberth-Ktschenko (EK) layer, located between the stratum spongiosum and stratum compactum and also in irregular deposits in stratum spongiosum They concluded that the EK layer of *B. ictericus* is a discontinuous layer, which is formed by hyaluronic acid, and a sulfated GAG different from chondroitin sulfate, heparin and heparan sulfate, and keratan sulfate. It is discontinuous in the region of ascending dermal connective fibers arranged perpendicularly to animal body surface. Thus, all components of the EK layer are essential for integument integrity and functionality. Porto (1936) also reported the same characteristics in *Bufo arenarum*. Sampson *et al.* (1987), studying the *Bufo marinus* integument, affirmed that when decalcifying substances are added to the integument, like EGTA (ethylene glycol tetra-acetic acid), the layer is no longer visualized after staining with hematoxylin indicating the removal of the GAGs along the calcium. In *B. ictericus,* after the removal of dermal calcium from the tissue and subsequent staining with HE, the EK layer still exhibits its basophilic staining characteristic. These results indicated that the acid treatment did not remove GAGs. The dermal calcium was also not detected when the tissues received the enzymatic pretreatment. These results suggest that calcium is linked to dermal GAGs, that is, predominantly hyaluronic acid.

Goncalves and de Brito- Gitirana (2008) showed that the iliac gland is a specialized region of the ventrolateral integument of *Cycloramphus fuliginosus* males (Amphibia, Leptodactylidae), in which two kinds of glands occur: the mucous merocrine gland and the tubuloalveolar syncytial apocrine gland. The tubulo-alveolar gland is the main glandular component and is responsible for the macroscopic elevation. After employing the histochemical techniques (PAS and AB), the mucous glands reveal a secretion rich in neutral glycoprotein. The end product released by the iliac gland represents a mix of secretions elaborated by both glandular types. Thus, the final secretion plays an important role in the biology of this cycloramphid, and may act not only as pheromone, but also in chemical defense, such as parental care. Further studies should be carried out in order to clarify the iliac gland secretion activity. Other anuran, *Physalaemus nattereri*, has a pair of black and round inguinal glands located on the lumber region of the dorsal integument of male and female, and the glands are emarginated by a white contour giving the impression of two black eyes (Vizotto, 1964; Sazima and Caramaschi, 1986).

The presence of multicellular mucous and serous (granular) exocrine glands in the dermis of metamorphosed skin is a synapomorphy for extant Amphibia (Houck and Sever, 1994). Among the more unique types of breeding glands are adhesive glands in the pectoral region of certain male frogs that cause the venter of the male to adhere to the skin of the dorsum of the female during amplexus. Such glands were first reported in the Microhylidae for Kaloula conjuncta from the Philippines by Taylor (1920), who stated that males adhere to females by virtue of a slimy secretion from the belly. Inger (1954) later reported "belly glands" from *K. picta* and *K. rigida*, and noted that they were absent in other members of the genus. In Kaloula, Inger (1954) describes adhesive glands as single celled epidermal aggregation on the ventors that vary in distribution depending on the species. Fitch (1956) described adhesion during amplexus of the North American microhylid *Gastrophryne olivacea*, and subsequently, Conaway and Metter (1967) described adhesive glands in *G. carolinensis*. Conaway and Metter (1967) reported that the adhesive glands secrete a protein rather than a mucoid substance. Adhesive glands are also known from male *Breviceps* in the South African family Brevicipitidae (Poynton, 1964; Visser *et al.*, 1982). Siegel *et al.* (2008) described the histology, histochemistry, and ultrastructure of the adhesive breeding glands of male *Gastrophryne carolinensis*. Adhesive glands are multicellular exocrine glands in the dermis of the sternum and forearm that cause the male to adhere to the female during amplexus. The epithelial cells have distinct plasma membranes, and the product consists of electron-dense secretory granules that fill the cytoplasm and are released intact by an apocrine process. Adhesive glands react positively for neutral carbohydrates and negatively for glycosaminoglycans and proteins. The ultrastructural results, the first on these organs, confirm that adhesive glands are derived from mucous glands and not serous glands.

Molecular Biology

Mangoni *et al*. (1997) had demonstrated that the expression of antimicrobial peptides in *Rana esculenta* is induced by the exposure to microorganisms and this induction is mediated through the NF-kB cascade.

Dube (2002) has studied the protein and peptide composition of four anuran species of Rajasthan, India, namely, *Bufo melanostictus, Rana tigerina, R. cyanophlyctus* and *Microhyla ornate*. In this study, he has compared protein composition of these four species and used them as a molecular tool in taxonomy of anurans of South Eastern Rajasthan.

Odierna *et al*. (2000), had studied the cytogenetic and molecular data on *Alytes muletensis* (Amphibia: Discoglossidae), compared with other representatives of archaebatrachian frogs.

Amphibian skin secretions are complex, species-specific cocktails of biologically-active molecules, including many uncharacterized peptides. The study of such for novel peptide discovery is time-limited as amphibians are in rapid global decline. Chen *et al*. (2002) discovered that polyadenylated mRNAs encoding dermal granular gland peptides are present in defensive skin secretions, stabilized by endogenous nucleic acid-binding amphipathic peptides. Thus parallel secretory proteome and transcriptome analyses can be performed without specimen sacrifice in this model amphibian system-a finding that has important implications in conservation of biodiversity within this threatened vertebrate taxon and whose mechanistics may have broader implications in biomolecular science.

Li *et al.* (2007) reported that peptidomics and genomics analyses were used to study an anti-infection array of peptides of amphibian skin. 372 c DNA sequences of antimicrobial peptides have been characterized from a single individual skin of the frog, *Odorrana grahami*, encoding 107 novel antimicrobial peptides. With respect to the development of antibiotics, these peptides provide potential new templates to further explore.

Miscellaneous

Rosenburg *et al.* (1978) reported the changes in structure of ventral epidermis of *Rana ridibunda* during metamorphosis. Denefle *et al.* (1990) reported the pigment cell localization in anuran ventral skin at climatic metamorphosis. In anuran amphibians, the specific colour pattern of the skin is expressed after metamorphosis, and its formation involves pigment cell migrations. Pigment cells are differently distributed in the tadpole, larval and froglet skin.

Hutchinson *et al.* (2004) had described the vasculature of the parotoid glands of four species of toads (bufonidae: bufo) – *B.alvarius*, *B. marinus*, *B. terrestris*, and *B. valliceps*.

Antimicrobial peptides in the skin secretion of anurans constitute a component of the innate immunity that protects the organism against invading pathogens. Conlon *et al.* (2005) isolated four peptides (Ranatuerin-2AUa, Brevinin-1AUa, Brevinin-1AUb and Temporin-1AUa) with antimicrobial activity in high yield from norepinephrine-stimulated skin secretions of the Northern red-legged frog *Rana aurora aurora* and their primary structures determined. The primary structures of the antimicrobial peptides are consistent with a close phylogenetic relationship between *R. aurora*, *Rana boylii* and *Rana luteiventris*.

Reichel (2006) had studied the differentiation of the opercular integument in *Rana pipiens*. They reported that moulting took place for the first time in tadpoles just before metamorphosis, and a well organized stratum granulosum was formed still containing the two main types of epidermal glands. The flask cells appear in the juveniles for the first time, greatly increasing in numbers in the adult epidermis.

In India, Gomes *et al.* (2007) reported that the amphibian skin secretion contains various bioactive molecules (peptides, proteins, steroids, alkaloids, opoids) that possess potent therapeutic activities like antibacterial, antifungal, antiprotozoal, antidiabetic, antineoplastic, analgesic and sleep inducing properties. Research on amphibian skin derived biomolecules can provide potential clue towards newer drug development to combat various pathophysiological conditions. Scientists throughout the world are now exploring the therapeutic potential of various toad and frog skin extracts and secretions. India, being a tropical country with diverse geographical variations, is home to wide species of toads, frogs and newts. There are about 200 species of frogs and toads in India. However, not much work has been carried out on toads and frog skin secretions in India as compared to the rest of the world. Gomes *et al.* (2007) provide an overview that is an attempt to enlighten the fact that amphibian skin is capable of providing a wide variety of bioactive compounds that may be turned to therapeutic advantage. Advanced knowledge on biotechnology and chemistry may be put to use to synthesize derivatives of the natural biomolecules, which may turn out to be more effective than the parent molecule. Thus, the multi-dimensional, multifunctional components of the amphibian skin warrant much more attention, which may lead to newer and more effective drug development in the near future.

References

Alexander, J., Christopher, J., and Andrew N., 1990. Immunoreactive Tamm-Horsfall protein in the kidney and skin of the frog *Rana temporaria*. *Cell and Tissue Research*, Springer Berlin Heidelberg, vol. 263, number.

Alibardi, L., 2001. Keratinization in the epidermis of amphibians and the lungfish: Comparison with amniote keratinization. *Tissue and Cell.*, 33(5): 439-449.

Almeida, P.G., Felsemburgh, F.A., Azevedo, R.A. and De Brito-Gitirana, L., 2007. Morphological re-evaluation of the parotoid glands of *Bufo ictericus* (Amphibia, Anura Bufonidae). *Contribution to Zoology*, 76 (3): 145-151.

Al-Adhami, M. A. and Qar J., 2005. A new type of cell in the epidermis of the premetamorphis skin of the green toad, *Bufo viridis viridis*. *Folia Biol.* (Krakow) 53: 179-181.

Azevedo, R.A., Santana, A.S.J. and de Brito-Gitirana, L., 2005. Hyaluronan in the epidermal and the dermal extracellular matrix: its role in cutaneous hydric balance and integrity of anuran integument. *Micron*.

Azevedo, R.A., Pelli, A.A., Ferreira-Pereira, A., Santana, A.S.J., Felsemburg, F. and de Brito-Gitirana, L., 2005. Structural aspects of the Eberth- Katschenko layer of *Bufo ictericus* integument: histochemical characterization and biochemical analysis of the cutaneous calcium (Amphibian, Bufonidae). *Micron*, vol. 36, pp. 61-65. Erratum in *Micron*, 36 (4): 385-386.

Azevedo, R.A., Carvalho, H.F. and de Brito-Gitirana, L., 2006. dermal collagen organization in Bufo ictericus and in *Rana catesbeiana integument* (Anuran, Amphibian) under the evaluation of laser confocal microscopy. *Micron*,37 (3): 223-228.

Baptiste, L., Gerard, T., Paul, F. and Ruddy, W., 2006. Identification and Characterization of New Protein Chemoattractants in the Frog Skin Secretome. *Molecular and Cellular Proteomics*, 5: 2114-2123.

Billet, F.S. and Gold, R.P. 1971. Fine structural changes in the differentiating epidermis of *Xenopus laevis* embryos. *J. Anat.*, 108: 465-480.

Blaylock, L.A., Ruibal, R. and Platt-Aloia, K., 1976. Skin structure and wiping behaviour of phyllomedusine frogs. *Copeia*, 2: 283-295.

Bovbjerg, A.M., 1963. Development of the glands of the dermal plicae in *Rana pipiens*. *J. Morph.*, 113: 231-243.

Brand, G.D., Leite, J.R., Silva, L.P., Albuquerque, S., Prates, M.V., Azevedo, R.B., Carregaro, V., Silva, J.S., Sa V.C., Brandao, R.A and Bloch, C.Jr., 2002. Dermaseptins from Phyllome-dusaoreades and *Phyllomedusa distincta*. Anti-Trypanosoma cruzi activity without cytotoxicity to mammalian cells. *J. Biol. Chem.*, 277: 49332.

Brizzi, R., Delfino, G. and Pellegrini, R., 2002. Specialized mucous glands and their possible adaptive role in the males of some species of Rana (Amphibia, Anura). *J. Morphol.*, 254: 328-341.

Brogden, K.A., 2005. Antimicrobial peptides: Pore formers or metabolic inhibitors in bacteria? *Nature*, 3: 238-250.

Burton, T.C., 1980. Phylogenetic and functional significance of cutaneous muscles in microhylid frogs. *Herpetologica*, 36: 256-264.

Cameron, J.A., 1936. The bodies of Eberth as a source of connective tissue ground substance in *Rana catesbeiana*, Shaw. *J. Morphol.*, 60: 279.

Cannon, M.S., Brindley, D.C. and Gill, M.M., 1978. The paracnemid gland of *Bufo alvarius. Texas, J. Sci.*, 30: 133-143.

Castro, M.S., Matsushita, R.H., Sebben, A., Sousa, M.V. and Fontes, W., 2005. Hylins: Bombinins H structurally related peptides from the skin secretion of the Brazilian tree- frog *Hyla biobeba. Protein and Peptide Letters*, 12: 89-93.

Catton, W.T., 1976. Cutaneous mechanoreceptors, in R. Llinas and W. Precht (eds.). *Frog Neurobiology*, Berlin: Springer-Verlag, pp. 629-642.

Cei, J.M., 1963.Some precipitin tests and preliminary remarks on the systematic relationships of four South American families of frogs, Serol. *Mus. Bull.*, 30: 4-6.

Cei, J.M. and Erspamer, V., 1972. "Biogenic amines". In: *Evolution in the Genus Bufo*, (Ed.) W.F. Blair. Univ. Texas Press, Austin, pp. 233-243.

Chapman, G.B. and Dawson, A.B., 1961. Fine structure of the larval anuran epidermis, with special reference to the figures of Eberth. *The Journal of Biophysical and Biochemical Cytology*,10: 425-435

Chen, T., Farragher, S., Bjourson, A.J., Orr, D.F. and Shaw, C., 2003. Granular gland transcriptomes in stimulated amphibian skin secretion. *Biochem. J.*, 371: 125-130.

Choi,B.T., Moon, D.Y., Choi, Y.H. and Jo, U.B., 1997. Seasonal variation in integument glycoconjugates of *Rana rugosa. Ant. Record*, 249: 24-31.

Clarke, B.T., 1997.The natural history of amphibian skin secretions, their normal functioning and potential medical applications. *Biological Review*, 72(3): 365 – 379.

Conaway, C.H. and Metter, D.E., 1967. Skin glands associated with breeding in *Microhyla carlinensis. Copeia*, 672-673.

Concaicao, K., Konno, K., Richardson, M., Antoniazzi, M.M., Jared, C., Daffre, S., Camargo, A.C. and Pimenta, D.C., 2006. Isolation and biochemical characterization of peptides presenting antimicrobial activity from the skin of *Phyllomedusa hypochondrialis. Peptides*, 27: 3092-3099.

Conlon, J.M., Al-Ghaferi, N., Abraham, B. and Leprince, J., 2007. Strategies for transformation of naturally-occurring amphibian antimicrobial peptides into therapeutically valuable anti-infective agents. *Methods*, 42: 349-357.

Conlon, J.M., Bevier, C.R., Coquet, L., Leprince, J., Jouenne and Vaudry, H., 2007. Peptidomic analysis of skin secretions supports separate species status for the tailed frog, *Ascaphus truei* and *Ascaphus montanus*. *Comp. Biochem. Physiol.*, 2D: 121-125.

Conlon, J.M., Demandt, A., Nielsen, P.F., Leprince, J. and Vaudry, H., 2009. The alyteserins: two families of antimicrobial peptides from the skin secretions of the midwife toad *Alytes obstericans* (Alytedae). *Peptides*, 30: 1069-1073.

Conlon, J.M., Kolodziejek, J. and Nowotny, N., 2004. Antimicrobial peptides from ranid frogs: taxonomic and phylogenetic markers and a potential source of new therapeutic agents. *Biochim. Biophys. Acta.*, 1696: 1-14.

Conlon, J.M., Sonnevend, A., Davidson, C., Demandt, A. and Jouenne, T., 2005. Host defence peptides isolated from the skin secretions of the Northern red-legged frog *Rana aurora aurora*. *Developmental and Comparative Immunology*, 29: 83-90.

Conlon, J.M., Woodhams, D.C., Raza, H., Coquet, L., Leprince, J., Jouenne, T., Vaudry, H. and Rollins-Smith, L.A., 2007. Peptides with differential cytolytic activity from skin secretion of the lemur leaf frog *Hylomantis lemur* (Hylidae: Phyllomedusinae). *Toxicon*, pp.1-9.

Croce, G., Gigliolo, N. and Bolognani, L., 1973. Antimicrobial activity in the skin secretions of *Bombina variedata* pachypus. *Toxicon*, 11: 99-100.

Damien, V., Francine, B., Pierre, N. and Mohamed, A., 2003. Antimicrobial peptides from hylid and ranin frogs originated from a 150-million-years old ancestral precursor with a conserved signal peptide but a hypermutable antimicrobial domain. *European Journal of Biochemistry*, 270 (9): 2068-2081.

Daly, J.W., Myers, C.W. and Whittaker, N., 1987. Further classification of skin alkaloids from neotropical poison frogs (Dendrobatidae), with a general survey of toxic/noxious substances in the amphibian. *Toxicon*, 25: 1023-1095.

Danguy, A. and Genten, F., 1989: Comparative lectin-binding affinity in the epidermis and dermal glands of *Bufo bufo* and *Xenpus laevis*. *Biol. Struct. Morphol.*, 2: 94-101.

Davidson, C., Benard, M.F., Shaffer, H.B., Parker, J.M., O'Leary, C., Conlon, J.M. and Rollins-Smith, L.A., 2007. Effects of chytrid and carbaryl exposure on survival growth and skin peptide defenses in foothill yellow-legged frogs. *Environ. Sci. Technol.*, 41: 1771.

Delfino, G., Brizzi, R. and Calloni, C., 1987. Differentiation of myoepithelial cells during the development of cutaneous serous glands in Anura. *Zoologische Anzeiger*, 218: 219-236.

Delfino, G., Brizzi, R. and Feri, L., 1995. Chemical skin defense in *Bufo bufo*: an ultrastructural study during ontogenesis. *Zool. Anz.*, 234: 101-111.

Delfino, G., Brizzi, R. and Kracke-Berndorff, Alvarez, B., 1998. Serous gland dimorphism, in the skin of *Melanophryniscus stelzneri* (Anura: Bufonidae). *J.Morphol.*, 237: 19-32.

Delfino, G., Brizzi, R., Alvarez, B.B. and Gentili, M., 1999. Granular cutaneous glands in the frog *Physalaemus biligonigerus* (Anura, Leptodactylidae): comparison between ordinary serous and 'inguinal' glands. *Tissue and Cell*, 31(6): 576-586.

Denefle, J.P. and Lechair, J.P., 1990. Pigment cell localization in anuran ventral skin at climatic metamorphosis. *American Journal of Anatomy*, 192(1): 89-95.

de Almeida, P.G., Felsemburgh, F.A., Azevedo, R.A. and de Brito-Gitirana, L., 2007. Morphological re-evaluation of the parotoid glands of *Bufo ictericus* (Amphibia, Anura, Bufonids). *Contribution to Zoology*, 76 (3): 145-152.

de Brito-Gitirana, L. and Azevedo, R.A., 2005. Morphology of *Bufo ictericus* integument (Amphibia, Bufonidae). *Micron*, 36 (6): 532-538.

de Brito Gitirana, L., Azevedo, R.A. and Pelli A.A., 2007. Expression pattern of glycoconjugates in the integument of *Bufo ictericus* (Anuran, Bufonidae): Biochemical and histochemical (lectins) profiles. *Tissue Cell*.

De Lima, C.G., Pastore, T.C., Schwartz, C.A., Cruz, J.S. and Sebben, A., 1991. Utilization of O-phthaladehyde-sulphuric acid as a spray reagent in thin- layer chromatographic detection of some indole alkylamines and application to cutaneous secretion extracts of toad species. *Talanta,* 38 (11): 1303-7.

de Lucas, I.M.S., Giarett, A.A., alberto-Rincon, M.C. and Bechara, I.J., 1996. Morphological study of the sexually dimorphic inguinal gland of *Cycloramphus dubius* (Amphibia, Anura, Leptodactylidae). *Braz. J.Morphol. Sci.,* 13 (1): 19-24.

Dube, P., 2002. Eco-biological Studies of Amphibians around South-Eastern Plateau of Rajastan, Ph.D. thesis, M.D.S. University, Ajmer, India.

Duda, T.F. Jr., Vanhoye, D. and Nicolas, P., 2002. *Mol. Biol. Evol.,* 19 (6): 858-864.

Duellman, W.R. and Trueb, L., 1994. *Biology of amphibians.* Johns Hopkins University Press, Baltimore and London, pp.367-531.

Dyrkacz, S., 1981. Recent incidences of albinism in North American amphibians and reptiles. *Herpetol. Circ.,* 11: 1-31.

Eberth, C.J., 1866. Zur Entwicklung der Gewebe im Schwanze der Froschlarven. *Arch. Mikr. Anat.,* 2: 490.

Elias, H. and Shapiro, J., 1957. Histology of the Skin of Some Toads and Frogs. *Amer.Mus.Movit.,* 1819: 1-27.

Elkan, E., 1968. Mucopolysaccarides in anuran defense against desiccation. *J. Zool.,* 155: 19-53.

Ellinger, M.S., 1980. Genetic and experimental studies on a pigment mutation, "pale" (P_a), in the frog, *Bombina orientalis. J. Embryol. Exp. Morph.,* 56: 125-137.

Ernst, V.V., 1973a. The digital pads of the treefrog *Hyla cinerea.* I. The epidermis. *Tissue and Cell,* 5: 83-96.

Ernst, V.V., 1973b. The digital pads of the treefrog *Hyla cinerea.* II. The mucous glands. *Tissue and Cell,* 5: 97-104.

Erspamer, V., 1971. Biogenic amines and active polypeptides of the amphibian skin. *Ann. Rev. Pharmacol.,* 11: 327-350.

Erspamer, V., 1994. Bioactive secretions of the amphibian integument. In: *Amphibian Biology,* (Eds.) G. Heatwole,

T. Barthalmus and A.Y. Heatwole. Surrey Beatty and Sons, Chipping Norton, p. 178-350.

Farquhar, M.G. and Palade, G.E., 1965. Cell junction in amphibian skin. *J. Cell Biol.*, 26: 263-291.

Faszewski, E.E. and Kaltenbach, J.C., 1995. Histology and lectin-binding patterns in the skin of the terrestrial horned frog Ceratophrys ornate. *Cell Tissue Res.*, 281: 169-177.

Felsemburg, F.A., Carvalho-e-Silva, S.P. and de Brito-Gitirana, L., 2006. Morphological characterization of the anuran integument of the Proceratophrys and Odontophrynus genera (Amphibia, Anura, Leptodactylidae). *Micron*, 38(5): 439-445.

Fitch, H.S., 1956. A field study of the Kanas and eating frog, *Gastrophryne olivacea*. University of Kanas publications, *Museum of Natural History*, 8: 275-306.

Forbes, M.S., Zaccaria, R.A., Dent, J.N., 1973. Developmental cytology of chromatophores in the red-spotted newt. *Amer. J. Anat.*, 138: 37-72.

Fox, H., 1983. The skin of Ichthyophis (Amphibia: Caecilia): An ultrastructural study. *J. Zool.*, 199: 223-248.

Fox, H., 1985. Changes in amphibian skin during larval development and metamorphosis. In: *Metamorphosis: A Problem in Developmental Biology*, (Eds.) M. Balls and M. Bowers. Springer, New York, p. 59-110.

Fox, H., 1986a. Epidermis. In: *Biology of the Integument Vol. 2: Vertebrates*, (Eds.) J. Bereiter-Hahn, A.G. Matoltsy and K.S. Richards. Springer-Verlag, Berlin/New York, pp. 78-110.

Fox, H., 1986b. Epidermis. In: *Biology of the Integument Vol. 2: Vertebrates*, (Eds.) J. Bereiter-Hahn, A.G. Matoltsy and K.S. Richards. Springer-Verlag, Berlin/New York, pp. 111-149.

Frost, D.R., 2008. "Amphibian species of the world 5.2, an online reference," American Museum of Natural History, New York, NY, USA, http: / /research.amnh.org/herpetology/amphibia/ index.php.

Frost, S.K. and Robinson, S.J., 1984. Pigment cell differentiation in the fire-bellied toad, *Bombina orientalis* I, structural chemical and physical aspects of the adult pigment pattern. *J. Morph.*, 179: 229-242.

Frost, 2003. Search the amphibian species of the word V2.21. Database (http: //research.amnh.org/cgibin/herpetology/amphibia?recordid=CQXUTEOHIKQDUE...), accessed on 8/9/03.

Garg, A.D., Kanitker, D.V., Hippargi, R.V. and Gandhare, A.N., 2007. Antimicrobial activity of skin secretions isolated from Indian toad, *Bufo melanostictus* Schneider 1799. *Nature Proceedings*: doi: 10.1038/npre.2007.1204.1.

Goncalves, V.F. and de Brito-Gitirana, L., 2008. Structure of the sexually dimorphic gland of *Cycloramphus fuliginosus* (Amphibia, Anura, Cycloramphidae). *Micron.*, 39: 32-39.

Goniakowska-Witalinksa, L. and Kubiczek, U., 1998. The structure of the skin of the tree frog (*Hyla arborea arborea* L.). *Anat. Anz.*, 180: 237-246 (abstract).

Gomes, A., Giri, B., Saha, A., Mishra, R., Dasgupta, S.C., Debnath, A. and Gomes, A., 2007. Bioactive molecules from amphibian skin: Their biological activities with reference to therapeutic potential for possible drug development. *Indian Journal of Experimental Biology*, 45: 579-593.

Green, D.M., 1979. Treefrog toepads: comparative surface morphology using scanning electron microscopy. *Canadian J. Zool.*, 57: 2033-2046.

Green, D.M., 1981. Adhesion and the toe-pads of tree frogs. *Copeia*, 1981: 790-796.

Greven, H., Zanger, K. and Schwinger, G., 1995. Mechanical properties of the skin of *Xenopus laevis* (Anura, Amphibia). *J. Morphol.*, 224: 15-22.

Hancock, R.E., 2001. Cationic peptides: Effectors in innate immunity and novel antimicrobials. *Lancet Infect. Dis.*, 1: 156-164.

Holloway, W.R. and Dapson, R.W. 1971. Histochemistry of the integumentary secretion of the narrow-mouth toad, *Gastrophryne carolinensis*. *Copeia*, 1971: 351-353.

Houck, L.D., D.M. Sever, 1994. Role of the skin in reproduction and behaviour, p. 351-381. In: *Amphibian Biology, Vol. 1*, (Ed.) H.

Heatwole. Surrey Beatty and Sons, Chipping Norton, NSW, Australia.

Hutchinson, D.A. and Savitzky, A.H., 2004. Vasculature of the parotoid glands of four species of toads (bufonidae: bufo). *J. Morphol.*, 260(2): 247-254.

Imamura, A., Takeda, H. and Sasaki, N., 1965. The accumulation of sodium and calcium in a specific layer of frog skin. J. Cell. Comp. Physiol. 66 (2): 221-225.

Inger, R.I., 1954. Systematics and Zoogeography of Philippine Amphibia. *Fieldiana Zoology*, 33: 181-531.

Kaltenbach, J.C., Harding, C.V. and Susan, S., 1980. Surface ultrastructure of the cornea and adjacent epidermis during metamorphosis of *Rana pipiens*: a scanning electron microscopic study. *J. Morphol.*, 166: 325-335.

Kierszenbaum, A.L., 2002. *Histology and Cell Biology: An Introduction to Pathology*. Mosby, St. Louis, Missouri, p. 55.

Kierszenbaum, A.L., 2004. *Histology and Cell Biology: An Introduction to Pathology*. Mosby Press, New York, p .536.

Kikuyama, S., Nakano, R. and Yasumasu, I. 1975. Synergist action of prolactin and androgen on the cloacal glands of the newt. *Comp. Biochem. Physiol. A.*, 51: 823-826.

Kossi, J., Vaha-Krula, M., Peltonen, J., Risteli, J. and Laato, M., 2004. Hexose sugars differentially alter collagen gene expression and synthesis in fibroblast derived from granulation tissue, hypertrophic scar andkeloid. *Arch. Dermatol. Res.*, 295 (12): 521-526.

Leite, J.R., Silva, L.P., Rodrigues, M.I., Prates, M.V., Brand, G.D., Lacava, B.M., Azevedo, R.B., Bocca, A.L., Albuquerque, S. and Bloch Jr., C., 2005. Phylloseptins: a novel class of antibacterial and anti-protozoan peptides from the Phyllomedusa genus. *Peptides*, 26: 565-573.

Lenzi-Mattos, R., Antoniazzi, M.M., Haddad, C.F.B., Tambourgi, D.V., Rodrigues, M.T. and Pared, C., 1995. The inguinal macroglands of the frog Physalaemus nattereri (Leptodactylidae): Structure, toxic secretion and relationship with deimatic behaviour. *J. Zool. Lond.*, 266: 385-394.

Le Quang Trong, Y., 1966. Histogenese et histochimie des glandes cutanees de l'Axolotl (*Ambystoma tigrinum* Green). *Arch. Zool. Exp. Gen.*, 108: 49-73.

Le Quang Trong, Y., 1967. Structure et developpement de la peau et des glandes cutanees de *Nectophrynoides occidentalis* Angel. *Arch. Zool. Exp. Gen.*, 108: 589-610.

Le Quang Trong, Y., 1974. Etude de la peau et des glands cutanees de *Xenopus tropicalis*. *Bull. I.F.A.N.*, 36 Ser. A, 407-426.

Lillywhite, H.B., Mittal, A.K., Garg, T.K. and Agrawal, N., 1997. Integumentary structure and its relationship to wiping behaviour in the common Indian tree frog, Polypedates maculates. *J. Zool.*, 243: 675-687.

Low, B.S., 1972. "Evidence from parotoid-gland secretions". In: *Evolution in the Genus Bufo*, (Eds.) W.F. Blair. Austin: Univ. Texas Press, pp. 244-264.

Lynch, J.D. 1971. Evolutionary Relationship, Osteology and Zoogeography of Leptodactyloid Frogs. University of Kansas Printing Service, Lawrence, pp. 130-135.

Macfoy, C., Danosus, D., Sandit, R., Jones, T. H., Garraffo, H. M., Spande, T. F., Daly, J. W.., 2005. Alkaloids of Anuran Skin: Antimicrobial Function. *Z. Naturforsch.*, 60c: 932–937.

Maciel, N.M., Schwartz, C.A., Pires Junior, O.R., Sebben, A., Castro, M.S., Sousa, M.V., Fontes, W. and Schwartz, E.N.F.., 2003. Composition of indolealkylamines of *Bufo rubescens* cutaneous secretions compared to six other Brazilian bufonids with Phylogenetic implications. *Comparative Biology and Physiology* Part B, 134: 641-649.

Mangoni, M.L., Marcellini, H.G. and Simmaco, M., 2007. Biological characterization and modes of action of temporins and bombinins H, multiple forms of short and mildly cationic anti-microbial and mildly cationic anti-microbial peptides from amphibian skin. *J. Pept. Sci.*, 13: 603-613.

Martenson, R.E., Deibler, E. and Kramer, A.J., 1974. The presence of cysteine in frog myelin basic protein. *Journal of Neurochemistry*, 24(5): 959-962, published 2006.

Matutte, B., Storey, K.B., Knoop, F.C., Conlon, J.M., 2000. *FEBs Lett.*, 483(2-3): 135-138.

Mignogna, G., Simmaco, M., Kreil, G. and Barra, D., 1993. Antibacterial and hemolytic peptides containing D-alloisoleusine from the skin of Bombina variegate. *EMBO J.*, 12: 4829-4832.

Mills, J.W., Prum, B.E., 1984. Morphology of the exocrine glands of the frog skin. *Am. J. Anat.*, 171: 91-106.

Mollay, C., Wechselberger, C., Mignogna, G., Negri, L., Melchiorri, P., Barra, D. and Kreil, G., 1998. Bv8, a small protein from frog skin and its homologue from snake venom induce hyperalgesia in rats. *European Journal of Pharmacology*, 374(2): 189-196.

Mor, A., Nicolas, P., 1994a. Isolation and structure of novel defensive paptides from frog skin. *Eur. J. Biochem*. 219: 145-154.

Muhse, E.F., 1909. The cutaneous glands of the common toads. *Amer. J .Anat.*, 9: 321-359.

Myers, C.W., Daly, J.W. and Malkin, B. 1978. A dangerously toxic new frog (phyllobates) used by Embera Indians of Western Colombia, with discussion of flowgun fabrication and dart poisoning. *Bull. Amer. Mus. Nat. Hist.*, 161: 307-366.

Nicolas, P., Amiche, M., 2006. The Dermaseptins. In: *Handbook of Biologically Active Peptides*, (Ed.) A.J. Kastin. Elesvier, San Diego, pp. 295-304.

Nielsen, H.I. 1978a. Ultrastructural changes in the dermal chromatophore unit of *Hyla arborea* during color change. *Cell Tissue Res.*, 194: 405-418.

Odierna, G., Andreone, F., Aprea,G., Arribas, O., Capriglione, T., Vences, M., 2000. Cytological and molecular analysis in the rare discoglossid species, *Alytes muletensis*. *Chromosome Res.*, 8: 435-42.

Parakkal, P.F., Matoltsy, A.G. 1964. Study of the fine structure of the epidermis of *Rana pipiens*. *J. Cell Biol.*, 20: 85-94.

Park, J.S. 1974. Histochemical study of the mucous gland of the frog (*Rana nigromaculata*) skin under dry conditions. *Korean J. Zool.*, 17, 43-50.

Pasteur, G., 1982. A classificatory review of mimicry systems. *Annual Review of Ecology and Systematics*, 13: 169-199.

Poynton, J.C., 1964. The Amphibia of Southern Africa. *Annals of the Natal Museum*, 17: 1-334.

Porter, K.R., 1972. *Herpetology*. V.B. Saunders Company, United States of America: 18-25.

Porto, J.., 1936. Contribution al studio de la Histofisiologia de tegumento de los Batrachios. La Prensa Argentina August, 1964-1971.

Pough, F.H., Andrews, R.M., Cadle, J.E., Crump, M.L., Savitzky, A.H. and Wells, K.D., 2003. *Herpetology*. New Jersey, Prentice Hall, p. 158-159.

Qar, J. and Al-Adhami, M.A., 2003. A histological study of the flank skin in the larval green toad, *Bufo viridis viridis* Laurenti. Dirasat. *Pure Science*, 30: 108-117.

Quay, W.B. 1972. Integument and the Environment: glandular composition, function, and evolution. *Am. Zoologist*, 12: 95-108.

Rabl, 1931. Integument der Anamnier. In: L.E. Bolk, E.Goppert, E. Kallius and W. Lubosch (eds), *Handbuch der Vergleichenden Anatomie der Wirbeltiere, Vol. I*, Berlin, pp 271-374.

Reichel, P., 2006. Differentiation of the opercular integument in *Rana pipiens*. *J. Differentiation*, 5(2-3): 75-83.

Richards, C.M., 1982. Toche alteration of chromatophore expression by sex hormones in the Kenyan reed frog, *Hyperolius viridiflavus*. *Gen. Comp. Endocrinol.*, 46: 59-67.

Rollins Smith, L.A., King, J.D., Neilsen, P.F., Sonnevend, A. and Conlon, J.M., 2005. An antimicrobial peptide from the skin secretion of mountain chicken frog *Leptodactylus fallax* (Anura: Leptodactylidae). *Regulatory Peptides*, 124(1-3): 173-178.

Rosenberg, M. and Warburg, M.R., 1992. Ultrastructure and Histochemistry of ventral epidermis in *Pelobates syriacus* (Anura: Pelobatidae) tadpoles. *Biol. Struct. Morphogen.*, 4: 164-170.

Rosenberg, M. and Warburg, M.R., 1995. Changes in structure and function of ventral skin in *Hyla arborea savignyi* Aud. (Anura; Hylidae). *Acta Zool.*, 76: 217-227.

Rudneff, M. 1865. Ueber die epidermoidale Schicht der Froschhaut. *Arch. Mikr. Anat.*, 1: 295.

Saguchi, S., 1913. Ueber Mitochondrien (Chondriokonten) und mitochondriale strange (sag. Eberthsche intrazellulare Gebilde) in den Epidermiszellen der Anurenlarven nebst Bemerkungen uber die Frage der Epidermis-Cutisgrenze. *Arch. Mikr. Anat.*, 83: 177.

Sakate, M., Lucas de Oliveira, P.C., 2000. Toad envenoming in dogs: effects and treatment. *Journal of Venom Animal Toxins*, 6: 46-58.

Sampson, H.W., Cannon, M.J. and Davis, R.W., 1987. The calcified amorphous layer of the skin of *Bufo marinus* (Amphibia: Anura). *J.Zool. Lond.*, 213: 63-69.

Sazima, I. and Caramaschi, U., 1986. Descricao de *Physalaemus deimaticus*, sp. N., e observacaoes sobre comportamento deimatico em *P. nattereri* (Steidn.)-Anura, Leptodactylidae. *Rev. Biol.*, 13 (1): 91-101.

Schwartz, E.F., Stucchi-Zucchi, A., Schwartz, C.A. and Salomao, L.C., 2003. Skin secretion of *Siphonops paulensis* (Gymnophiona, Amphibia) forms voltage-dependent ionic channels in lipid membranes. *Brazilian Journal of Medical and Biology Research*, 36 (9): 1279-1282.

Schwinger, G., Zanger, K. and Greven, H., 2001. Structural and mechanical aspects of the skin of *Bufo marinus* (Anura, Amphibia).*Tissue Cell.*, 33 (5): 541-547.

Siegel, D.S., Sever, D.M., Schriever, T.A. and Chabarria, R.E., 2008. Ultrastructure and Histochemistry of the adhesive breeding glands in male *Gastrophryne carolinensis* (Amphibia: Anura: Microhylidae). *Copeia*, 4: 877-881.

Simmaco, M., Boman, A., Mangoni, M.L., Mignogna, G., Miele, R., Barra,D. and Boman, H.G., 1997. Effect of glucocorticoids on the synthesis of antimicrobial peptides in amphibian skin. PMID: 9373168, 416(3): 273-5 [PubMed–indexed for MEDLINE].

Simon Pitman, 2008. Frog skin adds to growing list of animal-based anti-aging solutions; Formulation and Science, skincare. cosmeticsdesigneurope.com.

Speidel, C.C., 1926. Studies of hyperthyroidism. IV. The behaviour of the epidermal mitochondria and the pigment in frog tadpoles under conditions of thyroid-accelerated metamorphosis and of regeneration following wound infliction. *J. Morphol. and Physiol.*, 43: 57.

Taylor, E.H., 1920. Philippine Amphibia. *Philippine Journal of Science*, 16: 213-359.

Taylor, J.D., 1969. The effects of intermedin on the ultrastructure of amphibian iridophores. *Gen. Comp. Endocrinol.*, 12: 405-416.

Toledo, L.F. and Haddad, C.F.B., 2009. Review Article-Colors and Some Morphological Traits as Defensive Mechanisms in Anurans. *International Journal of Zoology*, 1-12.

Toledo, R.C. and Jared, C., 1993. Cutaneous adaptation to water balance in amphibians. *Comp. Biochem. Physiol.*, 105A: 593-608.

Toledo, R.C. and Jared, C., 1995. Cutaneous granular glands and amphibian venoms. *Comparative Biochemistry and Physiology*, 111A: 1-29.

Toledo, R.C., Jared, C. and Brunner, Jr. A., 1992. Morphology of the large granular alveoli of the parotoid glands in toad (*Bufo ictericus*) before and after compression. *Toxicon*, 30: 745-753.

Vanhoye, D., Bruston, F., Nicolas, P. and Amiche, M., 2003. Antimicrobial peptides from hylid and ranid frogs originated from a 150-million-years old ancestral precursor antimicrobial domain. *Eur. J. Biochem.* 270: 2068-2081.

Verma, M.N., 1969. Hydrobiological study of tropical impoundment, Tekampur.Reservoir, Gwalior, India, with special reference to the breeding of Indian carps. *Hydrobiol.*, 34: 358.

Villalba, J.M., Roldan, J.M. and Navas, P., 1993. Flask cells and flask-shaped glandular cells of amphibian skin specially produce fucose-rich glycoproteins. *Histochemistry*, 99 (5): 363-367.

Visser, J.J., Cei, J.M. and Gutierrez, L.S., 1982. The histology of dermal glands of mating Breviceps with comments on their possible functional value in microhylids (Amphibia: Anura). *South African Journal of Zoology*, 17: 24-27.

Vizotto, L.D., 1964. Observacoes preliminaries sobre glandulas inguinais de *Eupemphix nattereri* Steindachner (Amphibia, Salienta). *Cienc. Cult.*, 16: 168.

Warburg, M. R., Lewinson, D. and Rosenberg, M., 1994. Ontogenesis of amphibian epidermis. (In: Ontogenesis of Amphibian

Epidermis. H. Heatwole and G.T. Barthalmus eds, vol.1. The integument Surry Beatty and Sons. Chipping Norton Press, Sydney): 33-63.

Warburg, M.R. and Rosenberg, M., 1997. Ultrastructure of ventral epidermis in the terrestrial and aquatic phases of the newt *Triturus vittatus* (Jenyns). *Anat. Anz.*, 179: 341-347 (Abstract).

Warburgh, M.R., Rosenberg, M., Roberts, J.R. and Heatwole, H., 2000. Cutaneous glands in the Australian hylid *Litoria caerulea* (Amphibia, Hylidae). *Anat. Embryol.*, 201: 341-348.

Wechselberger, C., 1998. Cloning of cDNAs encoding new peptides of the dermaseptin family. *Biochem. Biophys. Acta.*, 1388: 279-283.

Weed, I.G., 1934. Cytological studies of the epidermis of *Rana Clamitans* tadpoles, with special reference to the figures of Eberth. *J. Morphol.*, 56: 213.

Weiss, L. and Greep, R.O. 1977. *Histology*. United States of American: McGraw-Hill Book Company: 140-144.

Willumsen, N.J., Amstrup, J.,Mobjerg, N., Jespersen, A., Kristensen, P. and Larsen, E.H., 2002. Mitochondria-rich cells as experimental model in studies of epithelial chloride channels. *Biochem. Biophys. Acta.*, 1566(1-2): 28-43.

Young, J.Z., 1985. *La vida de los vertebrados*. Ediciones Omega S.A. Barcelona.

Chapter 10

Human-Plants Interaction: A Case Study on Useful Plants of Dasigo Tribe from Mamberamo, Papua, Indonesia

Agustina Y.S. Arobaya[1]* and Freddy Pattiselanno[2]**

[1]Herbarium Manokwariense,
Biodiversity Research Centre,
University Negeri Papua, Manokurai, Indonesia
[2]Sub-laboratory,
Livestock and Wildlife Breeding–Animal Production Department,
Faculty of Animal Science,
Fishery and Marine Sciences (FPPK), Papua State University, Indonesia

ABSTRACT

Forests paly an important role in human life. It has been shown through the biodiversity richness that particularly specific plants have been ackowledeged as urgent resources by the local communities in past and the present as well. This chapter is aimed to compile the observations on ethnobotany aspects from the Dasigo ethnic group in Mamberamo, Papua. The results indicated about 40 plant species utilized by Dasigo tribe

E-mail: *agustinaarobaya@yahoo.com.au; **pattiselannofreddy@yahoo.com for daily need such as construction, food and beverage, fuel wood, traditional ornament and others.

Keywords: *Ethnobotany, Useful plants, Dasigo tribe, Mamberamo.*

Introduction

Study on biological and other natural resources have been conducted in Mamberamo to provide baseline information on development of this area as part of the Sarmi Regency. Collaboration survey between Pemda Kabupaten Sarmi and Universitas Negeri Papua was carried out to perform Natural Resources Mapping.

Three major tribes namely Dasigo and Airo – local people from Dabra and Dani – a migrant tribe from Jayawijaya regency occupied the site. Like any other forest-dwelling people, local communities of Dabra is closely integrated to the forest, and linked to the biodiversity of their forest environment. The interrelationship with the ecosystem is expressed on the traditional use of forest resources for multipurpose reasons. The form of interaction between human and environment clearly was depicted by the utilization of particular flora and fauna species by this ethnic group for numerous household needs. Sastrapradja and Rivai (1972) indicated in Indonesia 4.000 plant species that are currently directly utilized by people and approximately ¼ of them was cultivated.

The present chapter aims to compile observation on ethnobotany aspects of the Dasigo ethnic group at the Mamberamo, Papua, particularly focusing on the local condition and traditional knowledge of plant resource utilization.

Material and Methods

Survey was achieved from 4–28 September 2004 in the Dabra (03°16'S 138°36'E), Taiyeve (03°14.06'S 138°26.62'E) and Fokri-Baso (03°05.08'S 138°50.12'E) villages of the Mamberamo Hulu District of Kabupaten Sarmi, Papua. Dabra as the capital city of the Mamberamo Hulu was about 121 mile distance from Jayapura. It would be reached in an hour trip with an aircraft from Sentani Airport Jayapura.

The village of Dabra at the Mamberamo Hulu was the tropical rain forest, geographically remote with low human population level and lesser human impact on natural resources utilization. Polhemus and Richards (2002) described Dabra at the present time as reflected by the forest types and their associated aquatic habitats.

Information on ethnobotany aspect concerning the relationship between people and forest was obtained by the semi-structured interview by interviewing primary informants – villagers (chosen randomized among local people in the study site) and the key informants including highly respected and high status people within the villages, village leaders, tribe leaders, church leaders, highly educated people and the government officers. Direct observation to the plantation area around the study site to observe particular species growth and used by local people was also conducted to cross check the interview results. Supporting data was tracked trough secondary data by review of supplemented literature from previous study. Herbaria specimens were collected to identify anonymous plant species observed in the field. Identification was done in the Manokwariense Herbarium to complete checklist specimen found during the survey in Mamberamo.

The study site is lowland swampy area surrounded by primary rainforest along the Mamberamo river basin. Vegetation found in this area is much more varied, ranging from tall, mixed species forest near river to low, open canopy forest of mixed Pandanus species herbaceous swamp dominated by sedges, ridges and floating grasses. The climate is tropically dry from May to September signed by the period of crocodile hunting, followed by rainy season with the average of annually rainfall range from 180mm to 560mm. Daily temperature ranged from 29-32oC and relative humidity about 7 per cent and 80 per cent (Pattiselanno, 2003).

Results and Discussion

Nine species have been identified as construction material (house and fence), whereas two among those species have also been utilized as fuel wood. Particular species were commonly utilized for building material distributed fairly among the Papua region acknowledged as high quality wood (*Octomeles sumatrana, Terminalia complanata, Podocarpus blumei* and *Intsia bijuga*). The study of Arobaya and Pattiselanno (2007), Peday (2004) indicated seven species around the highland site of Baliem Valey utilized by the Dani ethnic group such as *Podocarpus papuana* (inside wall pannel) while the outside part constructed from *Araucaria cunninghamii*, *Paraserianthes* and other hardwood species that specifically found at the upland site. While people along the coastal site using mangrove species (*Sonneratia alba* and *Xeriops tagal*) for housing construction and fuel wood (Aibekob *et al.*, 2002; Mamoribo *et al.*, 2003).

Table 10.1: List of Useful Plants for Dasigo Tribe in Mamberamo

Family	*Species*	*Utilization*
Acanthaceae	*Abelmochus manihot* (L) Medik.	Vegetable
Acanthaceae	*Gendarusa vulgaris* Ness	Ornamental
Anacardiceae	*Dracontomellon edule*	Construction material
Arecaceae	*Arenga* sp.	Rope for binding fence
Arecaceae	*Areca catechu* Linn	Edible fruit
Arecaceae	*Calamus* sp.	String for fasten trap
Arecaceae	*Colocasia esculenta* (L) Schott.	Edible fruit
Arecaceae	*Metroxylon sago* Rottb.	Traditional food
Arecaceae	*Cocos nucifera* L.	Edible fruit, dry branch for fuel wood
Arecaceae	*Caladium bicolor* (W.Ait) Vent.	Ornamental
Arecaceae	*Xanthosoma sagittifolium* Schott.	Edible fruit
Brommeliaceae	*Ananas comoscus* (L). Merr.	Edible fruit
Burseraceae	*Canarium acutifolium* (DC). Merrr	Edible fruit
Caricaceae	*Carica papaya* L.	Vegetable, edible fruit
Combretaceae	*Terminalia complanata*	Construction material
Datiscaceae	*Octomeles sumtrana*	Construction material
Euphorbiaceae	*Antidesma montanum* Bl.	Garden fence, fuel wood
Euphorbiaceae	*Macaranga mappa* M.A.	Leaves for wrapping, fire wood
Euphorbiaceae	*Jatropha curcas* L.	Ornamental
Euphorbiaceae	*Codiaeum variagetum* (L.) Bl.	Ornamental
Fabaceae	*Intsia bijuga*	Construction material
Fabaceae	*Pterocarpus indicus*	Construction material
Gnetaceae	*Gnetum gnemon* L.	Vegetable
Lauraceae	*Cinnamomum culilavan* Bl.	Oil extract from bark
Lauraceae	*Cryptoria massoy* (Oken.) Kosterm.	

Contd...

Table 10.1--Contd...

Family	*Species*	*Utilization*
Maranthaceae	*Phacelophyrnium maximum* (Bl.) K. Schum	Roof construction
Meliaceae	*Aglaia sapindina* (F. and M.) Harms	Fuel wood
Moraceae	*Artocarpus communis* Forst.	Vegetable food
Moraceae	*Artocarpus integer* (Thunb.) Merr	Fruit
Moracea	*Ficus* sp.	Fuel wood
Moraceae	*Paratocarpus venosis* Becc.	Kitchen utensils
Musaceae	*Musa* spp	Fruit
Myrtaceae	*Psydium guajava* L.	Fruit
Nyctaginaceae	*Bougainvillea spectabilis* Wild.	Ornamental
Piperaceae	*Piper betle* L.	Chewing plants
Poaceae	*Zea mays* L.	Food
Podocarpaceae	*Podocarpus blumei*	Construction material
Rubiaceae	*Coffea robusta* Linden	Beverage
Rubiaceae	*Gardenia jasminoides* Ellis	Ornamental
Rubiaceae	*Morinda citrifolia* L.	Fruit medicinal
Rutaceae	*Citrus nobilis* Lour.	Fruit
Sapindaceae	*Pometia pinnata* J.R. and G. Frost	Fruit
Sterculiaceae	*Sterculia* sp.	Garden fence, fuel wood
Sterculiaceae	*Theobroma cacao* L.	Fruit, beverage
Verbanaceae	*Duranta erecta* L.	Ornamental
Zingiberaceae	*Alpinia galangal* (L.) Swartz	Spice, Medicinal
Zingeberaceae	*Curcuma domestica* Sw.	Food, spice
Zingiberaceae	*Zingiber officinalis* Rosc.	Spice, medicinal

Certain part of species that mostly used for construction (branch and small stem) can also be used for fuel wood. In this study we only noted four species that have been using for fuel wood. Fruit and leaves of two among four species recognized earlier, were also used for other purposes (food and wrap material). Differently, people in West Timor utilized approximately 21 species of plants as fuel wood sources (Pulunggono 1999).

Nineteen species have been consumed as edible fruit, vegetable and traditional food as well by the tribe. Some species were commonly used in Indonesia such as banana, cacao, citrus, pineapple, papaya and coconut, while others were locally consumed and utilized by certain ethnic group occupied the eastern part of Indonesia. For example, Colocasia, Xanthosoma, sago, canary, beetle nut and piper. Tuber crops were acknowledged as carbohydrate resources and according to Sastrapradja and Rifai (1989) in undeveloped and dry areas like in Nusa Tenggara and Maluku root of tuber crops utilized as food sources substituted by corn and sago.

Our findings is relatively similar to the study of Worabai, *et al.* (2001) that found twenty four plant species as food sources by Wondama tribe at Wasior. Uniquely, local communities in Biak and Inanwatan Papua particularly those who inhabited coastal sites, utilized mangrove (*Bruguiera gymnorhiza*) as carbohydrate sources for their household (Wanma, 2007; Prayitno *et al.*, 2002).

Rifai (1986) recognized around 329 fruit species including endemic and introduced species in Indonesia, and Uji (2007) compiled approximately 266 indigenous fruit species potency in Indonesia from various studies. In Gorontalo Province, Sunarti *et al.* (2007) recorded fifteen edible fruit consumed by local people around the Tangale Nature Reserve.

We recorded only three species used together as therapeutic items, spice and edible fruit as well. Arobaya and Pattiselanno (2007) have only noticed limited species used by Dani tribe at the Baliem Valley. Findings obtained from other studies in Papua evidenced that local communities were still dependent on medicinal product from particular forest sources (Hamzah *et al.*, 2003; Howay *et al.*, 2003; Suebu *et al.*, 2002). The use of medicinal plants in Indonesia is common such as in West Timor, Pulunggono (1999) recognized 22 plant species, and in North Sumatera it was relatively higher than West Timor (Simbolon, 1994).

Using plant for ornamental purpose was playing an important role among ethnic groups in Papua, because local people was dependently on local tradition and culture that require natural resources (plant and animals) for the traditional ritual and cultural ceremonies. During the survey, seven species have been identified using by the Dasigo for ornamental reason. Differently, people around the coastal site of the Bird's Head Area were more dependently on mangrove species (Leonard *et al.*, 2003). On the other hand, two palm species have been used commonly for culture and ritual activities by local community at the lowland forest of Bayeda Arguni Bay (Nega *et al.*, 2003).

In this survey, we also recognized three species used for spices and one species for beverage that widely used among other Indonesian ethnic groups. Other five species classified under other purposes usually use as rope, string, oil, utensils and chewing plants. Pinang (*Piper betle* L.) not only used by Dasigo, but also utilized by other ethnic groups in Papua as well.

References

Arobaya, A.Y.S and Pattiselanno, F., 2007. The useful plants of Dani Ethnic Group at the Baliem Valley of Papua. *Biota*, 12(3): 194-197.

Hamzah, P., Kesaulija, E.M. and dan Rahawarin, Y., 2003. Pemanfaatan Tumbuhan Obat Tradisional oleh Masyarakat Pulau Mansinam Kabupaten Manokwari. *Beccariana,* 5(2): 52-60.

Howay, M., Sinaga, N.I. and Kesaulija, E.M., 2003. Utilization of plants as traditional medicines by Maibrat Tribe in Sorong. *Beccariana,* 5 (1): 24-34.

Leonard, D., Wanggai, J. and Manusawai, J., 2003. The use of plants from mangrove forest by local people in Senebuay Village, District of Rumberpon Manokwari. *Beccariana,* 5(2): 97-108.

Mamoribo, S., Arwam, C.Y.H. and Yusuf, A., 2003. Utilization of mangrove by the community in Royori Kampong of South Supiori, Biak Numfor. *Beccariana,* 5 (1): 43-51.

Nega, L.B., Wasaraka, A.R. and Heatubun, C.D., 2003. Exploration of palm species in the lowland forest of Bayeda District, Arguni Bay. *Beccariana,* 5(2): 67-81.

Pattiselanno, F., 2003. Some fruit bats (Chiroptera, Pteropodiidae) of the Mamberamo River Basin, West Papua, Indonesia. *Asia Life Sciences,* 12 (1): 45-56.

Peday, H.F.Z., 2004. Analysis of vegetation of commercial trees in Ibele Village, District of Hubikosi Jayawijaya, the buffer zone of Lorentz National Park. *Beccariana,* 6: 33-39.

Polhemus, D.A and Richards, S., 2002. Geographic overview of Cyclops Mountains and the Mamberamo Basin, pp 32-37. *In:* Richards, S.J. and S. Suryadi (eds.). A biodiversity of Yongsu-Cyclops Mountains and the Southren Mamberamo Basin, Papua, Indonesia. RAP Buletin of Biological Assessment 25. Conservation International, Washington DC, USA.

Pulunggono, H.B., 1999. The ethnobotanical studies of people in Amarasi of Kupang, Mollo and Amanatun of South Central Timor, West Timor, Indonesia. *Media Konservasi,* 6: 27-38.

Prayitno, S.W.M., Manusawai, J. dan Witjaksono, W., 2002. Pemanfaatan Tumbuhan Mangrove bagi Kehidupan Masyarakat Suku Inanwatan di Kabupaten Sorong. *Beccariana,* 4(2): 79-92.

Rifai, M.A., 1986. Flora Buah-buahan Indonesia, Bogor. LBN-LIPI.

Sastrapradja, S.D. and M.A. Rifai. 1989. Mengenal sumber pngan nabati dan sumber plasma nutfahnya. Komisi Pelestarian Plasma Nutfah Nasional dan Puslitbang Bioteknologi, LIPI, Bogor.

Simbolon, H., 1994. Ethnobotany of people around the Dolok Sibuali-Buali Nature Reserve Area, North Sumatera, Indonesia. *Tropics,* 4: 69-78.

Suebu, J., Manusawai, J. and Ramandey, Y., 2002. Potensi Tumbuhan Berkasiat Obat pada Masyarakat Suku Wie-Khaya Kecamatan Arso Kabupaten Jayapura. *Beccariana,* 4(2): 68-78.

Sunarti, S., Rugayah, dan Djarwaningsih T., 2007. Tumbuhan berpotensi bahan pangan di daerah Cagar Alam Tangale. *Biodiversitas,* Vol. 8 (2): 88-91.

Uji, T., 2007. Keanekargaman jenis buah-buahan asli Indonesia dan potensinya. *Biodiversitas,* Vol. 8 (2): 154-164

Worabai, S., Kesaulija, E.M. dan Maturbongs, R.A., 2001. Pemanfaatan jenis tumbuhan pohon oleh suku Wondama di desa Tandia, Wasior Kabupaten Manokwari. *Beccariana,* 3(2): 19-30.

Chapter 11

Time Budget Activity Pattern of Behavioural Displays of Captive Axis Deer (*Axis axis*)

*Pradeep S. Khanpara and Kauresh D. Vachhrajani**
Division of Environment and Toxicology, Department of Zoology, Faculty of Science, The Maharaja Sayajirao University of Baroda, Vadodara – 390 002, Gujarat, India

ABSTRACT

In India, the ungulates in wild have been studied mostly in the tiger reserves, since they form the prey base for large carnivores. Studies so far have exhibited interest in the ungulate habitat, habitat utilization, density and distribution, social organization, group composition and dynamics, reproduction, ecology and conservation management etc. Several influences of wild are nonexistent in captivity and, therefore, general behavioural displays are different. In captivity, stress may be one of the factors resulting into disproportional display of certain behavioural patterns. Several studies have documented the behaviour of Axis deer (*Axis axis*, Chital or spotted deer, Schedule III of Wildlife Protection Act, India), mostly in wild; although, over a period of time the anthropogenic stress in various zoos has increased. Therefore, the behavioural patterns

* Corresponding author: E-mail: kauresh@gmail.com

of Axis deer were studies in Sakkarbaug Zoo, Junagadh, Gujarat, India to assess the influences of captivity on its behavioural displays.

The activities and displays were classified into three major categories as general behaviour patterns (feeding, rumination, resting, licking salt, short movement, long movement, running, territory marking and urination), reproductive behaviour patterns (smelling, flehming, scratch antler, rutting and conflict, chasing, mount and mating) and parental care behaviour patterns (suckling, licking fawn and playing with fawn). Each behavioural pattern was recorded for focal animal (one each male, female and fawn) at different times of the day and night for two years. Time spend on each activity mentioned herein was recorded and mean time invested per hour per day was calculated. Time budget activity (mean proportions of time spent active) was considered for noting behaviour displays and activities. Here time budget was considered for all the activities and therefore the data were recorded as actual time spent doing a particular activity (minutes per hour per day). In captivity, the high density of visitors during specific seasons at specified time of the day (morning and late noon to evening) is possibly the only major threat/disturbing activity to which the animals get acclimatized very soon and therefore, as compared to the responses in conditions of wild, the responses are almost absent in captivity. The behavioural displays are described in detail and the aspects of breeding biology in captivity are compared with observed in wild.

Keywords: *Axis axis, Breeding biology, Time budget activity, Captivity stress, Behaviour.*

Introduction

The ungulate diversity in India is represented by 2 orders, 7 families, 23 genera and 34 species. In India the ungulates are distributed in about 360 Protected Areas (Mathur *et al.*, 2001). Bibliographic survey of literature on Ungulates of Peninsular India contains references published between 1867 and 2005 where contributions of over 861 authors in fourteen subject categories have been indexed (Shankar and Goyal, 2004; Figure 11.1). Ungulates have been studied mostly in the tiger reserves, since they form the prey base for large carnivores (Schaller, 1967; Johnsingh and Shankar,

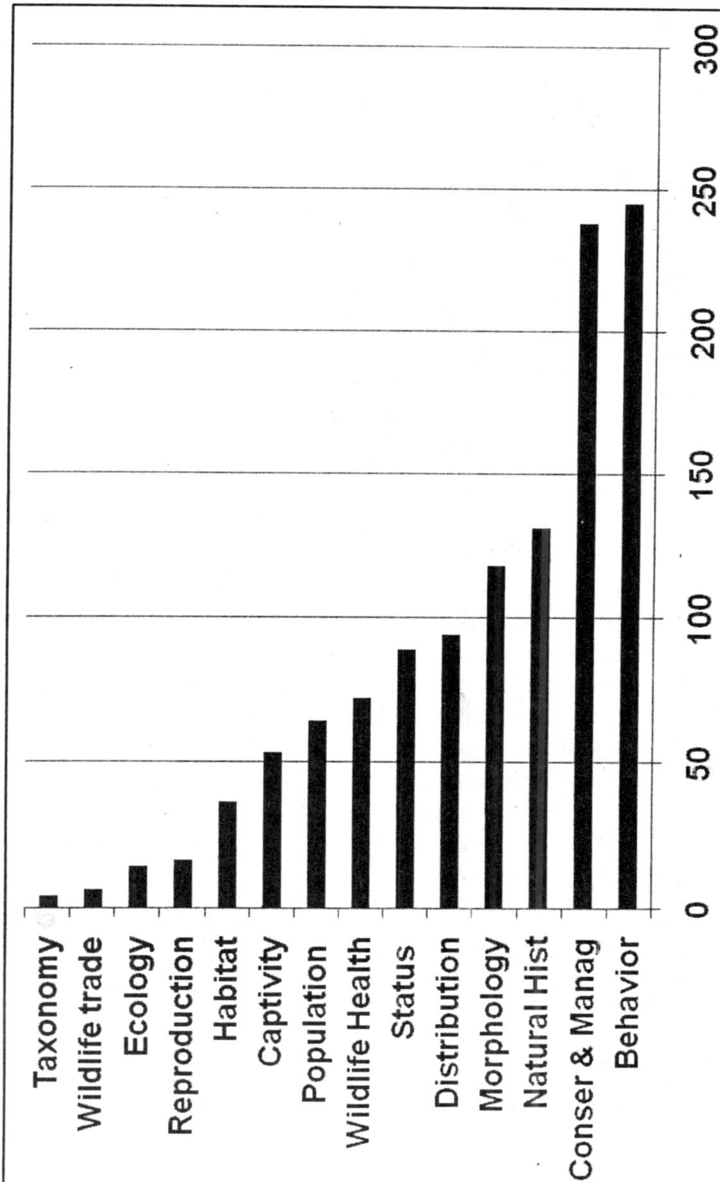

Figure 11.1: Categorization of Publications in Different Research Areas on Ungulates in India

1991; Khan *et al.*, 1995; Kotwal and Mishra, 2004; Edgaonkar, 2008). Other studies exhibited interest in the ungulate habitat, habitat utilization, density and distribution, social organization, group composition and dynamics, reproduction, ecology and conservation management etc (Dharmakumarsinhji, 1959; Ranjitsinh, 1982; Karanth and Sanquist, 1992; Gangadharan, 2005).

Chital or spotted deer (*Axis axis*) is an endemic ungulate species of south Asia, occurring in India, Sri Lanka, Nepal and Bangladesh (Prater, 1934; Schaller, 1967). It is included in Schedule III of Wildlife Protection Act, India but not listed in IUCN Red Data Book or CITES. Routine behavioural patterns of ungulates have been studied both in wild and captivity in India (Khan *et al.*, 1995; Gangadharan, 2005). In wild, these animals form social groups during foraging, migration and other daily activities where animal density, food availability and dispersion, social and environmental factors etc. influence overall behavioural patterns (Clutton- Brock, 1980; Raman, 1997). However, in captivity many of these influences are nonexistent and, therefore, general behavioural displays, calving pattern, birth weight, sex ratio, neonatal mortality etc. are different as compared to wild. Variations in mating behaviour have been noted for captive bovids and cervids (Isvaran, 2005). In captivity, stress may be one of the factors resulting into disproportional display of certain behavioural patterns. The food type and availability, total feeding time, overall climatic conditions and disturbances in captivity play significant role in behavioural responses of animals particularly with reference to breeding. Several reports suggested that variations in reproductive behaviour are common among ungulates, although alternative mating tactics are not numerous and some general patterns can be identified. The overall behaviour of an animal is influenced not only by environmental factors but may also be affected by social interactions (Isharvan, 2005). In wild, studies have generally documented some seasonality (Schaller, 1967). On the other hand, many reports on studies of captive herds have been conflicting.

Several studies have documented the behaviour of Axis deer in wild however, over a period of time the anthropogenic stress in various zoos has increased. Therefore, the behavioural patterns of Axis deer were studied in Sakkarbaug Zoo, Junagadh, Gujarat, India to assess the influences of captivity on its behavioural displays.

Materials and Methods

Study Area

Sakkar baug zoo, Junagadh (21:31: N latitude, E longitude, 82 m to 92 m above MSL) is one of the major cities of Saurashtra province of Gujarat state, India. The climate is generally hot and dry with temperature ranging from 43°C in summer to 7°C in winter. Average rainfall is about 80 cm. Sakkarbaug zoo, spreads over about 192 hectares in the foot hills of mount Girnar; it is the second largest and third oldest zoo in India (Figure 11.2). The animals are housed in sufficient large cages (20m x 18m) which are as per the specifications of Central Zoo Authority, India.

Water and Fodder Supplies

The bore well water was supplied during noon every day into the water tank/turf which was regularly cleaned. The animals were fed regularly as per the diet chart prepared by veterinarian. Some of the fodder varieties were grown in the farm facilities of the zoo and fresh items were supplied to animals. Seasonal variations were made in the quantity and types of ingredients, fortified with vitamins, and were verified by trained head animal keeper and the veterinary officer. Dry grasses were added to the feed supplement during winter to match with the natural feeding variations. To compensate for the salt loss especially during summer, in each cage salt licks were supplied.

Health Status Monitoring

A daily visit of veterinarian was scheduled in the morning for a close and personal observation of the animals. Further, based on the information of cage keeper, additional visits or care was taken for particular animal. In case of any ailment the animal was usually shifted to the zoo hospital for treatment. During the study period none of the study animals had any kind of health problem and such emergency never arrived. The cages were regularly cleaned to remove leaf litter and the excreta of animals. Following monsoon, the soil (cage bed) were heated using gas burners to clean it up from possible ecto-parasite load.

Animal Handling and Labeling

None of the animal was ever directly handled by the investigator. The zoo regulations and permission criteria were strictly followed.

The selected animal, one each adult male, adult female and fawn were marked on the rump using specific permissible paint by injection spray method. This was done while the animals were feeding and thus were least disturbed.

Observation Schedule

Two observation schedules were fixed; each one of 3 hours during day and night. The time period was changed periodically during different seasons to cover entire day and night over the year and to note any specific variation in the activity pattern of animal. The general time schedule was 0800 to 1100 hrs and 2000 to 2300 hrs. This was periodically changed to 1200 to 1500 hrs and 0000 to 0300 hrs, 1600 to 1900 hrs and 0400 to 0700 hrs. Each time schedule was fixed for one month. These schedules permitted a complete 24 hr study.

Sampling Method

For present studies direct focal animal sampling was used (Altman, 1974). The selected and marked animals (male, female and fawn) were continuously observed for the time period as detailed above. Time budget (mean proportions of time spent active) activity was considered for noting behaviour displays and activities. Here time budget was considered for all the activities and, therefore, the data were recorded as actual time spent doing a particular activity (minutes per hour per day). Present observations, therefore, do not simply indicate active bouts and inactive stages but elaborately describe different activities individually.

Behavioural Patterns

The activities and displays were classified into three major categories as general behaviour patterns, reproductive behaviour patterns and parental care behaviour patterns. The movement in cages was further sub divided into short and long distance movements and running since the cage size was large in present case and therefore the animal had an opportunity of exhibiting near natural locomotory activities. Each behavioural pattern was recorded for focal animal at different times of the day and night. Time spend on each activity mentioned herein was recorded and mean time invested per hour per day was calculated. General behaviour patterns included feeding, rumination, resting, licking salt, short

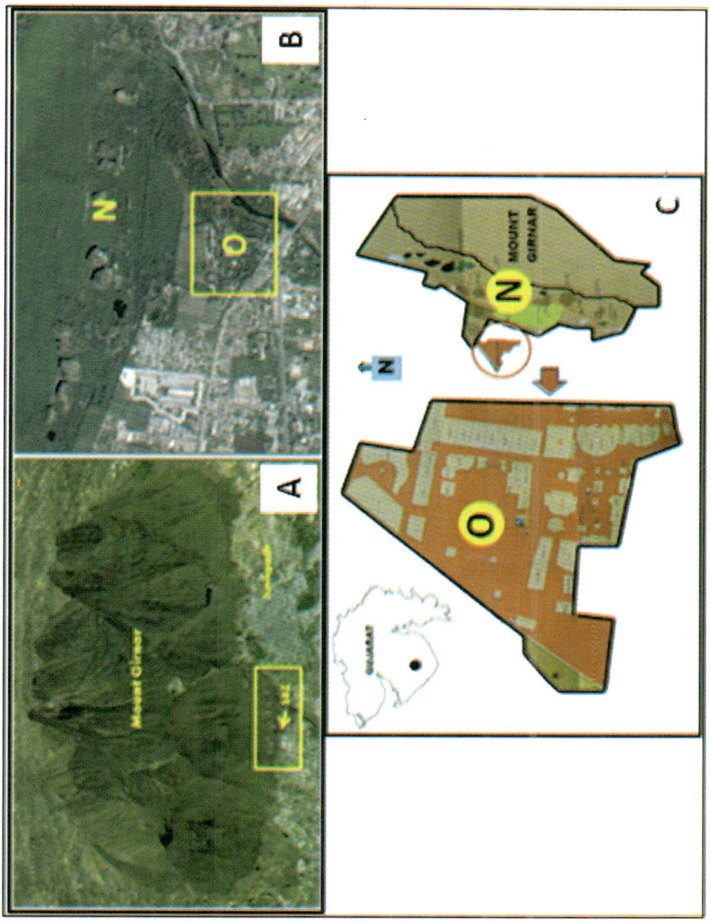

Figure 11.2: A: Showing Location of Zoo in the Foot Hills of Girnar in Junagadh City; B: Location of Old (O) and New (N) Regions of the Zoo, C. Layout of Sakkarbaug Zoo

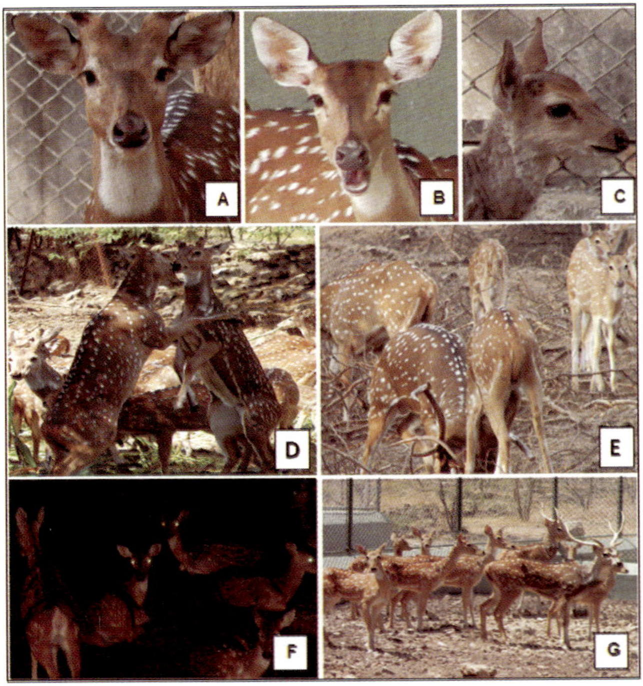

Figure 11.3: Behavioural Displays of Axis Deer

A: Features of adult male represented as presence of antler during the breeding season, prominently dark coat color, darker nostril region and white colored anterior neck region. The head region is also darker compared to doe; B: Photograph showing features of adult doe where the head region has lighter color; the coat color is much light than the buck even during breeding season. The white coloration covers small portion of the neck and it does not appear prominent; C: Features of the young fawn represented as light coat color with prominent white spots. Coloration wise sexual dimorphism was not seen in fawn; D: The adult buck exhibiting dominance fight at feeding point following the antler shedding. The antler development has just begun in one of them; E: The adult bucks exhibiting rutting to establish territoriality and dominance. The antlers are almost fully grown. The adult doe watches the act interestingly; F: Nocturnal activity is shown where most of the doe are resting while one of the adult doe is vigilant for security; G: The exhibition of response to threat due to excessive traffic of visitors. The animals move deeper in to the cage where the adult male leads the group, generally the fawn are almost in the center of the group.

movement, long movement, running, territory marking and urination. Reproductive behaviour patterns included smelling, flehming, scratch antler, rutting and conflict, chasing, mount and mating. Parental care behaviour patterns included suckling, licking fawn and playing with fawn.

Statistical Analysis

Statistical analysis of time activity budget was done using standard software. Pearson's correlation coefficient and One Way ANOVA were calculated for effective interpretation of the data.

Results and Discussion

Focal sampling of labeled animals during pilot survey was conducted for a three hour schedule four times a day, daily for one month. The final selection of parameters was done based on these studies. In routine the behaviour displays or activities are categorized into feeding, resting, locomotion, alert and others including reproductive displays. Here they are sub categorized into various others to precisely understand the behavioural description. Since feeding and rumination are complementary activities they need to be considered as two parameters. Inclusion of the total feeding and rumination time into one activity would not give actual idea of time spent for feeding and at times may be misleading. Locomotion includes short and long movements and running. Short movements are exhibited variably during feeding, post feeding, breeding or non breeding seasons and also under the influence of people. The long movements are almost always seen post feeding; even the distance travelled is variable if quantity of food consumed is different. Further the long movements can be correlated with temperature since more frequent long movements are seen during early morning and late evening hours, more so during winter, probably to generate heat by locomotion. Similarly, running is also variable during pre rut, antler shedding phase and as a play activity with the young fawn. Therefore, sub categorization of all these was essential to appropriately understand the behaviour in captivity. The behaviour parameters to evaluate reproductive and parental care displays were also segregated into specific activities since these are very peculiar and sex specific activities.

The feeding activity exhibited seasonal and sex specific variations (Figure 11.4). Prior to onset of winter the feeding rate was higher in females as compared to males. However, during this time

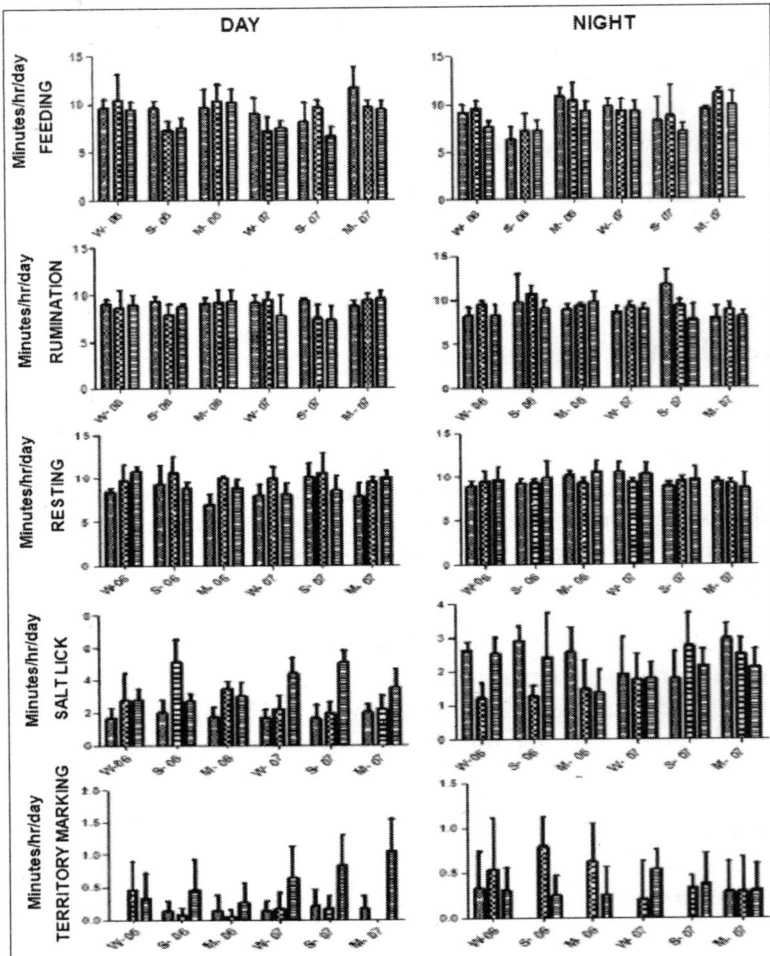

Figure 11.4: Time Budget Activity of Axis Deer Displayed During Day and Night During the Study Period

W: Winter: S: Summer; M: Monsoon. The bars from left to right represent buck, doe and fawn, respectively.

much variation was not noted between day and night feeding of females. In fawns the feeding time spent was equivalent to that spent by adult ones. The time spent for feeding and rumination collectively formed a larger share of daily activity (Figure 11.4). Separate male and female groups are formed in early winter and at this time also females feed more, correlated with nutritional enrichment, as fetal development is energy demanding phenomena if successful mating is there. Antlers of the males shed during monsoon so females become dominant for short period and will drive away the males from feed point. This gives ample time and opportunity to females to spend more time in feeding. This will also permit the fawn, particularly the males, to feed more. This is probably selective support to fawn, specifically males, for growth promotion. In captivity, behavioural modifications may help maximize survival in an environment widely variable from which the animals evolved.

Females continue to ruminate standing also and need not sit on the ground resting. Generally males do that. The rate of jaw movement for rumination is also variable immediately after feeding and following a prolonged period of rumination. In adults the rate is usually 45 movements per minutes initially for half an hour followed by less than 25-30 per minute. While in the fawn the initial rate is above 60 per minute followed by less than 40 per minute. If the animal is disturbed while ruminating the pattern also disturbs and abrupt changes may be seen.

The salt licking was not a prominent or time consuming activity for females or fawn particularly during winter and monsoon. They exhibited, however, irregular pattern throughout the year (Figure 11.4). The males spent extensive time period, almost thrice the females, specifically during summer at salt lick sites (Figure 11.4). It was high both during day and night. As compared to the adult ones, the requirement of salt lick by the fawn was very low. Summer season is marked with mineralization of antlers. The adult male may fulfill its requirements of minerals by spending more time at salt licks.

Very brief territory marking activity was exhibited by male during the day and it was totally absent during night, while the female and fawn spent some time doing territory marking (Figure 11.4). Fawn spent more time as compared to female considering 24 h period. Therefore, significant variation was noted both sex wise and age wise. The young fawn during 2007 spent more time as compared to the other fawn during 2006. In wild the male has to defend his territory from other males and express dominance. However, in captivity only two males coexisted and one of the male was much dominant than the other younger one. Therefore, territory marking was probably not required. The number of females was more per cage. In wild they spent least time in territory marking but in captivity it was seen. Similarly, the fawn also spent comparable time in this activity probably to secure and identify its routine place in the cage (Figure 11.4).

A distinct pattern of increase in short movement in males is seen from summer to winter in both the study years (Figure 11.5). Generally the activity was higher in male and fawn during night hours in monsoon and winter. The time spent for short movements by females was at average range through the day and night, the entire study period. The time activity budget for long movement shows specific pattern in female and fawn but not in male. A total of 24 h activity indicate that female spend overall more time than male and the fawn. The running is also an activity of game and playing between the fawn and female (Figure 11.5). The running activity in males may be because of disturbances, to push away the fawn or sub adult females from the vicinity of adult female or exhibiting dominance in the group during breeding season. Since the activity of male is not directly associated with the activity of other animal, no significant positive correlation is established between male and other animals (Figure 11.5).

Smelling is an activity almost equivalently done by male, female and fawn (Figure 11.5). Very little variations were noted among them. Even no specific seasonal or annual variations were noted (Figure 11.5). The smelling activity is a daylong activity and also associated with other activities. While feeding, locomotion, resting, urination and breeding displays the smelling activity is carried out. In wild this forms a significant activity as the olfactory cues are important for protection, routine movement and breeding. In captivity threat of predation is not at all there so the activity is much reduced as compared to wild. Further, in captivity the cages of different animals; herbivore or carnivore are nearby and therefore, the olfactory cues may be stereotype also. The movement of other animals outside the cage (like cats and monkeys), particularly during night and the presence of visitors during day induce smelling activity also, specifically in male and the fawn.

Flehming is very peculiar breeding associated activity, although overall time spent during the day is less. In wild the flehming is most prominent in males during pre breeding and breeding season.

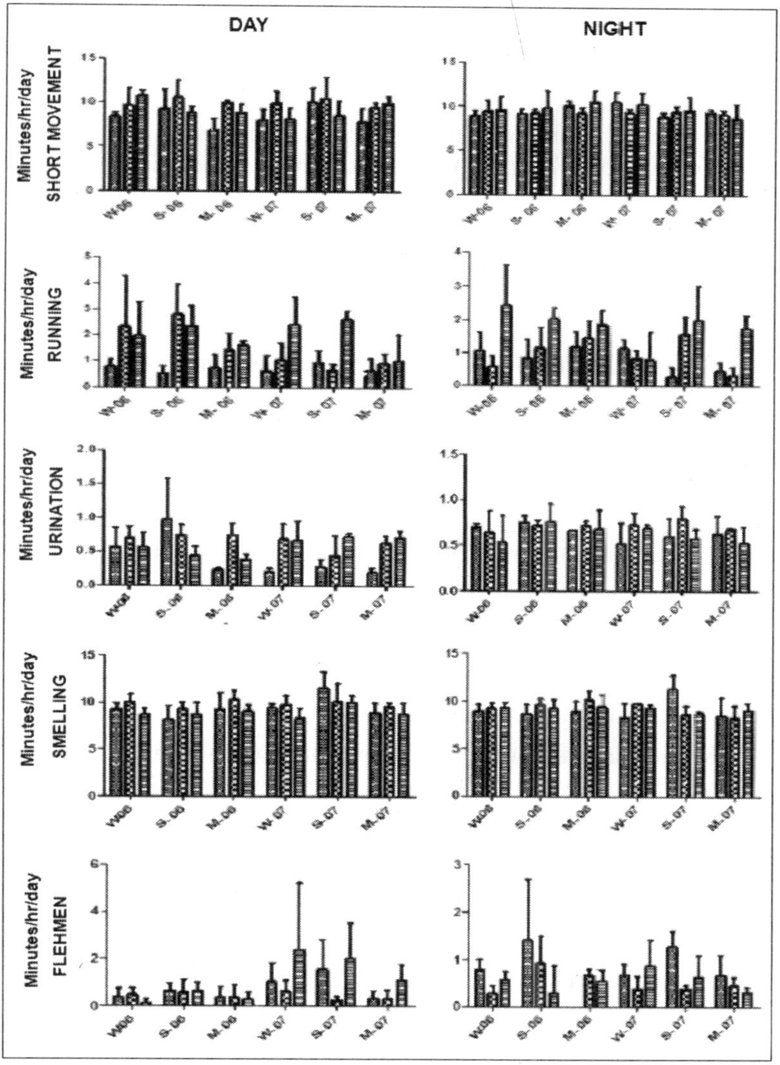

Figure 11.5: Time Budget Activity of Axis Deer Displayed During Day and Night During the Study Period

W: Winter; S: Summer; M: Monsoon. The bars from left to right represent buck, doe and fawn, respectively.

In captivity the males spent least time as compared to that by female and fawn (Figure 11.5). Probably the male easily identifies adult female suitable for mating and therefore, flehming of different females is not required. The male fawn which stays with the female carries out this activity more frequently. The adult females flehmens the sub adult female following urination and if the female is in heat then it will be chased and separated from the group so that opportunity of mating with dominant male is secured.

Scratching antler is a direct breeding associated activity. During early winter the male scratches the antler to remove the velvety skin of antler and then gradually sharpens the tip of main axis of antler. The initial scratching is carried out by rubbing the antlers with the fencing of the cage. Later on this is done by scratching the antler with the stem of the trees. The activity in wild is time consuming and depends on modes of establishing dominance, the number of males and the season. The male in wild scratch the antlers at various places and also by doing so establish territory. However, in captivity such peculiarity of ethogram is not seen. During present study, an adult female had delivered a fawn in late winter and therefore, subsequently the female was in heat during late winter to early summer period the next year. Correspondingly in the male, the antler scratching activity was a bit delayed and the sharp and hard antlers were ready following the onset of summer.

Rutting is pre conflict activity in adult males and at times a play activity in fawn and sub adult. The growing male fawn learns the tactics by indulging in such activities. Rutting in winter is mainly pre conflict act. The average of annual activity suggested that during the two years of study the overall pattern and time spent for the activity was almost equivalent. The fawn at a younger stage did not show any such activity but when the antlers grew in about six months after birth, the activity was seen.

The conflict is a specific feature prominently seen in wild. The conflict during winter is for establishing dominance during breeding season and to attract the female. In captivity, however, the conditions totally differ and therefore wide variations are noted. In present study, during first year two adult males were housed in the cage and hence conflict was seen among them, while during second year only one male was present in the cage and the size of cage was also bigger. Therefore, no sign of conflict were seen at all for adult male, the activity with female, in absence of male conflict, can be considered only a game activity.

Mounting is preparatory activity for mating. The adult male does mounting on adult female when it is in heat. However, it may also do so on sub adult female during summer or any other time of the year. The fawn carries out this activity for game and play. It usually tries to mount sub adult female, although may try out on adult female also. In present case mounting by adult was mostly evening specific activity and during the day when visitors are present in front of the cage, it avoided mounting. Further, the mounting was seen maximally during summer day and night as per the heating period schedule of the female. The average time spent between two mount is usually 5-7 min during the breeding season.

A very peculiar observation was noted in present study with reference to mounting an animal. The peak breeding season of female was delayed in present case leading to delayed expression of characteristic behaviour by the male. The mounting was significantly delayed by the male and therefore, the female tried to mount the male several times and thus excite the male.

Suckling is a phenomenon of bondage between the female and its fawn. The fawn usually sucks the mother for almost 14 months after birth. However, it starts feeding at its own after 3 weeks of birth. In summer the suckling activity is maximum time consuming as the solid feed supplied may not be utilized by the fawn to any greater extent. Moreover, the requirement of specific nutrients and water is received through the milk. In captivity, the female offers suckling opportunity to fawn of other female also. The year wise activity budget showed that the suckling activity was comparatively more in case of first fawn than the second one.

The mating season varies depending on geographical location. In more tropical areas like India there is no distinct mating season and breeding can take place throughout the year. In areas with more seasonal climates there will be a distinct breeding season. During the mating season males compete with each other for the possession of small groups of females known as harems. Males will compete with each other using bellowing, and sometimes fighting using their antlers. Usually the strongest most dominant males obtain harems and so get to mate.

The females have a 220-day long gestation period, after which normally a single calf is born, although twins can also sometimes occur. The calf is weaned at 6 months of age, and becomes sexually mature from 12 months of age. However, in several studies, captive ungulates did not exhibit any significant differences compared to their counter parts in the wild (Meng *et al.*, 2003; 2008).

Resting is closely associated and inter-bridging activity with feeding, rumination, short/long movements and running. It was observed in present studies that the animals generally selected specific site for resting; although this was not much restrictive for both antelope species. The group size and composition and the group varied particularly during breeding and non-breeding seasons.

In wild, resting largely depends on predation threat and therefore, variations may be observed on day to day basis. Seasonally this is associated with other activities. Generally, the ungulates feed for a while rest for some time and reinitiate feeding. If they are not resting then they exhibit short movements. At times, disturbance other than predation threat also cause running. Collectively, feeding and rumination, resting, long and short movements and running are allocated most time during a day which is then followed by alert responses including simple vigilant posture, standing alert or threat-specific actively (*e.g.* running). In captivity, the high density of visitors during specific seasons at specified time of the day (morning and late noon to evening) is possibly the only major threat/disturbing activity to which the animals get acclimatized very soon and therefore, as compared to the responses in conditions of wild, the responses are almost absent in captivity.

Although, studies for wild populations were not carried out in present studies, outcomes of several previous studies were compared with our findings in captivity and suggested that where in wild various factors influenced and induced behavioural responses variations; and seasonal activities, some of such factors (*e.g.* Climatic/ environmental) although existed in captivity had no significant influences.

References

Altmann, J., 1974. Observational study of behaviour: Sampling methods. *Behaviour*, 49: 227-267.

Clutton-Brock, Ô.Ç., Albon, S.D. and Harvey, Ñ.Ç., 1980. Antlers, body size and breeding group size in Cervidae. *Nature* (*London*), 285: 565–567.

Dharmakumarsinhji, K.S., 1959. A field guide to big game census in India. *Indian Board for Wildlife*, New Delhi, 2: 62-66.

Edgaonkar, A., 2008. Ecology of the Leopard (*Panthera Pardus*) in Bori Wildlife Sanctuary and Satpura National Park, India. *Ph.D. Dissertation*, University of Florida.

Gangadharan, A., 2005. Density Estimation and Time Trend Analysis of Large Herbivores in Nagarhole, India. Page 82. University of St. Andrews.

Isvaran, K., 2005. Female grouping best predicts lekking in blackbuck (*Antilope cervicapra*). *Behav Ecol Sociobiol.*, 57: 283-294.

Johnsingh, A.J.T. and Sankar, K., 1991. Food plants of chital, sambar and cattle on Mundanthurai plateau, Tamil Nadu, South India. *Mammalia*, 55:57-66.

Karanth, K.U. and Sunquist, M.E., 1992. Population structure, density and biomass of large herbivores in the tropical forests of Nagarahole, India. *J. Trop. Eco.*, 8: 21-35.

Khan, J.A., Chellam, R. and Johnsingh, A.J.T., 1995. Group size and age-sex composition of three major ungulate species in Gir lion Sanctuary, Gujarat, India. *J. Bombay Natl. Hist. Soc.*, 92: 295-302.

Kotwal, P.C. and Mishra, R.P., 2004. Ecobiology of Indian wild buffalo *Bubalus arnee* L. in Udanti Wildlife Sanctuary. *J. Bom. Nat. Hist. Soc.*, 101: 252-254.

Mathur, V.B., Kathayat, J.S. and Rath, D.P., 2000. Directory of wildlife protected areas in India. *Envis Bulletin* Vol. 3, No.1. Wildlife Institute of India, Dehradun, 236p.

Meng, X., Yang, Q., Feng, Z., Xia, L., Jiang, Y. and Wang, P., 2003. The temporal estrous patterns of female alpine musk deer in captivity. *Appl. Ani. Behav. Sci.*, 82: 75-85.

Meng, X., Yang, Q., Feng, Z., Xu, H., Perkins, G.C., Zhao, C., Hui, C., Feng, J. and Zhou, Y., 2008. Gender specific behavioural patterns of captive alpine musk deer (*Moschus sifanicus*). *Belg. J. Zool.*, 138: 101-105.

Prater, S.H., 1934. The wild animals of the Indian Empire. *J. Bombay Nat. Hist. Soc.*, 37: 76-79.

Raman, T.R.S., 1997. Factors influencing seasonal and monthly changes in the group size of chital or axis deer in southern India. *J. Bio.*, 22: 203-218.

Ranjitsinh, M.K., 1989. *The Indian Blackbuck*. Natraj Publishers, Dehradun.

Sankar, K. and Goyal, S.P. (Eds), 2004. *Ungulates of India*. Wildlife Institute of India, India.

Schaller, G.B., 1967. *The Deer and the Tiger: A Study of Wildlife in India*. The University of Chicago Press, Chicago.

Chapter 12

Alleviation of Obesity Induced Oxidative Stress in Heart by Triphala

B. Kalaivani[1] and G. Vanithakumari[2]*

*[1]*Department of Zoology, Sri Sarada College for Women, Salem – 636 016, Tamil Nadu, India*

[2]Division of Endocrinology, Department of Zoology, Bharathiar University, Coimbatore – 641 046, Tamil Nadu, India

ABSTRACT

Obesity has been shown to be one of the conditions that decrease antioxidant capacity. The aim of the present study was to investigate the obesity induced oxidative stress in heart and amelioration by triphala. This was compared with standard herbal (ayurslim) and synthetic (sibutrex10™) anti-obesity drugs. Albino rats were divided in to three groups. Group I: Control group–the rats received normal standard diet orally, Group II: Short duration group–The animals were fed individually with triphala, ayurslim and sibutrex10™ at12 hours intervals for thirty consecutive days. Group III: Long duration group–The animals groups were fed individually with triphala, ayurslim and sibutrex10 ™ at12 hours intervals for sixty consecutive days. Group II and Group III were further sub-divided into six sub groups, each group consisting of five animals. 1. Obesity control–The animals received vanaspathi

* Corresponding author: E-mail: kalai03win@yahoo.co.in

(hydrogenated oil), 200mg/Kg. body weight/day as an oral dose. 2. Obesity + Triphala–The animals received 200mg. of vanaspathi + 200 mg of triphala/Kg. body weight/day, as an oral dose. 3. Obesity + Ayurslim–The animals received 200mg. of vanaspathi + 250mg of ayurslim/Kg. body weight/day, as an oral dose, 4. Obesity + Sibutrex10™–The animals received 200mg. of vanaspathi + 10mg. of sibutrex10™/Kg. body weight/day, as an oral dose. The present study showed that obesity had caused an increase in lipid peroxidation and decrease in superoxide dismutase, catalase and glutathione in heart. Triphla, and ayurslim were more effective in the restoration of obesity induced oxidative stress in the heart.

Keywords: *Obesity, Oxidative stress, Heart, Lipid peroxidation, Superoxide dismutase, Catalase, Glutathione.*

Introduction

Obesity is a global nutritional concern. The increasing prevalence of overweight, obesity and its consequences promoted the World Health Organization (WHO) to designate obesity as a global epidemic (WHO, 1998). Oxidative stress has been repeatedly addressed as an important mechanism of cytotoxicity and indirect genotoxicity that may be considerably increased in certain pathologies (Kirkland and Muller, 2000; Pratt and Barron, 2003). It is triggered by exposure to exogenous factors or by chemicals producing reactive oxygen species and is associated with an over production of ROS, as well as impairment of anti-oxidant defensive capacity. Obesity has been shown to be one of the conditions that decrease anti-oxidant capacity (Carmiel Haggai *et al.*, 2003).

Patients with type 2 diabetes mellitus showed an increase in lipid peroxidation from the onset of disease (Sundaram *et al.*, 1996). Previous reports indicate that lipid peroxidation is elevated in both liver and plasma in humans and obese animals (Desci *et al.*, 1997). Furthermore, diets rich in fats (either saturated or unsaturated) are also associated with increased lipid peroxidation in several tissues, such as aorta, liver and plasma (Folch *et al.*, 1957; Koneru *et al.*, 1995). Obesity is associated with lower plasma or tissue levels of anti-oxidants and/or increased susceptibility to injury during oxidative changes *in vitro* (Koneru *et al.*, 1995; Vincent *et al.*, 1998).

The present study is an attempt to investigate the obesity induced oxidative stress in heart and restoration by triphala.

Materials and Methods

Animals

Adult female albino rats of Wistar Strain weighing about 180 – 200g were procured from Kerala Agricultural University, Kerala and acclimatized to our animal house conditions for 2 weeks. The animals were housed in well-ventilated animal house with constant 12 ±1 hours light and dark schedule. They were provided with standard diet and clean water *ad libitum.*

Experimental Design

The following experimental design was as per the guidelines of SPCA and was approved by the Institutional Animal Ethical Committee (IAEC) (No. 722/02/a/CPCSEA)

The animals were divided into three groups as follows.

Group I: Control Group

The rats received normal standard diet orally.

Group II: Short Duration Group

The animals groups were fed individually with triphala, ayurslim and sibutrex10™ at12 hours intervals for thirty consecutive days.

Group III: Long Duration Group

The animals groups were fed individually with triphala, ayurslim and sibutrex10™ at12 hours intervals for sixty consecutive days.

Group II and Group III were further sub-divided into six sub groups, each group consisting of five animals. The animals received the following regimen of treatment, all the treatments were constructed on the basis of adult dosage prescribed by the physicians to humans and extrapolated to animal body weight.

1. Obesity Control

The animals received vanaspathi (hydrogenated oil), 200mg./ Kg. body weight/day as an oral dose.

2. Obesity + Triphala

The animals received 200mg. of vanaspathi + 200 mg. of triphala/Kg. body weight/day, as an oral dose.

3. Obesity + Ayurslim

The animals received 200mg. of vanaspathi + 250mg. of ayurslim/Kg. body weight/day, as an oral dose.

4. Obesity + Sibutrex10™

The animals received 200mg. of vanaspathi + 10mg. of sibutrex10™/Kg. body weight/day, as an oral dose.

Suitable controls were maintained for each duration of treatment. However, as there was no obvious difference in any parameter among control groups, a common control was employed in the present study.

Animal Sacrifice

The animals were weighed before and after treatment. Twenty four hours after the last treatment schedule the animals were sacrificed by decapitation method. Serum was separated immediately after the sacrifice by centrifugation of blood at 3000 x g for 30 minutes and stored at –20°C until used for hormone assays and biochemical parameters. The animals were dissected out and heart was removed based on the guidelines of Hamilton (1975). The organs were cleaned off adhering connective tissues and blood stains, washed in cold physiological saline thrice, blotted on a filter paper and weighed using electronic balance, wrapped in aluminum foil and stored at –20°C in air tight glass containers until assayed for biochemical parameters. The levels of lipid peroxidation (Nichens and Samuelson, 1968), oxidative enzymes like catalase (Sinha, 1972), superoxide dismutase (Kakkar *et al.*, 1984) and non–enzymatic anti-oxidant glutathione (Beutler and Kelly, 1963) were estimated in the heart tissue.

Results and Discussion

Lipid peroxidation is a free-radical generating process which occurs in every membranous structure of the cell. Free radicals are known to be involved in a number of human pathologies including atherosclerosis (Steinberg, 1997), cancer (Cerutti, 1994) and hypertension (Russo *et al.*, 1998). Hyperlipemia leads to increased production of oxygen free radicals, which exert their toxicity effects by causing lipid peroxidation and the resulting formation of malondialdehyde (MDA). Obesity increases the mechanical and metabolic load on the myocardium, thus increasing myocardial oxygen consumption. It is likely that, obesity induced increased myocardial oxygen consumption directly contributes to elevated lipid peroxidation (Girotti, 1998; Reid *et al.*, 1992). A potential mechanism for increased lipid damage in obesity seen in this study might be the increased lipid substrate within the myocardium that can serve as a larger target for oxidation by free radicals (Girotti, 1998).

Table 12.1: Effect of Triphala and Standard Anti-obesity Drugs on Lipid Peroxidation and Superoxide Dismutase in the Heart of Albino Rats

Treatments	*Lipid Peroxidation (nmoles/min/mg protein)*	*Superoxide Dismutase (nmoles/min/mg protein)*
Group I – Control	3.520 ± 0.03[j]	8.360 ± 0.02[c]
Group II – Short duration		
Obesity	7.420 ± 0.03**[b]	4.860 ± 0.02**[i]
Obesity + Triphala	4.880 ± 0.03**[fg]	7.380 ± 0.03**[d]
Obesity + Ayurslim	4.500 ± 0.04**[h]	8.280 ± 0.33**[c]
Obesity + Sibutrex10™	3.980 ± 0.07**[I]	4.840 ± 0.02**[j]
Group III – Long duration		
Obesity	9.480 ± 0.03**[a]	3.380 ± 0.03**[k]
Obesity + Triphala	5.820 ± 0.03**[d]	9.560 ± 0.03**[a]
Obesity + Ayurslim	5.000 ± 0.04**[ef]	8.860 ± 0.33**[b]
Obesity + Sibutrex10™	4.860 ± 0.02**[g]	6.060 ± 0.07**[g]

Each value is the Mean ± SE of five animals

** Control Vs Treatment, significant at 1 per cent level by ANOVA

Means ± SE followed by a common letter are not significantly different at the 5 per cent level by DMRT (a, b, c etc).

A negative consequence of the elevated myocardial oxygen consumption is the production of ROS such as superoixde, hydroxyl radical and hydrogen peroxides from the increased mitochondrial respiration (Turrens, 1997). Indeed, leakage of electrons out of the mitochondrial electron transport chain promotes a one-electron reduction of molecular oxygen resulting in the formation of superoxide radicals (Kukraja and Hess, 1992). The second mechanism by which obesity can independently cause increased lipid peroxidation is by progressive and cumulative cell injury observed histologically and resulting from pressure from the large body mass. Lachieitner *et al.* (2000) have shown that cell injury causes the release of cytokines, especially tumor necrosis factor alpha (TNF-α) which generates ROS from the tissues, which inturn cause lipid peroxidation. A third possible mechanism to explain this observation is through the diet. Nutritional obesity which is the predominant form implies the consumption of hyperlipidemic diets which may be involved in oxygen metabolism. Double bonds in the fatty acids molecules are vulnerable to oxidation reactions and may consequently cause lipid peroxidation. All the three mechanisms suggested above are operating in the obese of the present study.

Table 12.2: Effect of Triphala and Standard Anti-obesity Drugs on Catalase and Glutathione in the Heart of Albino Rats

Treatments	*Catalase (nmoles/min/mg protein)*	*Glutathione (nmoles/min/mg protein)*
Group I – Control	4.602 ± 0.02[bc]	4.844 ± 0.004[b]
Group II – Short duration		
Obesity	3.604 ± 0.02**[g]	3.458 ± 0.008**[i]
Obesity + Triphala	4.444 ± 0.009**[de]	4.820 ± 0.01**[b]
Obesity + Ayurslim	4.400 ± 0.03**[e]	4.880 ± 0.004**[a]
Obesity + Sibutrex10™	4.656 ± 0.01**[ab]	4.562 ± 0.01**[e]
Group III – Long duration		
Obesity	3.048 ± 0.05**[h]	2.776 ± 0.008**[j]
Obesity + Triphala	4.478 ± 0.02**[de]	4.548 ± 0.01**[e]
Obesity + Ayurslim	4.710 ± 0.03**[a]	4.762 ± 0.01**[c]
Obesity + Sibutrex10™	4.536 ± 0.006**[cd]	4.630 ± 0.006**[d]

Each value is the Mean ± SE of five animals

** Control Vs Treatment, significant at 1 per cent level by ANOVA

Means ± SE followed by a common letter are not significantly different at the 5 per cent level by DMRT (a, b, c etc).

Recent evidence indicates that obesity is associated with increased myocardial lipid peroxidation and susceptibility to oxidative damage *in vitro* also (Vincent *et al.*, 1998). Investigators examining oxidative stress induced cellular injury can be lost due to oxidatively modified lipids and proteins (McDufee *et al.*, 1997). In the heart significant oxidative injury can ultimately lead to cardiac arthmias, poor contractibility, infraction, cardiac failure or sudden death (Yu, 1994).

At least four general potential mechanisms could contribute to the obesity-induced myocardial lipid peroxidation (*a*) increased myocardial work and subsequent radical production via mitochondrial respiration (Yu, 1994), (*b*) decreased myocardial antioxidant defense (Desci *et al.*, 1997; Ohrvall *et al.*, 1993), (*c*) increased fat deposition within myocardial tissue (1991; Lamers *et al.*, 1987) and (or) (*d*) increased rates of radical formation such as superoxide (O_2) or the hydroxyl radical (Braddy *et al.*, 1985).

In the present investigation, obesity induction had caused an increase in lipid peroxidation and consequent free radical production and indicate low-antioxidant defense in heart. Further increased fat deposition within the myocardial tissue was also observed histologically leading to oxidative stress within the tissue. Previous reports indicate that lipid peroxidation is elevated in both liver and plasma in humans and obese animals (Desi *et al.*, 1997; Koneru *et al.*, 1995). Furthermore, diets enriched in fats (either saturated or unsaturated) are also associated with increased lipid peroxidtion in several tissues such as aorta, liver and plasma (Folch *et al.*, 1951; Koneru *et al.*, 1995; Montilla *et al.*, 2006) reported that the cholesterol enriched diet caused clear increase in lipid peroxidation products in the brain kidney and erythrocytes. Triphala, trikatu and their combinations had effectively lowered the lipid peroxidation in the obese animals. Administration with ayurslim and Sibutrex10™ seem to be more effective in lowering the lipid peroxidation levels when compared to triphala and trikatu.

The SOD catalyses the removel of superoxide radicals, thus reducing the degree of oxidation (Bannister, 1987). SOD activity is undoubtedly important to the regulation of oxidative status in diabetes. Some studies have reported decreased SOD activity (Obrosova *et al.*, 2000) while others have shown increase (Rauscher *et al.*, 2001) in the enzyme activity in diabetic rats. Santiago *et al.* (1993) showed an increase in SOD in the brain regions of aged rats. There is strong evidence that the oxidative metabolism pathway of catecholamines exert their neurotoxic effect mainly due to the generation of highly reactive quinines and superoixde radicals (Haque *et al.,* 2003).

In the present study, the enzymatic activity of SOD was considerably decreased in the obese animals. The reason might be due to the increase in oxidative stress by obesity induction and probable utilization of the enzyme to scavenge H_2O_2 radicals. Increased lipid peroxidation might have led to cardiomyocytes damage and degeneration of cellular membranes and tissues as seen histologically, such an observation was made by Sies and Packer (2000) in human heart. The two key enzyme SOD and CAT have been shown to decrease during the peak period of infraction due to peroxidiative insult as reported by Manjula *et al.* (1994).

Administration of triphala and trikatu combination was more effective in restoring the obesity induced oxidative stress by eliminating excess superoxide or hydrogen peroxide ions. When compared to individual treatment of triphala and trikatu. Ayurslim, seemed to be more effective in its restorative action compared to other treatments.

Catalase decomposes hydrogen peroxide and protects the tissue from highly reactive hydroxyl radicals (Chance *et al.,* 1952) and is thought to be the first line of defence against oxidative damage caused by hydrogen peroxide and other radicals induced by high fat diet. The decreased activities of CAT and SOD may be a response to increased production of H_2O_2 and O_2 by the auto-oxidation of glucose and non-enzymatic glycation (Aragno *et al.,* 1997). These enzymes have been suggested as playing an important role in maintaining physiological levels of oxygen and hydrogen peroxide by hastening the dismutation of oxygen radicals and eliminating organic peroxides and hydroperoxides generated from obesity induction.

In the present study, it was noted that catalase activity was lowered by induction of obesity at both durations of treatment. The decreased level of CAT activity observed may be due to the utilization of this enzyme in the removal of hydrogen peroxide radicals caused by obesity induction. Increased lipid peroxidation and extensive necrosis of cell membrane (seen in histology) is evidence to the oxidative stress of damaged myocardial tissue because of high fat diet. Administration with combination of triphala and trikatu was effective in restoring the catalase activity. Both Ayurslim and

Sibutrex10™ had effectively restored the catalase activity to normalcy at both durations of treatment. These observations suggest the minimizing of necrosis in heart tissues by the herbs their cardioprotective properties.

Glutathione (GSH) is an endogenous antioxidant in the human body. It may however delay the oxidation of LDL enabling it to leave the sub endothelial space before oxidation occurs. This may reduce the incorporation of LDL into the foam cells, thereby decreasing the atheroma development and progression (Perwaiz Iqbal *et al.*, 2006). Under *in vivo* conditions, GSH acts as an antioxidant and its decrease was reported in diabetes mellitus by Rotruck *et al.* (1973). In the present study, it was noted that glutathione concentration was lowered by induction of obesity. The decrease in GSH levels represents increased utilization due to the oxidative stress as reported by Matcovis *et al.* (1982). Reduction in glutathione might indicate the damage to the heart tissues and increased oxidative stress because of lowered anti-oxidant, non-enzymatic mechanisms. Administration with triphala, trikatu and their combination were moderately effective in restoring the glutathione concentrations to normalcy. Both ayurslim and Sibutrex10™ were effective in restoring the glutathione concentration to normalcy at both the durations of their treatments.

Polyphenols have been reported to have a major role in reducing oxidative-stress associated diabetes which in turn helps the regulation of plasma glucose concentration and hepatic glucose metabolism (DU Thie and Crozier, 2000). There are several lines of evidence that polyphenolic compounds contained in fruits and vegetables have been beneficial effect on cardiovascular system function (Zenebe *et al.*, 2001). This effect is mediated mainly by the oxygen free radical scavenging properties and stimulation of nitric oxide production in vascular endothelium by the polyphenols. The polyphenols isolated from red wine were shown to improve vascular functions and morphology in the rat experimental model of NO-deficient hypertension (Bernatova *et al.*, 2002; Pechanova *et al.*, 2004).

Obesity induction had caused an increase in lipid peroxidation and consequent decrease in superoxide dismutase, catalase and glutathione at both durations. Triphala, trikatu, and their combination were effective in restoring the above parameters. Ayurslim seems to be more effective in restoring lipid peroxidation and SOD activities. Siburex10™ was effective in restoring catalase and glutathione.

Triphala, being a mixture of *Terminalia chebula*, *Terminalia bellerica* and *Phyllanthus emblica*, has a greater reportoire of active components such as vitamin C, polyphenols tanins, saponins, carbohydrate derivatives, gallic and ellagic acids as well as anthroquinones (Deep *et al.*, 2005). The extracts of *T. chebula* in triphala exhibits negative inotropic and chronotropic effect on the heart muscle and hence recommended for heart diseases (Srivastava *et al.*, 1991). The rich ascorbic acid content of the herbs like amla extract inhibits radiation –induced lipid peroxidation in microsomes and SOD in mitochondria as shown by Khopde *et al.* (2001). High anti-oxidant activity of trikatu might be due to the presence of capsanthin in pepper and gingerol in ginger both of them being its constituents (Kikuzaki and Nakatani, 1993).

The ethanolic extract of *Piper longum* (Pippali) fruits was found to protect mice against the radiation induced decline in WBC, bone marrow cells, α-esterase positive cells and GSH. Pippali extract also reduce the elevated levels of glutathione pyruvate transaminase (GPT), alkaline phosphatase (ALP), and lipid peroxidation in liver and serum of irradiated animals (Sunila *et al.*, 2005). Ginger has been reported to increase glutathione, reduce lipid peroxidation *in vivo* and scavenging various free radicals *in vitro* (Jagetia *et al.*, 2002).

Effect of Ayurslim on lipid peroxidation might be due to the antioxidant activity of *T. chebula* and *Trigonella foenum graecum*. Earlier studies have shown that the protective effect of *T. chebula* fruit extracts against oxidative and peroxidative tissue damage might be attributed to its antioxidant potential (Thatte and Dahanukar, 1997). The anti-oxidant property of fenugreek inhibits lipid peroxidation of the erythrocytes as reported by Thirunavukkarasu *et al.* (2003). Fenugreek seeds have antioxidant activity and have been shown to produce beneficial effects such as neutralization of free radicals and enhancement of antioxidant apparatus (Anuradha and Ravikumar, 1998, 2001). Furthermore, the polyphenolic fraction of the seeds was found to inhibit peroxide-induced oxidative damage and prevent haemolysis of erythrocytes in vitro (Kaviyarasan *et al.*, 2004).

Epidemiological studies have shown that consumption of food and beverages rich in phenolic content can reduce the risk of heart diseases by slowing the progression of atherosclerosis by acting as anti-oxidants towards low-density lipoprotein (LDL) (Frankel *et al.*, 1995). The anti-oxidant activity of phenolics is mainly because of their redox properties which allow them to act as reducing agents, hydrogen donars, singlet oxygen quenchers and metal chelators (Rice – Evans *et al.*, 1997). Sumithra *et al.* (2001) reported that arjuonolic acid from *T. arjuna* prevents the decrease of SOD in isoproterenol induced myocardial necrosis in rats. Siburex10™ shows weight reducing effect which in turn helped reduce oxidative stress.

Thus, in the present study it was found that obesity had caused an increase in lipid peroxidation and decrease in superoxide dismutase, catalase aand glutathione in the heart. Triphala administration had recover the above said parameters like ayurslim. This might be due to the antioxidative property of the triphala.

References

Beutler, E. and Kelly, B.M., 1963. The effect of sodium nitrate on RBC glutathione. *Experimentia*, 29: 96–97.

Brady, L.J., Brady, P.S., Romosos, D.R. and Hoppel, C., 1985. Elevated hepatic mitochondrial and peroxysomal oxidative capacities in fed and starved adult obese (ob/ob mice). *Bicohem J.*, 231: 439–444.

Carmiel-Haggai, M., Cederbaum, A.I. and Nieto, N., 2003. Binge ethanol exposure increases liver injury in obese rats. *Gastroenterology*, 125: 1818- 1833.

Cerutti, P.A., 1994. Oxy-radicals and cancer. *Lancet.*, 344: 796–798.

Chance, B., Green Stein, D.S. and Roughton, R.J.W., 1952. The mechanism of catalase action-1-steady state analysis. *Arch. Biochem. Bio. Phys.*, 37: 301–339.

Desci, T., Molnar, D. and Koletzko, B., 1997. Reduced plasma concentrations of alpha-tocopherol and beta-carotene in obese boys. *J. Pediat.*, 130: 653–655.

Folch, D.J., Lees, M. and Stanely, G.H.S., 1957. A simple method for the isolation and purification of total lipids from animal tissues. *J. Biol. Chem.*, 226: 496–509.

Frankel, E.N., Waterhouse, A.L. and Tessdre, P.L., 1995. Principal phenolic phytochemcials in selected California wines and their antioxidant activity in inhibiting oxidation of human low-density lipoprotein. *J. Agriculture and Food Chemistry*, 43: 890–894.

Girrotti, A.W., 1998. Lipid hydroperoxide generation, turnover and effector action in biological systems. *J. Lipid Res.*, 39: 1529–1542.

Jagetia, G.C., Baliga, M.S., Malagi, K.J. and Sethukumar, K.M., 2002. The evaluation of the radio protective effect of triphalā (an ayurvedic rejuvenating drug) in the mice exposed to gamma radiation. *Phytomedicine*, 9: 99–108.

Kakkar, P., Das, B. and Visvanathan, P.N., 1984. A modified spectrophotometric assay of superoxide dismutase. *Ind. J. Biochem. Biophys.*, 211: 131–132.

Khopde, S.M., Indira Priyadarsini, K., Mohan, H., Gawandi, V.B., Satav, J.G., Yakhmi, J.V., Banavaliker, M.M. Biyani, M.K. and Mittal, J.P. Characterizing the antioxidant activity of amla (*Phyllanthus emblica*) extract. *Curr Sci.*, 18(2): 185–190.

Kirkland, D.J. and Muller, L., 2000. Interpretation of the biological relevance of genotoxicity test results: the importance of thresholds, *Mutat Res.*, 464: 47–147.

Koneru, B., Reddy, M.C., Dela Torre, A.N., Patel, D., Ippolito, T. and Ferranate, R.J., 1995. Studies of warm ischemia in the obese zucker rat. *Transplant.*, 59: 942–946.

Lamers, J.M.J., Hartog, J.M., Verdouw, P.D., Hulsmann, W.C., 1987. Dietary fatty acids and myocardial function. *Basic Res. Cardiol.*, 81: 209–221.

Mc Duffee, A.T., Senisterra, G., Huntley, S., Lepock, J.R., Sekhar., K.R., Meredith, M.J., Borrell, M.J., Morrow, J.D, and Freeman, M.L., 1997. Proteins containing non-native disulfide bonds by oxidative stress can act as signals for the induction of the heart shock response. *J. Cell Phy.*, 171: 143–151.

Montilla, P., Espejo, I., Munox, M.C., Bujalance, I., Munoz-Castaneda, J.R. and Tunez, I., 2006. Protective effect of red wine on oxidative stress and antioxidant enzyme activities in the brain and kidney induced by feeding high cholesterol in rats. *Clin. Nutr.*, 25: 146–153.

Nichens, W.G. Jr. and Samuelson, B., 1968. Formulation of malondialdehyde from phospholipids arachidonate during microsomal lipid peroxidation. *Eur. J. Biochem.*, 6: 126–130.

Ohrvall, M., Tengblad, S. and Vessby, B., 1993. Lower tocopherol serum levels in subjects with abdominal adiposity. *J. Intern. Med.*, 234: 53–60.

Pratt, I.S. and Barron, T., 2003. Regulatory recognition of indirect genotoxicity mechanisms in the European union. *Toxicol. Lett.*, 140–141: 53–62.

Reid, M.B., Shoji, T., Mody, M.R. and Entman, M.L., 1992. Reactive oxygen in skeletal muscle. II. Extra cellular release of free radicals. *J. Appl. Physiol.*, 73: 1805–1809.

Rice-Evans, L.A., Millar, N.J. and Paganga, G., 1997. Antioxidant properties of phenolic compounds. *Trends in Plant Sci.*, 4: 304–309.

Russo, C., Oliviri, O., Girelli, D., Faccini, g., Zenari, M.L., Lombardi, S. and Corrocher, R., 1998. Anti-oxidant status and lipid peroxidation in patients with essential hypertension. *J. Hypertens.*, 16: 1267–1271.

Sinha, K.A., 1972. Colorimetric assay of catalase. *Anal Biochem.*, 47: 389–394.

Srivastava, R.D., Dwivedi, S., Sreenivasan, K.K. and Chandrasekar, C.N., 1991. Cardiovascular effects of *Terminalia* species of plants. *Indian Drugs*, 29(4): 144–149.

Steinberg, D., 1997. A critical look at the evidence for the oxidation of LDL in atherogenesis. *Antheroscelerosis*, 13: 5–7.

Sundaram, R.K., Bhaskar, A., Vijayalingam, S., Viswanathan, M., Mohan, R. and Shanmugasundram, K.R., 1996. Anti oxidant status and lipid peroxidation in type 2 diabetes mellitus with and without complications. *Clin. Sci.* 90: 255–260.

Turrens, J.F., 1997. Superoxide production by the mitochondrial respiratory chain. *Biosci. Res.*, 17: 3–8.

Vincent, H.K., Powers, S.K., Stewart, D.S., Demirel, H., Shanely, A. and Naito, H., 1998. Obesity and myocardial oxidative stress. *Int. J. Obes. Relat. Metab. Disord.*, 22: 1–8.

WHO, 1998. *World Health Report, Life in the 21st century: A Vision for All*. Geneva, pp. 132.

Yu, B., 1994. Cellular defense against damage from reactive oxygen species. *Phys. Rev.*, 74: 139–162.

Chapter 13

Study of Age Related Changes in the Activity of Some Metabolic Enzymes in *Cyprinus carpio* as Biomarkers

K.L. Jain, Meenakshi Jindal and Simmi*

Department of Zoology and Aquaculture,
Haryana Agricultural University, Hisar – 125 004, Haryana, India

ABSTRACT

Age and growth related changes in liver composition and metabolic enzyme activities are interlinked with toxicity in various water resources. The activity of metabolic enzymes, Succinate dehydrogenase (SDH), Glutamate dehydrogenase (GDH) and Pyruvate dehydrogenase (PDH) in liver and serum of fish *Cyprinus carpio* showed a significant variation with different growth periods. The SDH enzyme activity increased rapidly from 70 days old fish to 100 days old fish, as indicated by the mean values of 0.244 µg and 0.394 µg of formazan formed/mg of protein/h, respectively, which was almost double in 100 days. Likewise activity of GDH, increased from 0.199 µg in 70 days old fish to 0.229 µg of formazan formed/mg of protein/h in 100 days old fish, the increase was only from 11.3 to 41.1 per cent in this growth period. In liver, PDH showed a significant increase from 40 days old fish to 70 days old fish. The mean values were 0.205 µg in 40 days and 0.240 µg

---

* Corresponding author: E-mail: meenjind@gmail.com

of formazan formed/mg of protein/h in 70 days, with an increase of 17.1 per cent. The PDH activity in serum, however, remained similar during the growth period from 70 to 100 days. The mean activity values for a 40 days old fish was 0.209 μg and 0.329 μg of formazan formed/mg of protein/h for130 days old fish, *i.e.* an increase from 19.6 per cent in 40 days to 57.4 per cent in 130 days old fish. The increase and decrease in the activity of metabolic enzymes is a clear cut evidence of changes in the metabolic environment of the fish which may be due to age or stress as both these parameters influence dietary intake.

Keywords: *Age, Growth, SDH, GDH, PDH, Liver, Serum.*

Introduction

Waste generation due to the expansion of industrial activity in India has a serious impact on the water resources. Rivers, lakes, reservoirs close to the industries continue to be dirty and contaminated resulting in the decline of the quality of the water. This problem is persisting and cannot be ignored given that it can have a serious long-term impact on the national economy and human health, particularly due to global fisheries which is facing constant decline in fish population. Several environmental factors known to affect fish condition vary throughout the year. Early life stage mortality and decreasing reproductive success are of special importance because their occurrence is not easily detected and alterations in population structures and abundance may only be perceived over the long term. Growth in fishes and pollution are the inter-related terms. As the growth and size of fish increases the impact of pollutants also increases. Growth in mass, infect is likely to influence metabolic capacity when growing fish restores protein stores including some soluble enzymes, but enzymes which actually increase as a result of growth may not be directly involved in the growth process, although their increased activities may facilitate future growth. Growth in length partially involves different physiological processes than growth in mass, as the former employees the synthesis of structural molecule, while the important part of growth in mass may be due to the restoration and accumulation of energy resources.

Age and growth related changes in liver composition and metabolic enzyme activities are interlinked with toxicity in various water resources. Physiological parameters tell us how the various enzyme activities change in different tissues of vertebrates according to their age and growth. Changes in enzymatic activities with age are thus evident and these could be well correlated with metabolic requirement of the fish as well as with the environmental stress or any other such factor, which needs to be worked out in fish commonly employed as test animals. This study was aimed to study activity of some enzymes in *Cyprinus carpio* being applied as biomarkers.

The activity of metabolic enzymes, Succinate dehydrogenase (SDH), Glutamate dehydrogenase (GDH) and Pyruvate dehydrogenase (PDH) in liver and serum showed a significant variation with different growth periods. The SDH enzyme activity increased rapidly from 70 days old fish to 100 days old fish, which was almost double. Likewise, the GDH and PDH enzymes also showed an increase in activity with age. The increase and decrease in the activity of metabolic enzymes is a clear cut evidence of changes in the metabolic environment of the fish which may be due to age or stress as both these parameters influence dietary intake.

Materials and Methods

The fish seed of approximately 3 to 5 cm were cultured in a local fish farm located at Hindwaan village, in months of June to October. The fish sampling at different periods of growth starting after 40 days were first made in the month of June until October. The healthy specimens of *C. carpio* of variable age as depicted by their size ranging from 10 to 25cm were procured and their length and weight were measured. The fish were anesthetized with MS-222 and dissected for liver, for the estimations of activity of enzymes *i.e.* SDH, GDH and PDH in liver and the blood serum, following the methods, given by Nachlas *et al.* (1960) and using enzyme specific substrates.

Results and Discussion

Succinate dehydrogenase (SDH), Glutamate dehydrogenase (GDH) and Pyruvate dehydrogenase (PDH) in liver and serum (Tables 13.1 and 13.2) showed a significant variation with different growth periods.

Table 13.1: Age Related Changes in Succinate Dehydrogenase (SDH), Glutamate Dehydrogenase (GDH), Pyruvate Dehydrogenase (PDH) (µg of formazan formed/mg of protein/h) in Liver of Fish *Cyprinus carpio*

Age (Days)	*SDH*		*GDH*		*PDH*	
	Mean	*S.E*	*Mean*	*S.E*	*Mean*	*S.E*
40	0.196	0.006	0.184	0.003	0.205	0.004
70	0.244* (24.5)	0.016	0.199 (8.15)	0.002	0.240 (17.1)	0.004
100	0.394 (101.0)	0.037	0.229 (24.4)	0.007	0.268 (30.7)	0.004
130	0.503 (156.6)	0.016	0.258 (40.2)	0.006	0.321 (56.5)	0.012
CD (5 per cent)		0.045		0.008		0.014
F-cal		100.92		200.07		126.0

* Values in parentheses are percent increase in SDH, GDH and PDH enzyme activity in liver over the 40 days growth.

Table 13.2: Age Related Changes in Succinate Dehydrogenase (SDH), Glutamate Dehydrogenase (GDH), Pyruvate Dehydrogenase (PDH) (µg of formazan formed/mg of protein/h) in Serum of Fish *Cyprinus carpio*

Age (Days)	*SDH*		*GDH*		*PDH*	
	Mean	*S.E*	*Mean*	*S.E*	*Mean*	*S.E*
40	0.206	0.008	0.185	0.004	0.209	0.005
70	0.242* (17.5)	0.005	0.206 (11.3)	0.004	0.250 (19.6)	0.005
100	0.346 (67.9)	0.007	0.231 (24.8)	0.005	0.259 (23.9)	0.006
130	0.425 (106.3)	0.013	0.261 (41.08)	0.005	0.329 (57.4)	0.006
CD (5 per cent)		0.011		0.003		0.003
F-cal		910.25		1430.60		2475.08

* Values in parentheses are percent increase in SDH, GDH and PDH enzyme activity in liver over the 40 days growth.

The enzyme activity of SDH in liver increased rapidly from 70 days old fish to 100 days old fish; as indicated by the mean values of 0.244 µg and 0.394 µg of formazan formed/mg of protein/h, respectively, which has been almost double (Table 13.1). Likewise, in serum SDH also showed rapid increase from 70 days old fish *i.e.* 0.242 µg to 0.346 µg of formazan formed/mg of protein/h in100 days (Table 13.2). Likewise activity of GDH, increased from 0.199 µg in 70 days old fish to 0.229 µg of formazan formed/mg of protein/h in 100 days old fish, the increase was only from 11.3 to 41.1 per cent in this growth period. In liver, PDH showed a significant increase from 40 days old fish to 70 days old fish. The mean values were 0.205 µg in 40 days and 0.240 µg of formazan formed/mg of protein/h in 70 days, with an increase of 17.1 per cent. The PDH activity in serum, however, remained similar during the growth period from 70 to 100 days. The mean activity values for a 40 days old fish was 0.209 µg and 0.329 µg of formazan formed/mg of protein/h for130 days old fish (Table 13.2), *i.e.* an increase from 19.6 per cent in 40 days to 57.4 per cent in 130 days old fish.

Metabolic enzymes studied in liver and serum such as SDH, GDH and PDH showed a strong relationship of their activity with growth rate both in length and mass, than with condition factor (Tables 13.3 and 13.4). SDH varied with growth in length 89 per cent and 87 per cent growth in mass in liver and varied with growth in mass up to 93.2 per cent and in length up to 92 per cent as compared to condition factor (R^2=0.553, p<0.0001) in serum. The condition factor, however, also increased significantly, but up to 64 per cent only variability, in enzyme activity in liver. Among the metabolic enzymes in liver and in serum, PDH alone showed highest variability of 95 per cent with growth in length in serum and 68 per cent variability with condition factor in serum. All the variables examined, showed a positive correlation with growth rate in serum (Table 13.4). Condition factor showed the highest variability with GDH in serum (R^2=0.553, p<0.0001). In liver, GDH showed the same percent of variability in growth rate in length and in mass *i.e.* 89 per cent. Regression line represents the regression equation between dehydrogenases enzyme activity and growth in length and mass are shown in Figure 13.1 and 13.2 in liver and Figures 13.4 and 13.5 in serum. The regression lines for condition factor vs SDH, GDH and PDH were shown in Figure 13.3 in liver and Figure 13.6 in serum of fish *C. carpio*.

Figure 13.1: Regression Line for Growth in Length and Activities of Succinate Dehydrogenase (SDH), Glutamate Dehydrogenase (GDH), Pyruvate Dehydegenase (PDH) in the Liver of Fish *Cyprinus carpio*

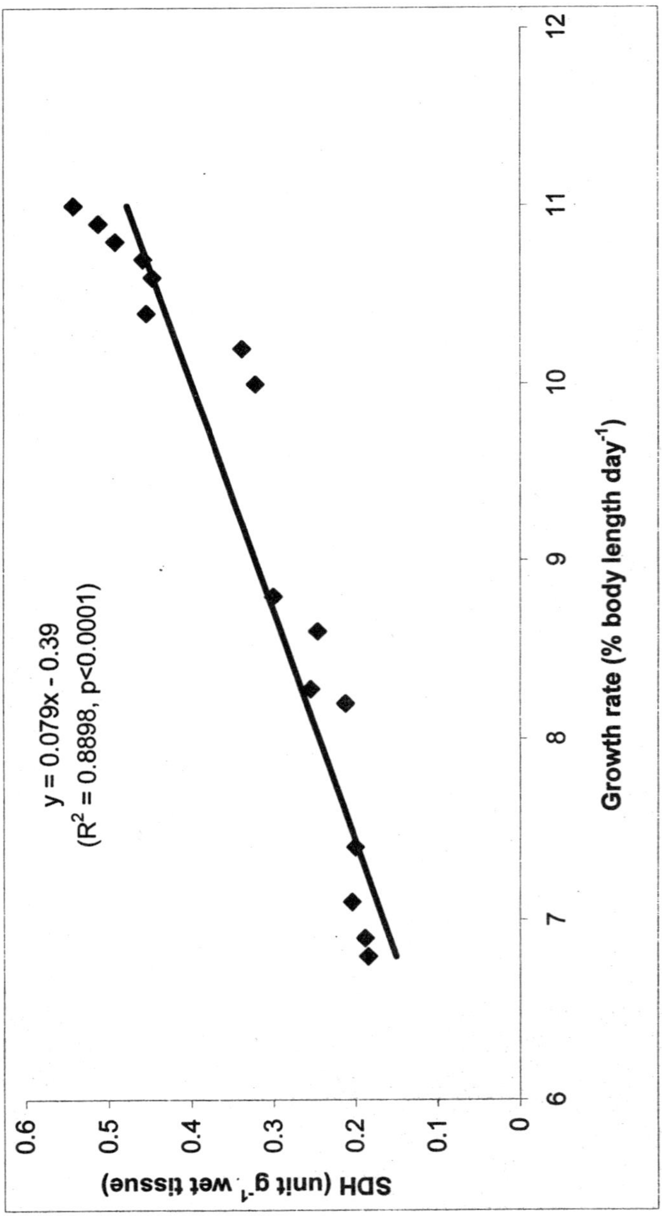

Contd...

Figure 13.1–Contd...

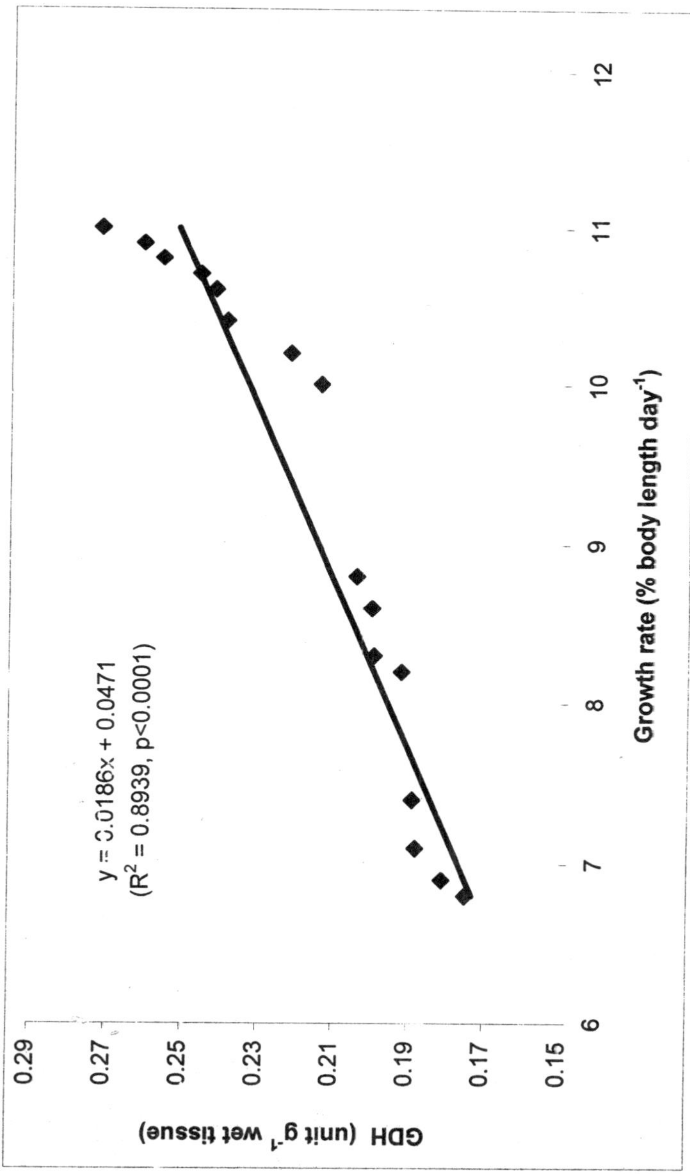

Contd...

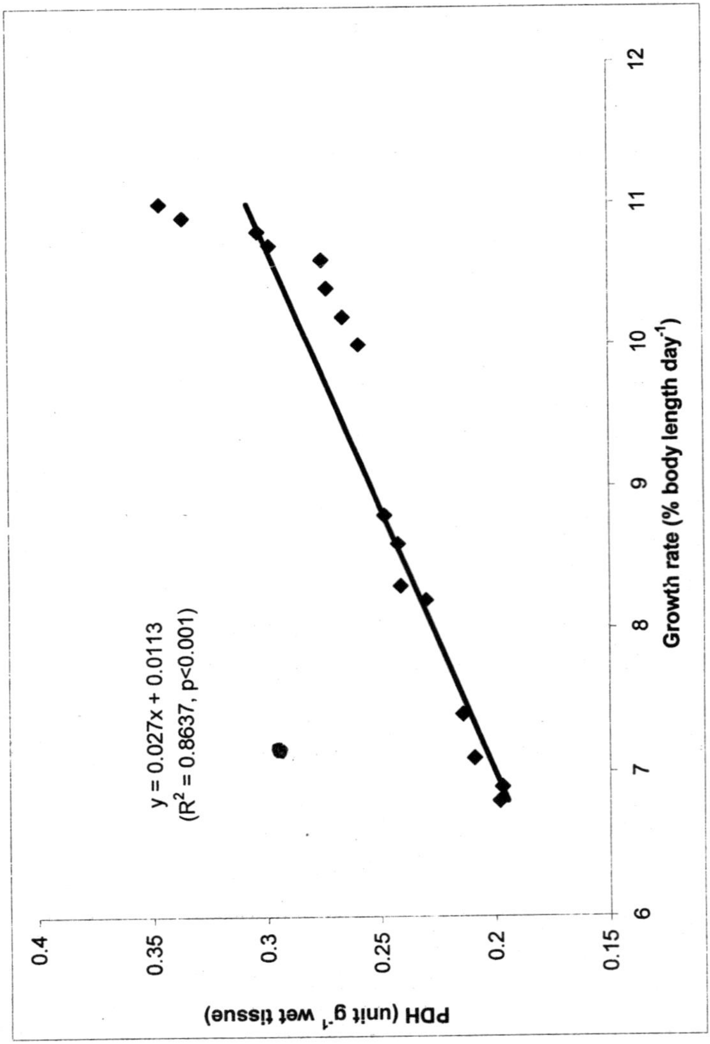

Figure 13.1–Contd...

Figure 13.2: Regression Line for Growth in Mass and Activities of Succinate Dehydrogenase (SDH), Glutamate Dehydrogenase (GDH), Pyruvate Dehydegenase (PDH) in the Liver of Fish *Cyprinus carpio*

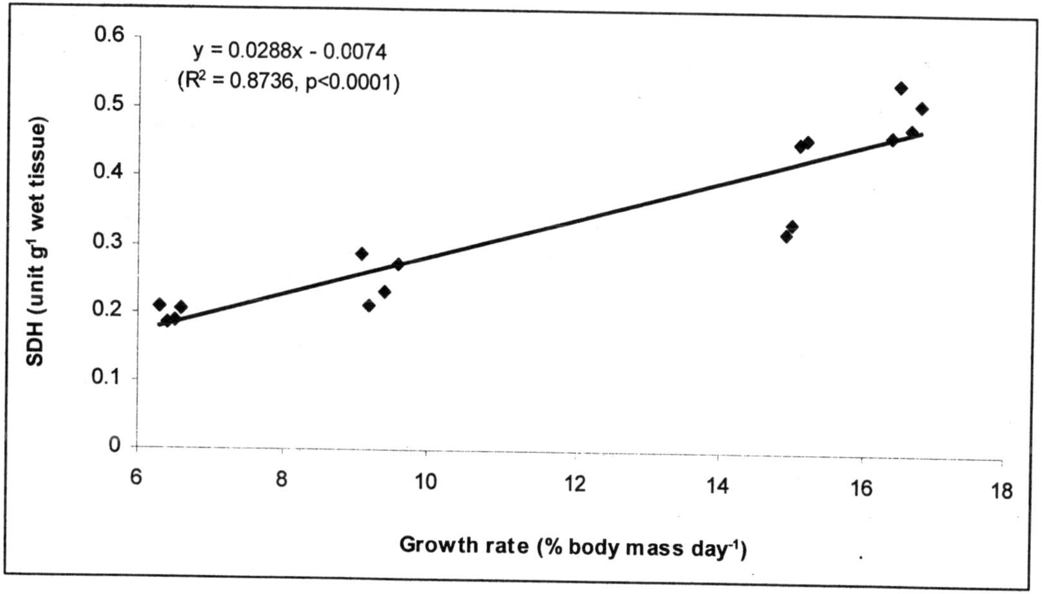

Contd...

Contd...

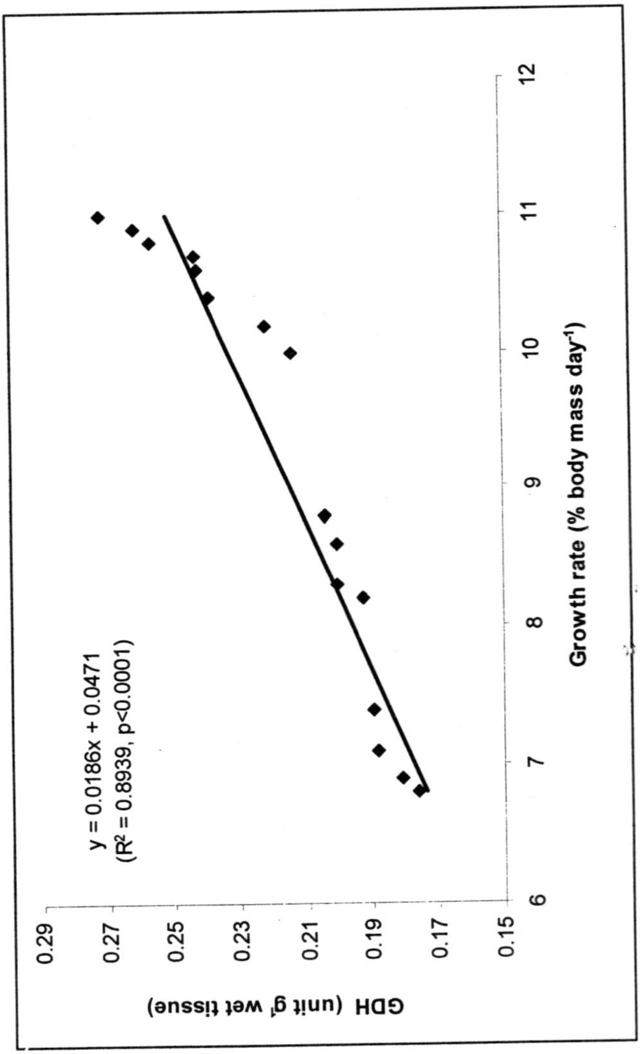

Figure 13.2–Contd...

Figure 13.2: Regression Line for Growth in Mass and Activities of Succinate Dehydrogenase (SDH), Glutamate Dehydrogenase (GDH), Pyruvate Dehydegenase (PDH) in the Liver of Fish *Cyprinus carpio*

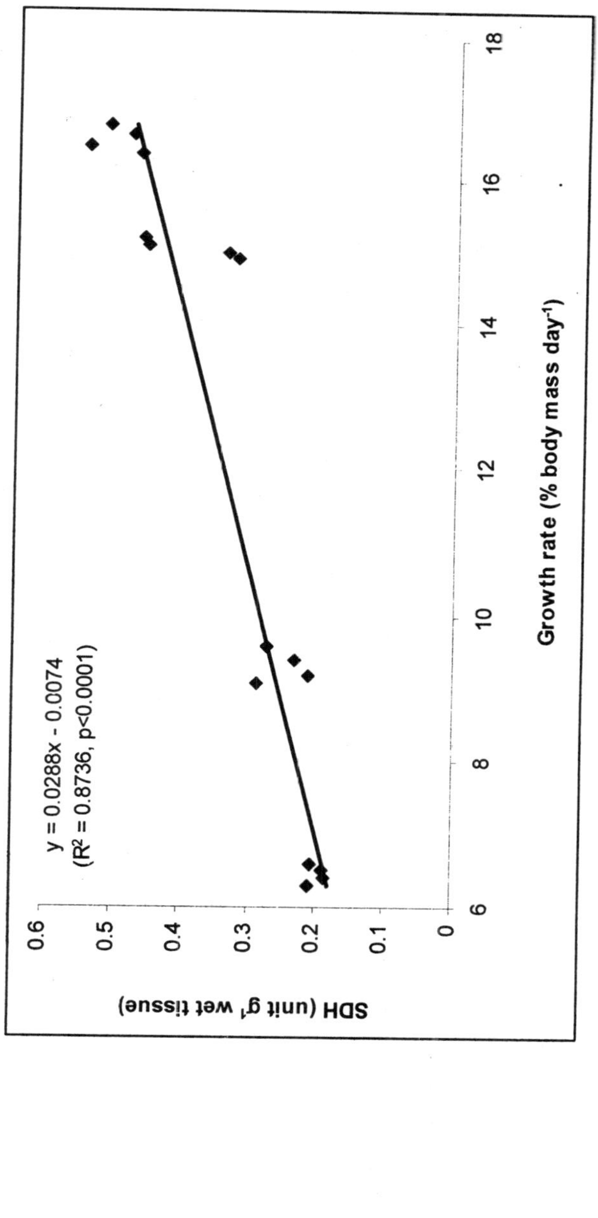

Contd...

Figure 13.2–Contd...

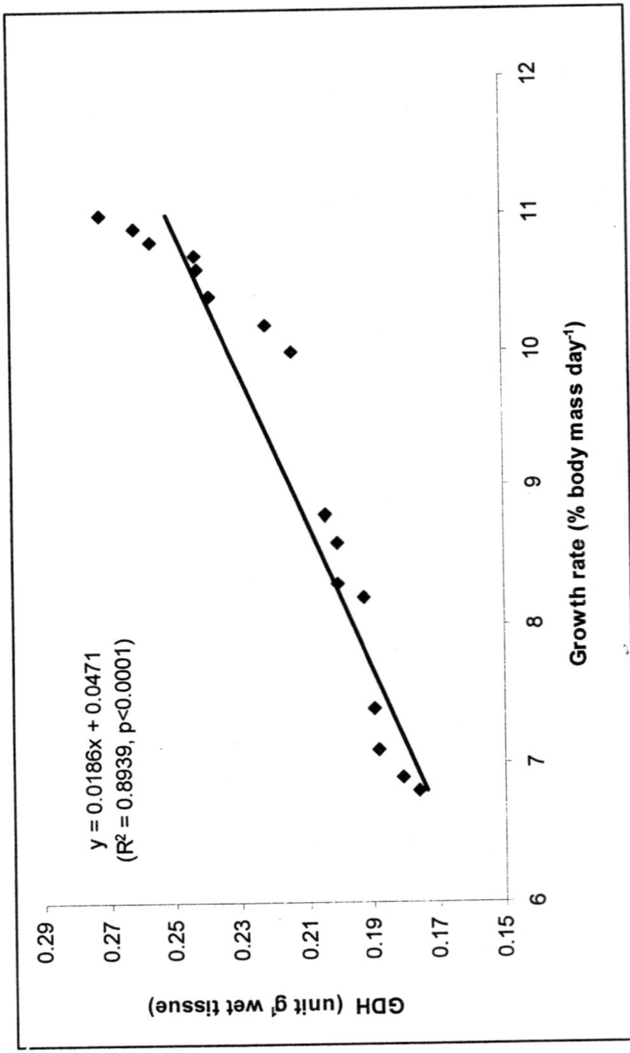

Contd...

Figure 13.2–Contd...

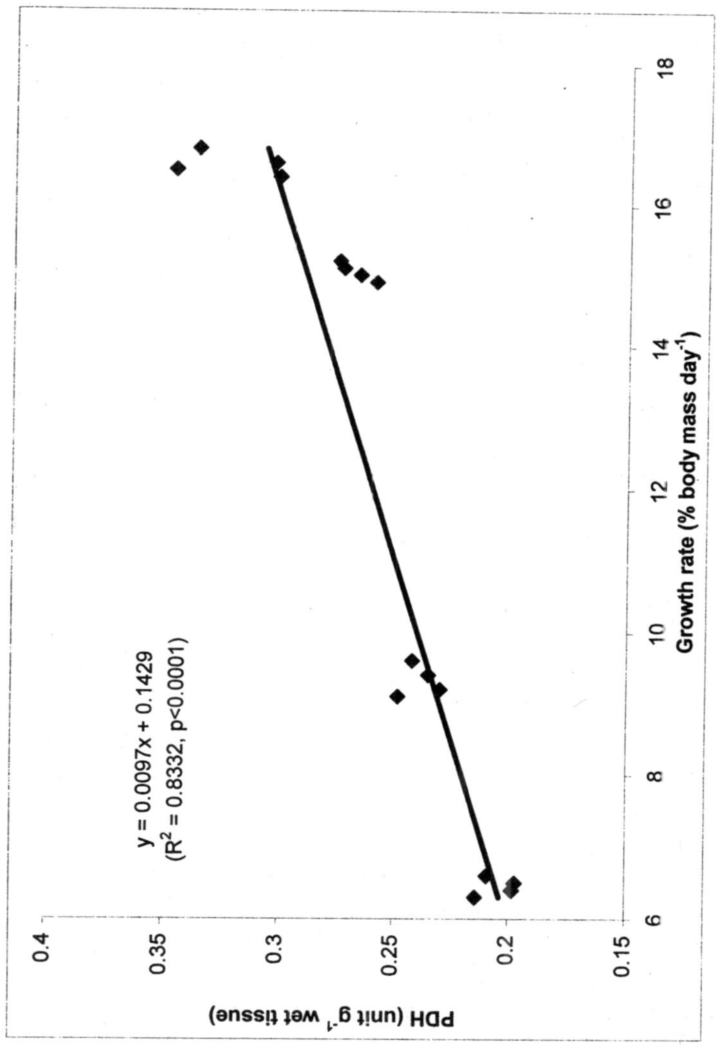

Table 13.3: Linear Regression Between the Dehydrogenases Enzyme Activity (units/g wet tissue) and Growth in Length, Mass and Condition Factor in Liver of Fish *Cyprinus carpio*

Variables	*Growth in Length (per cent gain/day)*	*Growth in Mass (per cent gain/day)*	*Condition Factor*
Succinate dehydrogenase	Y=-0.390+0.079GL (R^2=0.889)*	Y=-0.007+0.029GM (R^2=0.873)	Y=0.725-0.232CF (R^2=0.521)
Glutamate dehydrogenase	Y=0.047+0.0185GL (R^2=0.894)	Y=0.047+0.018GM (R^2=0.894)	Y=0.312-0.056CF (R^2=0.554)
Pyruvate dehydrogenase	Y=0.011+0.127GL (R^2=0.863)	Y=0.143+0.009GM (R^2=0.833)	Y=0.484-0.089CF (R^2=0.641)

* Level of significance is $p<0.0001$.

* Values in parentheses are percent increase in SDH, GDH and PDH enzyme activity in serum over the 40 days growth.

Table 13.4: Linear Regression Between the Dehydrogenases Enzyme Activity (units/g wet tissue) and Growth in Length, Mass and Condition Factor in Serum of Fish *Cyprinus carpio*

Variables	*Growth in Length (per cent gain/day)*	*Growth in Mass (per cent gain/day)*	*Condition Factor*
Succinate dehydrogenase	Y=-0.204+0.055GL (R^2=0.922)*	Y=0.062+0.020GM (R^2=0.926)	Y=0.582-0.165CF (R^2=0.553)
Glutamate dehydrogenase	Y=0.051+0.018GL R^2=0.913)	Y=0.142+0.006GM (R^2=0.869)	Y=0.320-0.059CF (R^2=0.631)
Pyruvate dehydrogenase	Y=0.0005+0.029GL (R^2=0.956)	Y=0.144+0.010GM (R^2=0.916)	Y=0.430-0.095CF (R^2=0.689)

* Level of significance is $p<0.0001$.

* Values in parentheses are percent increase in SDH, GDH and PDH enzyme activity in serum over the 40 days growth.

Fish Growth and Enzyme Activity

The study evidence highest increase in SDH, GDH and PDH enzyme activities in 130 days old fish in both in the liver and the serum of *C. carpio* (Tables 13.1 and 13.2) thereby, showing a maximum increase up to 156.6, 40 and 56.5 lowest in liver SDH, GDH and PDH enzyme activity respectively and 106.3, 41.1 and 57.4 lowest respectively in serum enzyme activity. Likewise the activities of

Figure 13.3: Regression Line for Condition Factor and Succinate Dehydrogenase (SDH), Glutamate Dehydrogenase (GDH) and Pyruvate Dehydegenase (PDH) in the Liver of Fish *Cyprinus carpio*

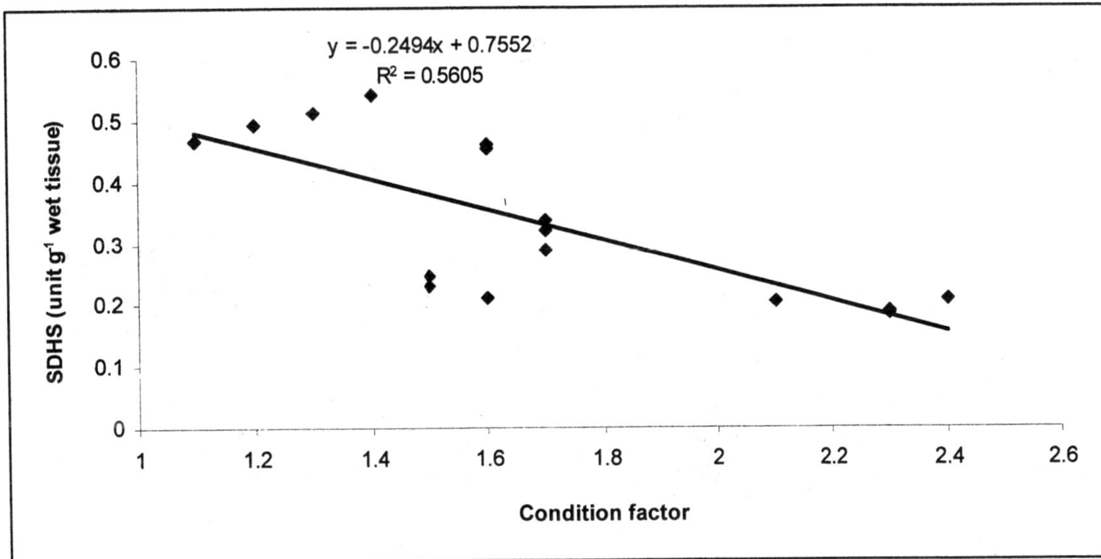

Contd...

Contd...

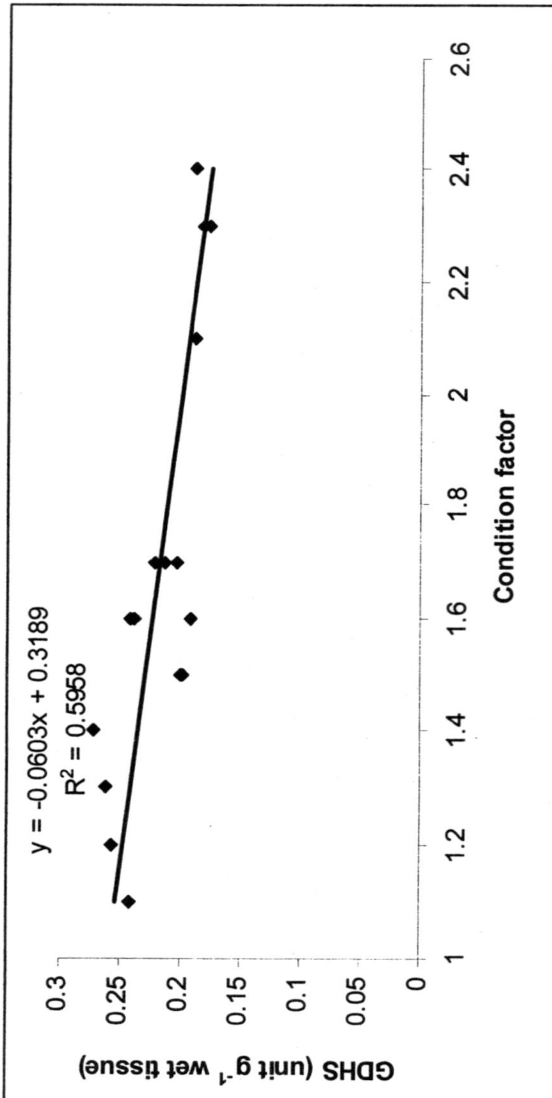

Figure 13.3–Contd...

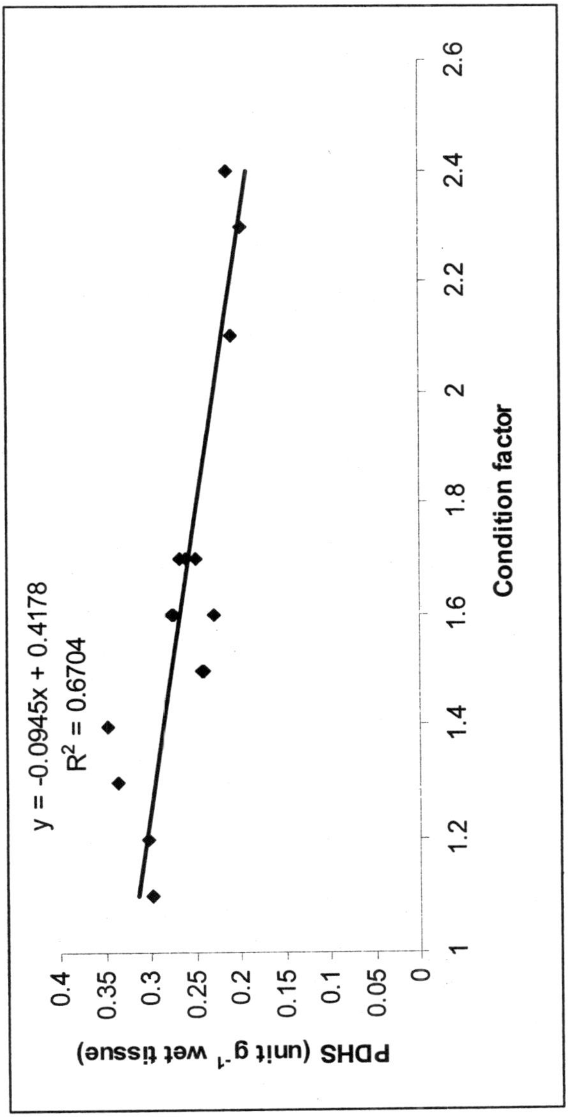

Figure 13.3–Contd...

Figure 13.4: Regression Line for Growth in Length and Succinate Dehydrogenase (SDH), Glutamate Dehydrogenase (GDH), Pyruvate Dehydegenase (PDH) in the Serum in Fish *Cyprinus carpio*

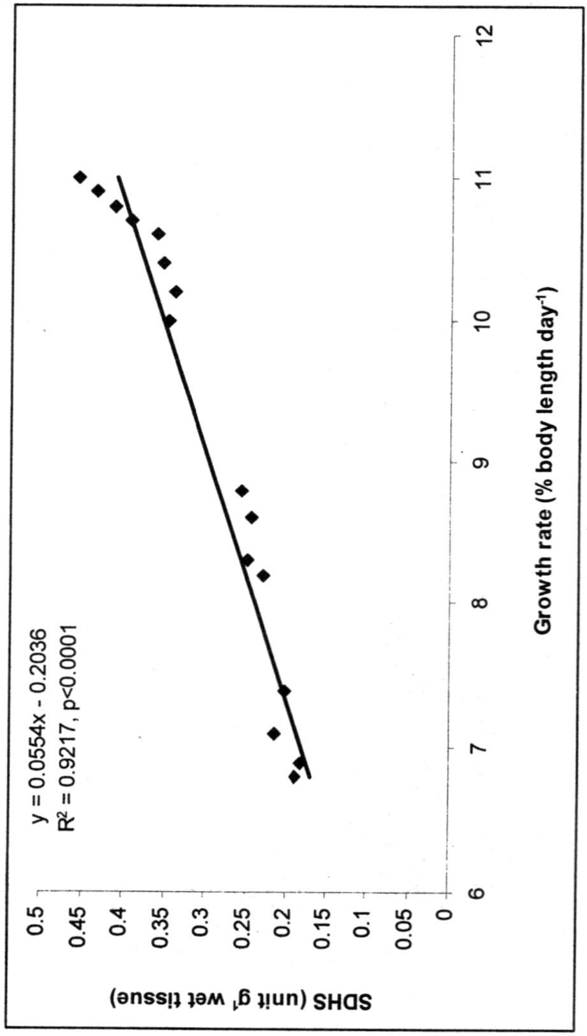

Contd...

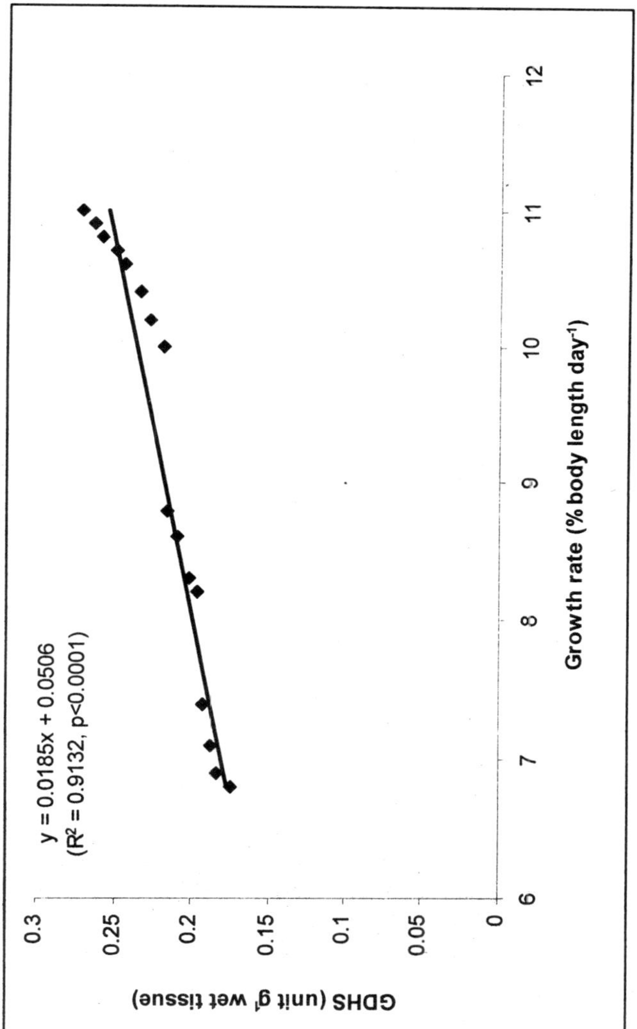

Figure 13.4–Contd...

Contd...

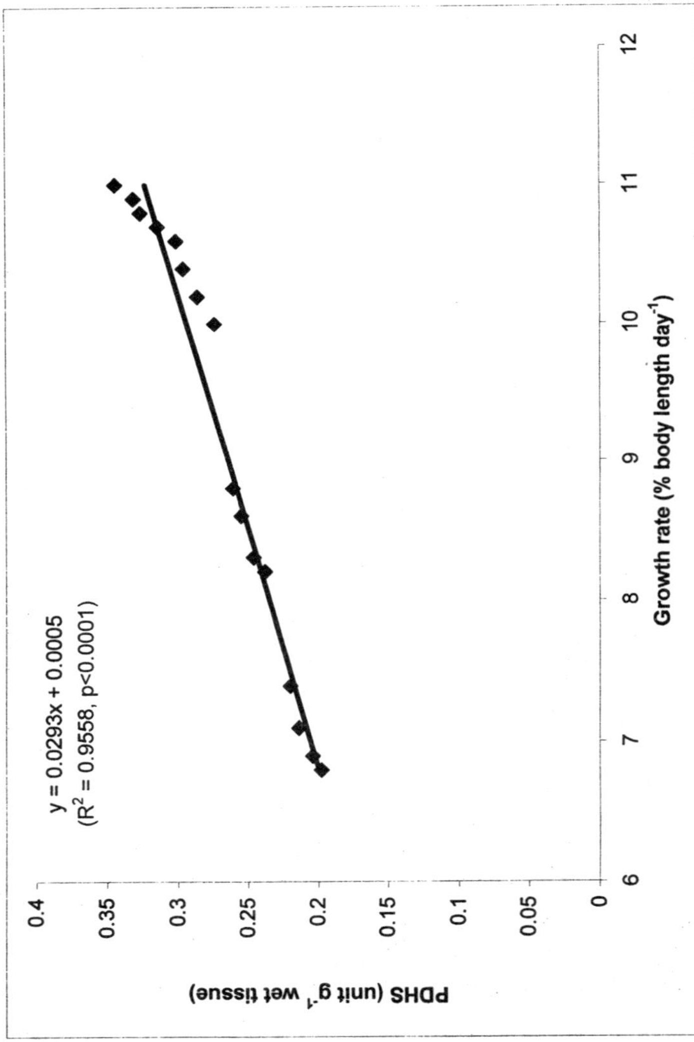

Figure 13.4–Contd...

Figure 13.5: Regression Line for Growth in Mass and Succinate Dehydrogenase (SDH), Glutamate Dehydrogenase (GDH), Pyruvate Dehydegenase (PDH) in the Serum of Fish *Cyprinus carpio*

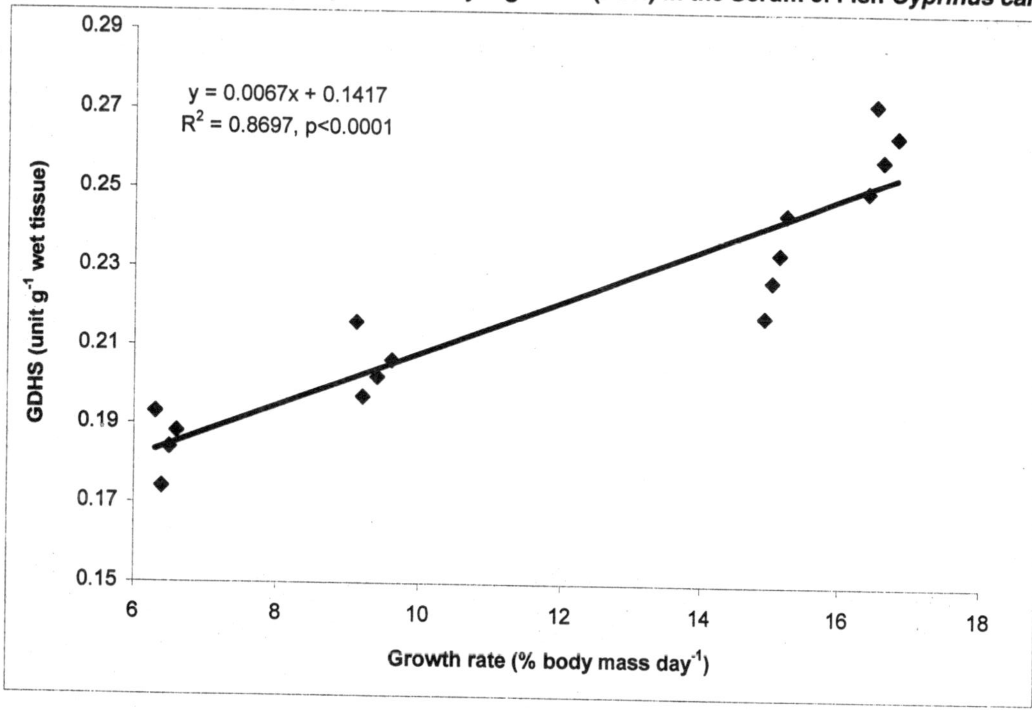

Contd...

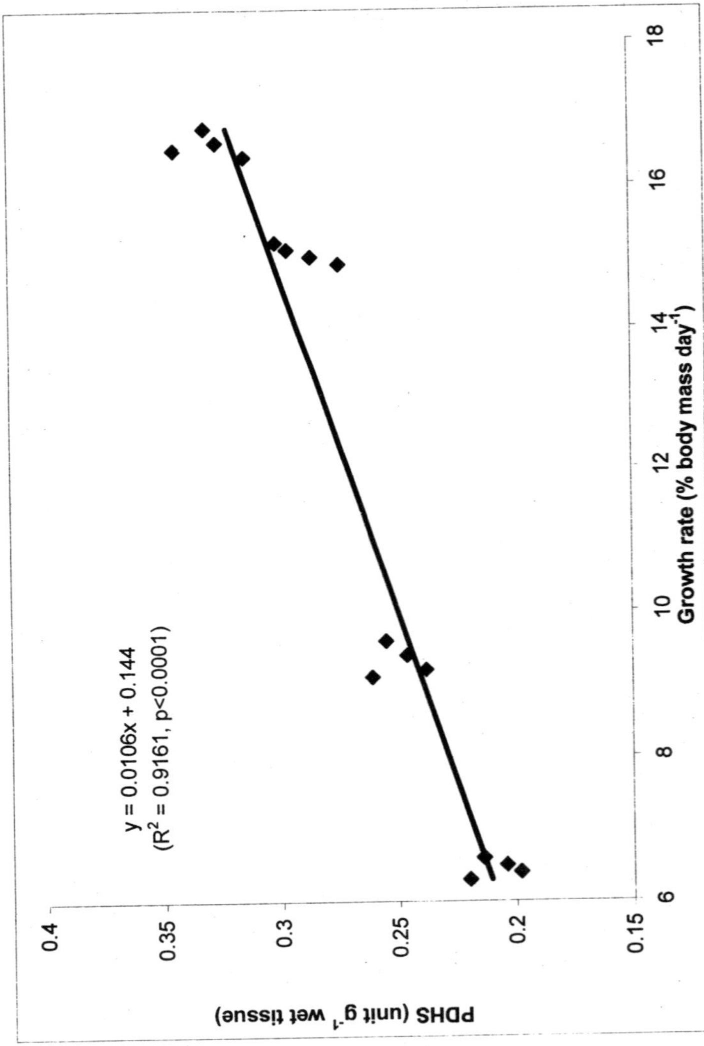

Figure 13.5–Contd...

Figure 13.6: Regression Line for Condition Factor and Succinate Dehydrogenase (SDH), Glutamate Dehydrogenase (GDH) and Pyruvate Dehydegenase (PDH) in the Serum of Fish *Cyprinus carpio*

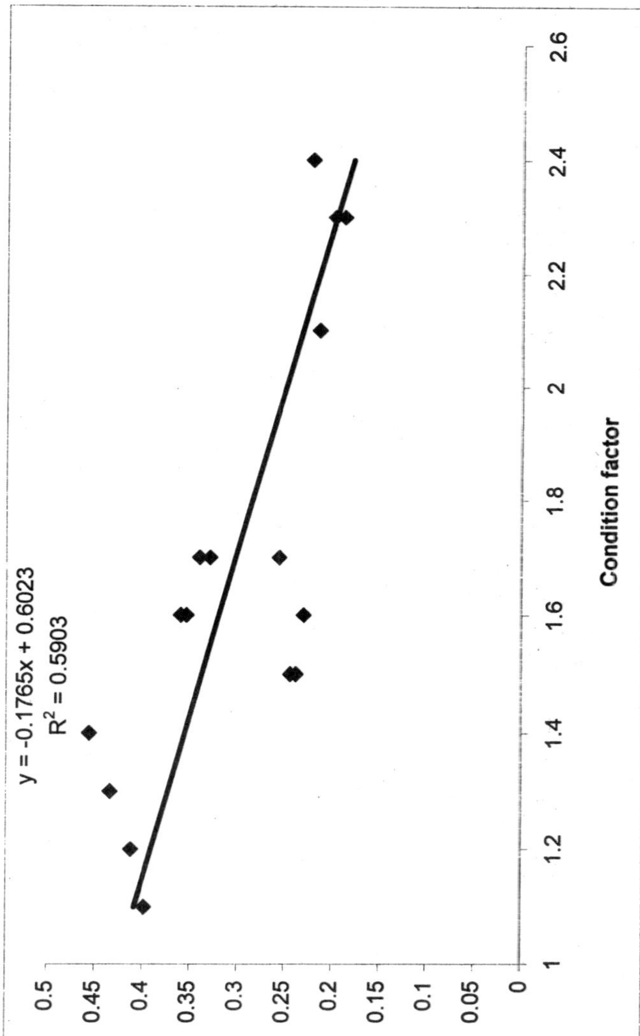

Contd...

Figure 13.6—Contd...

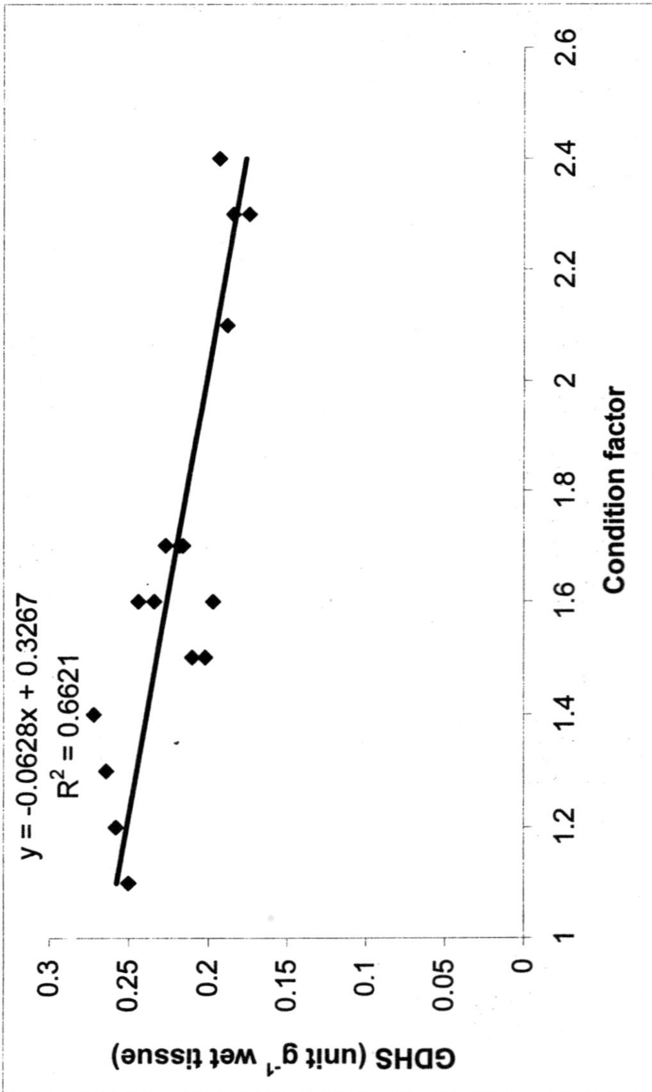

Contd...

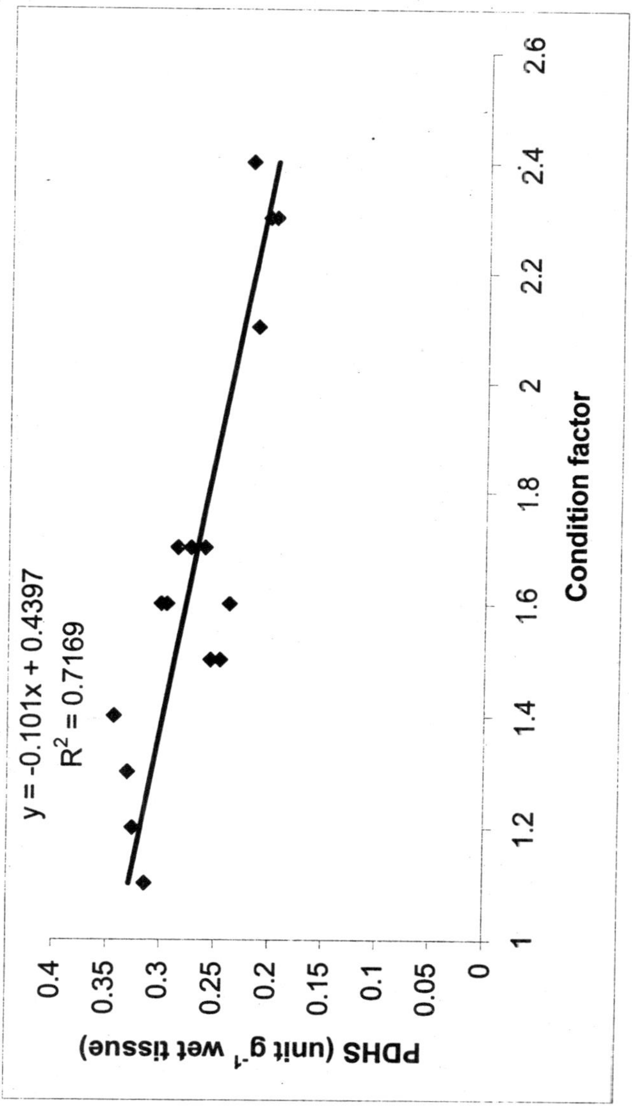

Figure 13.6–Contd...

phosphatases (Table 13.5) also revealed significantly high increase in acid and alkaline phosphatase activities after 100 days fish growth of *C. carpio*. The regression models for the activity of these enzymes and growth in length and mass further evidenced variability up to 89 per cent in dehydrogenases (Figures 13.1 and 13.2) and 95 per cent of phosphatases (Figures 13.7 and 13.8) in liver due to growth in the length of *C. carpio* fish. The variability explained for the changes in CF vs these enzymes was however, less correlated as it explained variability only up to 64 per cent due to dehydrogenases and 60 per cent due to phosphatases in liver of *C. carpio*. A similar pattern of variability and correlation were evident for these enzyme activity in the serum of the fish suggests that anaerobic metabolism was favoured over aerobic oxidation of glucose through Kreb's cycle in order to mitigate the energy crisis for survival.

Table 13.5: Linear Regression Between Phosphatases Enzyme Activity (units/g wet tissue) and Growth in Length, Mass and Condition Factor in Liver of Fish *Cyprinus carpio*

Variables	*Growth in Length (per cent gain/day)*	*Growth in Mass (per cent gain/day)*	*Condition Factor*
Acid phosphatase	Y=0.073+0.035x (R^2=0.952)*	Y=0.240+0.013x (R^2=0.945)	Y=0.564-0.103CF (R^2=0.568)
Alkaline phosphatase	Y=0.102+0.0341x (R^2=0.927)	Y=0.102+0.034x (R^2=0.927)	Y=0.592-0.105CF (R^2=0.595)

* Level of significance is $p<0.0001$.

Moon and Johnston (1980) determined changes in body index parameters and liver, red muscle and white muscle enzyme profiles in fed and four month starved fish plaice, *Pleuronectes platessa*. The results are compared to other vertebrates to estimate specific tissue metabolic patterns and changes in these patterns with starvation. Liver demonstrates the lowest glycolytic but highest gluconeogenic capacity of the three tissues. Red muscle has little, if any, gluconeogenic potential, based upon low activities of phosphoenol pyruvate carboxykinase and glucose-6-phosphatase and no detectable activities of pyruvate carboxylase. Plaice white skeletal muscle has the highest glycolytic potential of the tissues studied. Plaice starved for four months demonstrate significant reductions in liver-somatic index and red muscle-somatic index, and increases in tissue water contents. Enzyme activities generally decline in both

Figure 13.7: Regression Line for Growth in Length and Activities of Acid Phosphatase and Alkaline Phosphatase in the Liver of Fish *Cyprinus carpio*

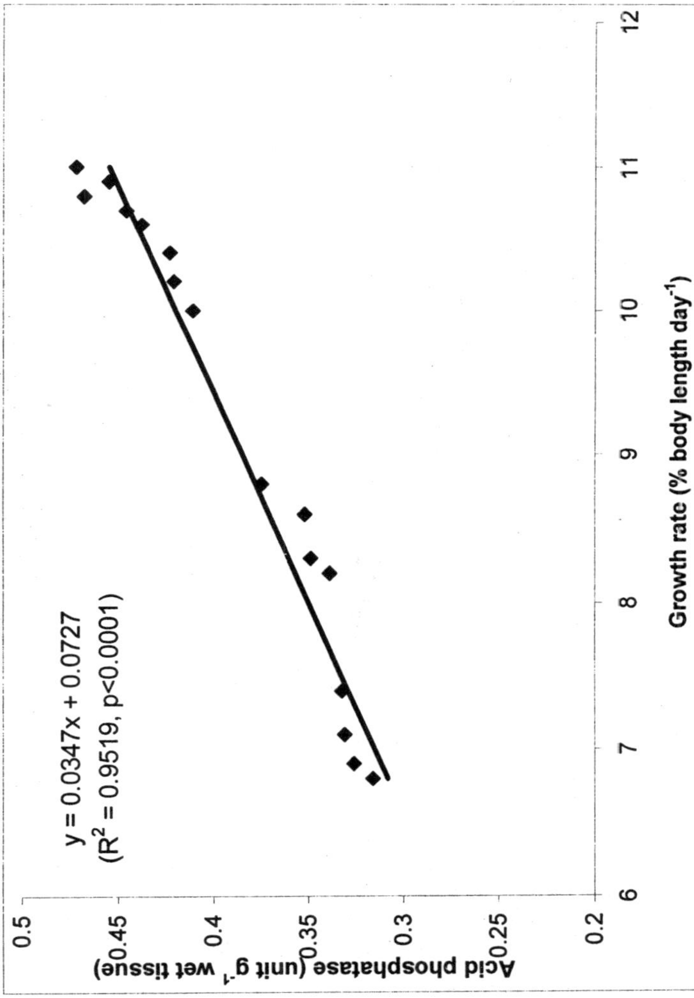

Contd...

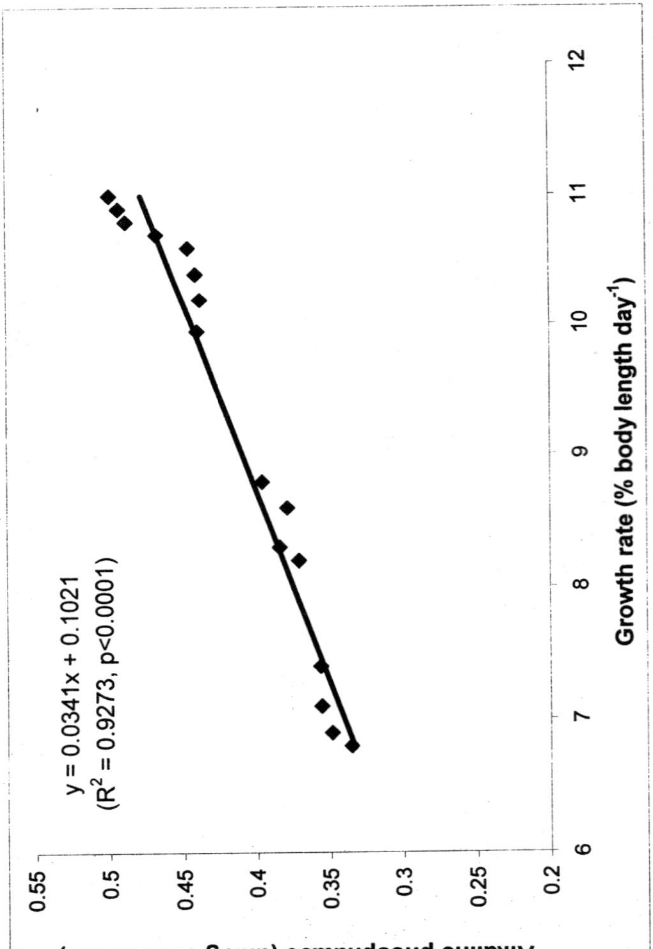

Figure 13.7–Contd...

Figure 13.8: Regression Line for Growth in Mass and Acid Phosphatase and Alkaline Phosphatase in the Liver of Fish *Cyprinus carpio*

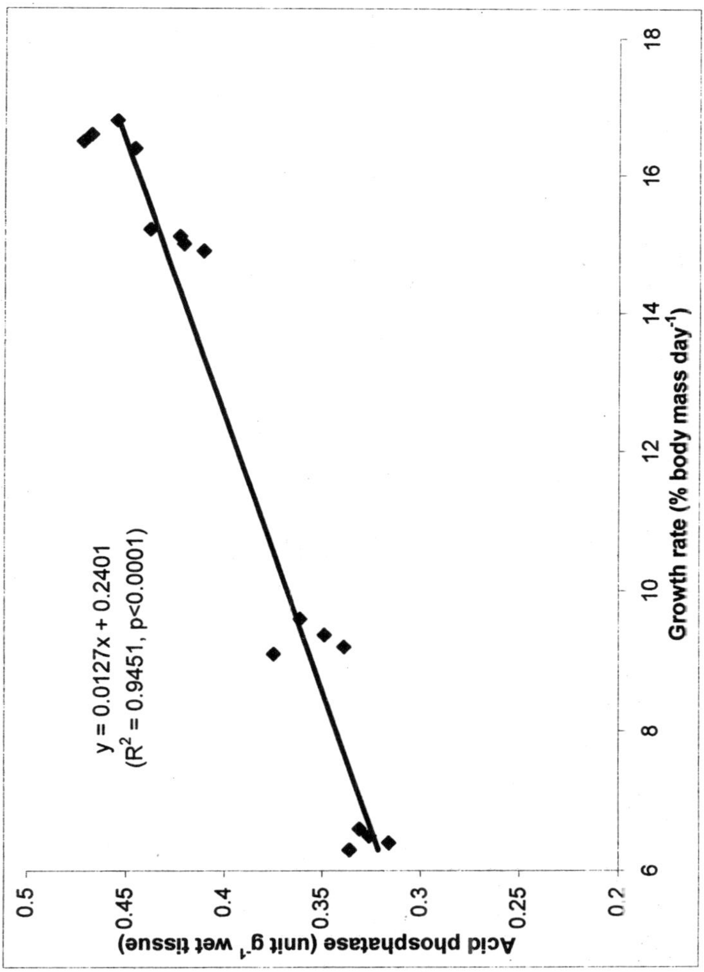

Contd...

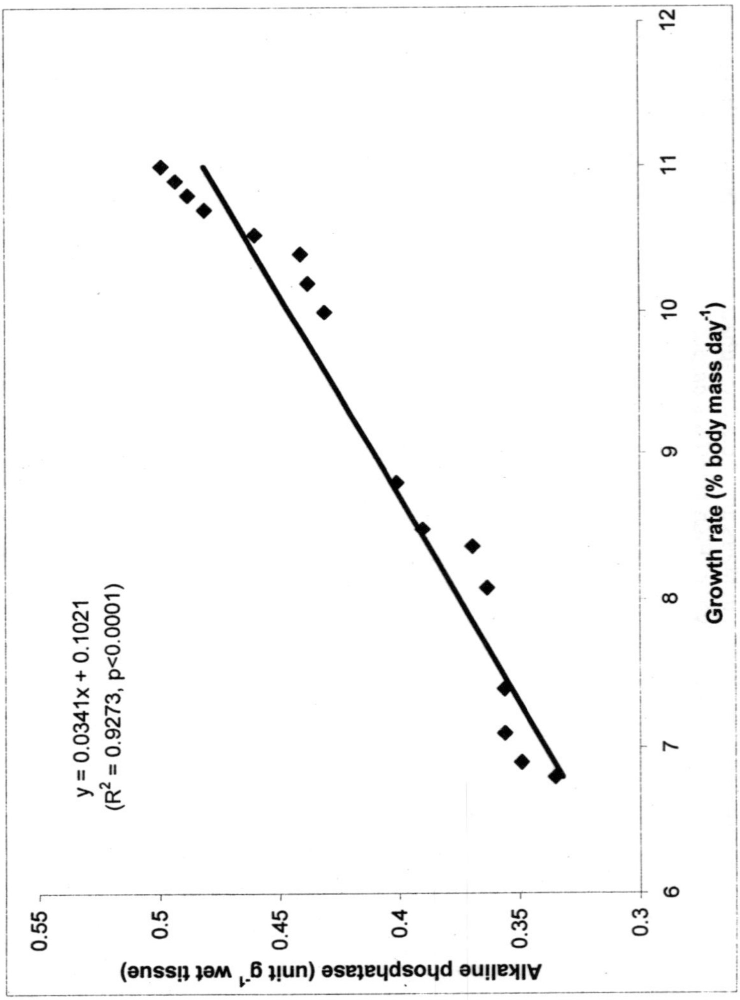

Figure 13.8–Contd...

muscle types, but are maintained in the liver. Activities of liver soluble phosphoenol pyruvate carboxykinase increased by approximately 8-fold, suggesting that the enzymatic response to starvation in plaice is similar to that of mammals.

The increase and decrease in the activity of metabolic enzymes a clear cut evidence of changes in the metabolic environment of the fish may be due to age or stress as both these parameters influence dietary intake. Sastry and Sharma (1980) observed increase in the level of serum enzymes namely glutamate-oxaloacetate transaminase and glutamate-pyruvate transaminase after acute exposure to mercury in *Channa punctatus*. Increased activities of these enzymes may be due to the damage of liver. Age and growth related changes in liver composition and metabolic enzyme activities are interlinked with toxicity in various water resources. Physiological parameters tell us how the various enzyme activities change in different tissues of vertebrates as according to their age and growth. Gould (1977) recorded increase in carbonic anhydrase activity in flounders, after their exposure to cadmium, probably because of increased requirement for CO_2 transportation through blood under stress. Christesen and Tucker (1976) however, reported a strong inhibition by heavy metals including Cadmium of carbonic anhydrase from mild fish erythrocytes when measured in erythrocytes. This enzyme inhibition was attributed to replacement of Zinc from the enzyme by the toxic metal, thereby reducing their enzyme activity. Gill *et al.* (1991) observed heterogeneity in the response of alkaline phosphatase in various organs in the freshwater sybarite fish on exposure to Cadmium. They demonstrated that alkaline phosphatase was unaffected in liver and gills, stimulation in kidney and ovary and inhibited in the gills. Bay *et al.* (1990) in marine scorpion fish on long term exposures to Cadmium was also said to show more changes in the alkaline phosphatase, succinate dehydrogenase, glyceraldehydes phosphate dehydrogenase in several tissues. Heterogeneity in enzyme activity was also reported by Shaffi, 1993 who recorded greatest inhibition in LDH, SDH and MDH in certain freshwater fishes in liver with progressively less inhibition in muscles, brain, kidney and gill after their exposure to mercury. Seasonal variations in condition indices and in liver metal concentrations have been reported for metal-polluted yellow perch (*Perca flavescens*) from the Sudbury area (Eastwood and Couture, 2002).

Conclusions

The increase and decrease in the activity of metabolic enzymes in fish liver and serum as indicated in this study is a clear evidence of changes in the metabolic environment of the fish as affected by its age since it influence dietary intake as well as change in body structure and function. This study shall provide a good evidence to apply these parameters as an index for estimating fish age in their juvenile stage and to correlate correctly with any health parameter in toxicological studies.

References

Bay, S., Greenstein, D., Szalay, P. and Brown, D., 1990. Exposure of scorpion fish (*Scopaena guttata*) to cadmium: Biochemical effects of chronic exposure. *Aquat. Toxicol.*, 16: 31.

Christesen, G.M. and Tucker, J.H., 1976. Effect of selected water toxicants on the *in vitro* activity of fish carbonic andydrase. *Chem. Biol. Interact.*, 13: 181-197.

Eastwood, S. and Couture, P., 2002. Seasonal variations in condition and liver metal concentrations of yellow perch (*Perca flavescens*) from a metal-contaminated environment. *Aquat. Toxicol.*, 58: 43–56.

Gill, T., Tewari, H. and Pande, J., 1991. *In vivo* and *in vitro* effect of cadmium on selected enzymes in different organ of the fish *Barbus conchonius* Ham. (Rosy barb). *Comp. Biochem. Physiol.*, 100C: 501.

Gould, E., 1977. Alteration of enzyme in winter flounder, *Pseudopleuronectes americanus*, exposed to sublethal amounts of cadmium chloride. In: *Physiology Responses of Marine Biota to Pollutants*, (Eds.) F.J., Vernberg, A. Calabese, F.P. Thurberg and W.B. Vernberg. Academic Press, New York, p. 209.

Moon, T.W. and Johnston, I.A., 1980. Starvation and the activities of glycolytic and gluconeogenic enzymes in skeletal muscles and liver of the plaice, *Pleuronectes platessa*. *J. Comp. Physiol.*, 136: 31–38.

Nachlas, M.N., Margulies, S.I. and Seligman, A.M., 1960. A clorimetric method for the estimation of succinate dehydrogenase activity. *J. Biol. Chem.* 235: 499-503.

Sastry, K.V. and Sharma, S.K., 1978. The effect of *in vivo* exposure of endrin on the activities of acid, alkaline and glucose-6-phosphatases in liver and kidney of *Opheocephalus* and *Channa punctatus*). *Bull. Environ. Contam. Toxicol.*, 20(4): 456-460.

Shaffi, S., 1993. Comparison of the sublethal effect of mercury and lead on visceral dehydrogenase system in three inland teleosts. *Physio. Res.*, 33: 88.

Chapter 14

Biopesticides–Its Prospects and Limitations: An Overview

Shahnawaz A. Dar, Z.H. Khan, Akhtar Ali Khan and Sheikh Bilal Ahmad

Division of Entomology, Sher-e-Kashmir University of Agricultural Sciences and Technology of Kashmir, Shalimar Campus – 191 121, J&K

ABSTRACT

Biopesticides are major components of integrated pest management and potential alternative to their chemical counterparts. Biopesticides represent only 2.89 per cent of the overall pesticide market in India (Thakore, 2006). In India, so far only 12 types of biopesticides have been registered under the insecticidal act, 1968 (Sinha and Biswas, 2008). Biopesticide market is growing very rapidly. The growth rate of biopesticides over the next 10 years has been forecast at 10-15 per cent per annum, in contrast to 2 per cent of chemical pesticides (Menn, 1996). In India, the annual growth rate of biopesticides is estimated to be 2.5 per cent. It is also gathered that all baculoviruses developed so far occupy a share of only 0.2 per cent (Moscardi, 1999). Over the years more than 6000 species of plants have been screened and nearly 2400 plants belonging to 235 families were found to possess significant biological activity against insect pests (Grainge and Ahmad, 1988). About 700 products of microbials are currently available worldwide. In India,under microbials about 16 commerical *Bt* preparations, 38 fungi (based on *Metarhizium, Beauveria, Verticillium* and *Trigoderma*) and 45 viruses are available and it is expected to replace at least 10 per cent of chemical pesticides which means market of Rs. 60 corers annually (Abdul Kareem, 1996).

Keywords: *Biopesticides, Pest management, Insecticidal act, Biological activity, Microbials.*

Introduction

Biopesticides include in a broader sense, pesticides of biological origin, including microbial pesticides, entomopathogenic nematodes, baculoviruses, plant derived pesticides, insect pheromones, as alternatives to chemical pesticides and are key components of integrated pest management (IPM) system (Menn, 1997).The reality, however, is that biopesticides currently represent only a small fraction of the world pesticide market. The biopesticide share of the market was estimated to be around $380 million in 1995 (Menn, 1997). Although representing only 1.3 per cent of the total, and since the majority of biopesticides are currently marketed for insect control. The growth rate for biopesticides over the next 10 years has been forecast at 10-15 per cent per annum in contrast to 2 per cent for chemical pesticides (Menn, 1996).

In India, biopesticide science is not a new tool and is as old as human civilization back to prehistoric days. Though biopesticides cover only about 1 per cent of the total plant protection products globally, their number and the growth rate have been showing an increasing trend in the past two decades (Rao *et al.*, 2007). Neem based pesticides, *Bacillus thuringiensis*, NPV and *Trichoderma* are major biopesticides produced and used in India.The striking feature of biopesticides are eco- friendly and easy biodegradable thereby resulting in lower toxic residues and largely avoiding pollution problems associated with chemical pesticides. Further, use of biopesticides as a component of IPM programme can greatly decrease the use of conventional pesticides, while achieving almost the same level of crop yield.

Success Stories of Biopesticides in India

- ✰ Control of the Diamondback moth by *Bt* (*Bacillus thuringiensis*) (Biolep) in Ajmer and Najafgarh.
- ✰ Control of mango hoppers by *Beauveria* (Biorin) in Malihabad and Lucknow.
- ✰ Control of *Helicoverpa* on cotton, pigeonpea and tomato by *Bt* (Biolap) in Gujarat, Haryana, Punjab and West-Bengal.
- ✰ Control of *Helicoverpa* on gram by nuclear polyhedrosis virus (Biovirus-H) in Maharashtra and Rajasthan.
- ✰ Monitoring of *Helicoverpa* and *Spodoptera* by traps and lures (biotraps and biolures) in Gujrat, Haryana and Maharashtra.
- ✰ Control of sugar cane borers by *Trichogramma* (Biogramma) in Haryana and Rajasthan.
- ✰ Control of coffee pod borer by *Beauveria* in Karnataka.
- ✰ Control of sugarcane *Pyrilla* by *Epiricania sp.* in Karnataka.
- ✰ Control of white fly on cotton by neem products (Neemarin Grow, Neemazole) in Haryana, Punjab, Gujrat and West-Bengal.

(*Source*: Kalra and Khanuja, 2007)

Table 14.1: Annual Availability of Biopesticides in India

Biopesticides	*Quantity/Annum (Approx)*
Bt	50,000 kg
NPV (liquid)	500,000 LE
Beauveria	Meager
Neem 300 ppm	1,000,000 L
Neem 1500 ppm	250,000 L
Pheromone traps	500,000 no's
Lures	2 million
Trichogramma	10 lakh cards
Trichoderma	Over 500 T

Source: Kalra and Khanuja, 2007.

Biopesticides represent only 2.89 per cent (as on 2005) of the overall pesticide market in India and is expected to exhibit an annual growth rate of about 2.3 per cent in the coming years (Thakore, 2006). In India, so far only 12 types of biopesticides have been registered under the Insecticide Act, 1968. Neem based pesticides, *Bacillus thuringiensis*, NPV and *Trichoderma* are the major biopesticides produced and used in India. Whereas more than 190 synthetics are registered for use as chemical pesticides. Most of the biopesticides find use in public health, except a few that are used in agriculture. Besides, (*i*) transgenic plants and (*ii*) beneficial organisms called bioagents are used for pest management in India.

Table 14.2: Market Share of Biopesticides vis-à-vis Pesticides

Pesticides	*Market Share (per cent)*	
	World	*India*
Organochlorines	6	16
Organophosphates	37	50
Carbamates	23	4
Pyrethroids	22	18
Biopesticides (Bt, NPV, fungi, pheromones, attractants, repellents)	12	<1

Source: Ramarethinam, 1998.

The production and availability of microbials in India is low due to several limitations both at the industry and policy levels coupled with the low adoption by the farming community. The niche market for biopeticides, botanicals is only 12 per cent world wide and less than 1 per cent in India (Table 14.2). The current production in India is not even sufficient to cover 2 per cent of the area under any particular crop. The projected 15 per cent increase by the end of IX Plan will only be able to cover only few agroecological regions.

The Insecticide Act of 1968 has been amended accordingly to simplify the process of registration to allow speedier development and production of biopesticides. The National Farmer Policy 2007 has strongly recommended the promotion of biopesticides for increasing agricultural production, sustaining the health of farmers and environment. It also includes the clause that biopesticides would be treated at par with chemical pesticides in terms of support and promotion.

Table 14.3: Acts and Policies for Regulation and Promotion of Biopesticides in India

Acts/Policies	*Objectives*
Insecticide Act, 1968 (*Act*)	To regulate the import, manufacture, sale, transport, distribution and use of insecticides with a view to prevent risk to human beings or animals
Destruction Insect and Pest Act, 1914 (*Act*)	To prevent the introduction of any insect, fungus or other pests from one state to another in India.
Insecticides Rules, 1971 (*Rules*)	Functioning of CIB, licensing registration, production, packaging and transport of insecticides.
Promotion of IPM, 1991 (*Scheme*)	To promote use of biopesticides neem based pesticides, *Bacillus* based biopesticides, insect pathogen as alternative to chemical pesticides
National farmer policy, 2007 (*Policy*)	Recommended support and promotion of biopesticides as par with chemical pesticides.

Source: Sinha and Biswas, 2008.

Components of Biopesticides

Use of Organisms

About 60 per cent of insect pests are controlled naturally by their enemies such as parasitoids, predators, and insect pathogens. Only a few species have been intensively studied and utilized in IPM. There is ample score to develop many of them into useful products of IPM.

Use of Botanicals

Many plant species having selective action against a number of pests through a variety of biological activities including production of several behaviour-modifying chemicals such as pheromone analogues, antifeedant, repellents, attractants, direct toxicants, and insect growth regulators.

Use of Pheromones

Reduction in the load of pesticides on the basis of IPM. This can be achieved by monitoring pests through field surveys and surveillance, which help tackle the build up of pests/diseases, and use of pheromone traps and lures, which ensure minimum and need based application of pesticides instead of prophylactic and calendar-based pesticide spray schedules. These synthetic pheromones are being commercially exploited for monitoring insect populations, mass trapping, luring and killing, and mating disruption(MD) which disrupts communication between the sexes.

Advantages of Biopesticides

1. They are inherently less harmful
2. They are target spacific
3. Effective in small quantities
4. Decompose quickly and don't leave problematic residues
5. They are only eco-safe alternative
6. Development of resistance is less

Biopesticides: Industrial Overview

The biopesticide market is growing very rapidly. In 2005, biopesticides accounted for about 2.5 per cent of the total pesticide market, which was merely 0.2 per cent during 2000. This share is expected to grow to about 4.2 per cent by 2010 while the market value is estimated to reach more than US$ 1 billion (BCC Research). However, the overall growth rate of biopesticides is estimated to be about 10 per cent annum for the next 5 years.

In terms of use, orchards claim the largest share (55 per cent) of the total biopesticides used. Region-wise North America consumes the largest share (40 per cent) of the global biopesticide production followed by Europe and Oceanic countries accounting for 20 per cent.

The biopesticide R and D status presented here is based on two parameters, publications and patents. Total Indian publication on biopesticide stands at 443 papers which accounts for 13-23 per cent of the 3,348 global papers in the field. The share of India is biopesticide related patents is only 3.55 per cent of the global holdings. The average annual growth rate of global publications during the specified period is 51.1 per cent while that of India is 37.4 per cent. In terms of patenting, Indian condition appears to be very poor whereas in case of global patents it is showing a slight increase over the years. India has so far secured only 19 patents in biopesticides.

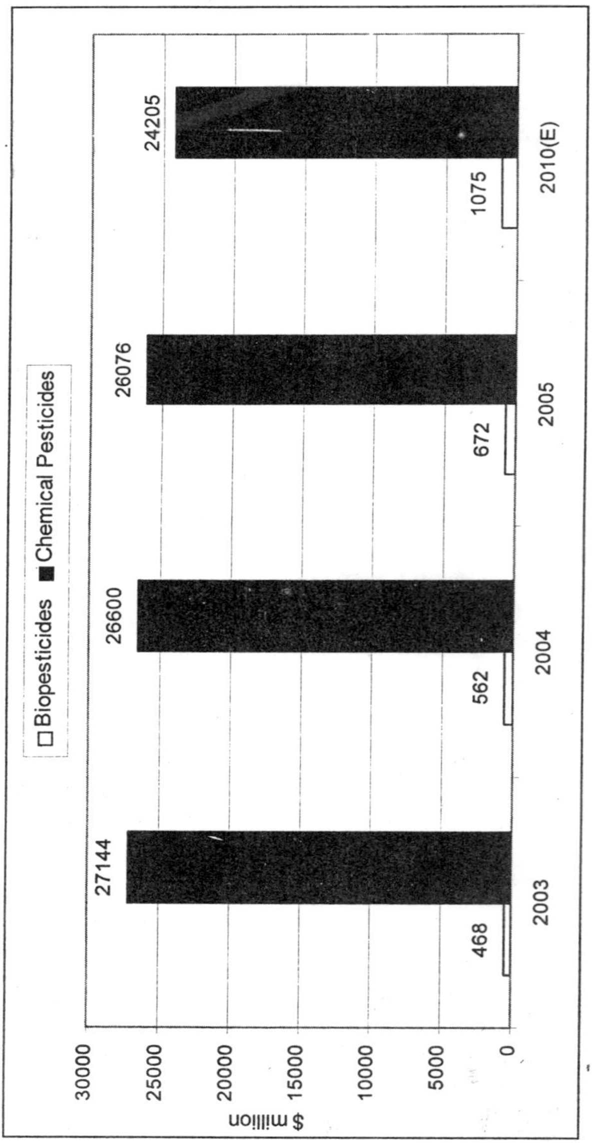

Figure 14.1: Trend of Global Pesticide vis-à-vis Biopesticide Market (Sinha and Biswas, 2008)

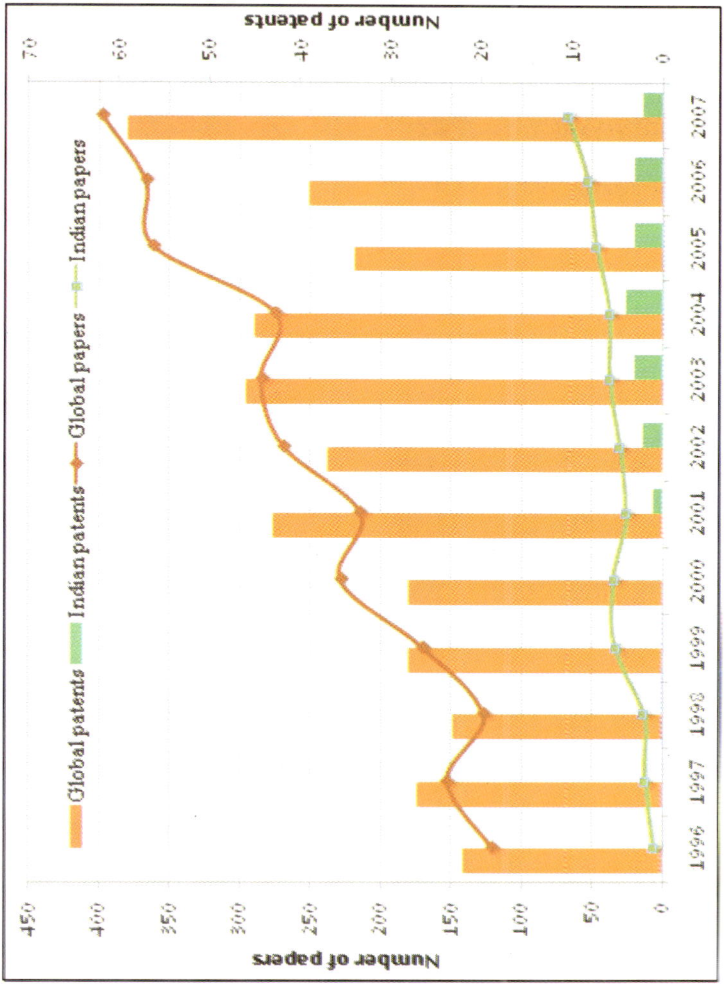

Figure 14.2: Trend of Biopesticide Research Outputs (Sinha and Biswas, 2008)

Over the years more than 6000 species of plants have been screened and nearly 2400 plants belonging to 235 families (Grainage and Ahmed, 1988) were found to possess significant biological activity against insect pests (Table 14.4).

Table 14.4: Type of Pest Control Action Reported in Plant Species

S. No.	*Pest Control Action*	*No. of Species of Plants*	*Sl.No.*	*Pest Control Action*	*No. of Species of Plants*
1.	Insecticidal	1053	9.	Fungicidal	100
2.	Antifeedant	230	10.	Bactericidal	4
3.	Repellent	225	11.	Molluscidal	6
4.	Growth inhibitor	32	12.	Herbicidal	14
5.	Attractant	27	13.	Antiseptic	35
6.	Rodenticidal	29	14.	Fish poison	147
7.	Acaricidal	2	15.	Arrow poison	90
8.	Nematicidal	58	16.	Poisonous	69

Graindge and Ahmed, 1988.

The seed oils of custard apple, *Annona squamosa* Linnaeus in combination with neem oil reduced the longevity of the rice green leafhopper, *Nephotettrix virescens* Distant (Mariappan and Saxena, 1984).

Derivatives from several tree species (Table 14.5) have also been found to possess pesticidal properties (Shankar and Solanki, 2000). Large number of plants have been screened and identified as a source of pesticide principles but most of the studies were limited to academic interest. Only few plants like tobacco, pyrethrum, neem, pungam, custard apple and mahua, were brought to field use because of obvious reasons and a plant like tobacco was discontinued from use because of toxicity to mammals and higher animals as well as high cost of production.

The studies have shown that sprays on lettuce, cabbage, strawberry and pepper, two or three times at weekly intervals with 1 per cent neem seed oil (20 ppm, AZA) or emulsifier only as a control could reduce the population of aphids to the extent of 40 to 98 per cent (Table 14.6). Generally, neem reduced aphid populations in a dose dependent manner.

Table 14.5: Trees with Insecticidal Activity

Tree Species (Common Name)	*Plant Part(s)/ Products(s)*	*Active Principles*	*Activity*
Albizia lebbeck (Troll.) (*desi siris*)	Seed, leaf, pod, bark and root	Caffeic acid, alkaloids and quercetin	Insecticide
Anacardium occidentale (Scarrone) (caṣhew)	Shell oil	Phenolic compounds	Insecticide
Annona squamosa (custard apple)	Stem, leaf and semi-ripe fruit	Annonine	Insecticide
Azadirachta indica (neem)	Leaf, seed and seed oil	Azadirachtin, nimbidin, salanin, meliantrol and other bitter principles (tetranorterpenoids)	Antifeedant, oviposition, deterrent, IGRs, insecticide
Butea moneosperma Koen Roxb. (flame of the forest)	Flower extract	Chalcones and aurones	Termiticidal
Hardwockia binata Roxb. (*Anjan*)	Heartwood	Mopanol and epicatechin	Antifeedant
Madhuca latifolia Roxb. (Mahua)	Seed and seed oil	Saponins	Repellent, insecticide
Melia azedarach (China tree, *bakain*)	Fruit and seed	Meliacin	Antifeedant, insecticide
Pongamia pinnata L. (pongam; *karanja*)	Seed and seed oil	Karanjin	Repellent, insecticide

(Shankar and Solanki, 2000)

Table 14.6: Population Reduction of Aphids in Fields Following Foliar Spray of 1 per cent Neem Seed Oil

Crop	*Aphid Species*	*Population Reduction (per cent)*
Cabbage	*Myzus persicae* (Sulzer)	87.7
	Brevicoryne brassicae (Linnaeus)	97.9
Pepper	*M. persicae* (Sulzer)	80.6
	Aphis gossypii Glover	80.7
Strawberry	*Chaetosiphon fragaefolii* (Cockerell)	55.1
	Fimbriaphis fimbriata Richards	73.4
Lettuce	*Nasonovia ribsngri* (Mosley)	39.5

Lowery and Isman, 1994.

Field evaluation of commercially available NPV of *H. armigera* as well as *Bt* based biopesticides particularly Dipel 8L either alone or in alternation with the recommended insecticides indicated low to moderate effectiveness against bollworms. Pooled analysis of data of 3 year's field trials on American cotton with Dipel 8L showed that seed cotton yield was 1426, 1640, 1819 and 1978 kg/ha in Dipel 8L alone, Dipel 8L alternated with endosulfan, recommended spray schedule and untreated control, respectively (Table 14.7). Field studies revealed that crude water extract of *vitex negundo* 10 per cent with NPV resulted in higher grain yield of chickpea than NPV alone. The studies on the combination of neem oil 4 per cent with HaNPV showed higher mortality with decreased LT_{50} values (Table 14.8).

The results show significant difference in the mortality recorded from the different treatments under laboratory conditions with the exception of quassin I and II significantly higher morality was detected in all the treatments compared with the untreated control (Table 14.9). *Bt aizawai* (Bta) + Need Azal (NA 58 per cent) and Bta alone (50 per cent) caused significantly higher mortality than that recorded in the NA, Neem blank and the three quassin treatments in 2nd instar larvae under laboratory conditions. Mortality tended to decline with increasing larval age and significant differences were recorded between the instars. 4th instar larvae suffered significantly lower mortality than that recorded for 2nd instar larvae (Table 14.9).

Table 14.7: Efficacy of *Bacillus thuringiensis* var. *kurstaki* (Dipel 8L) Against Cotton Bollworms Attacking American Cotton at Ludhiana

Treatment	*Dose per ha*	*Bollworm Infestation (per cent)*			*Seed Cotton Yield (kg/ha)*	*% Increase in Yield Over Control*
		Boll Basis	*Loculi Basis*	*% Reduction in Infestation*		
		Over control				
Bacillus thuringiensis var. *kurstaki* (Bt) Dipel 8L (alone)	750 ml	24.9 (27.9)	11.5 (19.7)	31.1	1426	32.3
Bt alternated with endosulfan (Thiodan 35EC)	750 ml/2.5 litre	19.6 (26.4)	8.2 (16.5)	50.9	1640	52.1
Recommended spray schedule	Recommended doses	15.1 (22.5)	6.1 (13.9)	63.8	1819	68.7
Control	Unsprayed	31.9 (36.0)	16.7 (24.0)	–	1078	–
LSD (p = 0.05)		(4.7)	(2.7)	NS	–	–

Butter *et al.*, 1995.

Table 14.8 Percent Mortality of Second Instar Larvae of *Helicoverpa armigera* Influenced by *Ha*NPV and Neem Oil

Treatment	*No. of Larvae Tested*	*Corrected Mortality (per cent)*	*LT_{50} (Days)*
HaNPV (5 x 10^6 PIBs/ml)	25	54.54	7.83
HaNPV (5 x 10^6 PIBs/ml) + 0.5 per cent neem oil	25	77.27	6.64
HaNPV (5 x 10^6 PIBs/ml) + 1.0 per cent neem oil	25	86.35	6.56
HaNPV (5 x 10^6 PIBs/ml) + 2.0 per cent neem oil	25	86.35	5.58
HaNPV (5 x 10^6 PIBs/ml) + 4.0 per cent neem oil	25	90.9	5.70
Untreated control	25	12.00	–

Pawar, 1998.

Table 14.9: Effect of Bio-rational Insecticides on the 2nd and 4th Instar Larvae of *H. armigera* Under Laboratory Conditions

Treatments	No. of Larvae Exposed	Mean Percentage Mortality (2nd instar) After			Mean Percentage Mortality (4th instar) After		
		24 h	48 h	72 h	24 h	48 h	72 h
Bta	25	37.0	46.0	50.0c	0.0	6.0	14.0b
Bta+NA	25	27.0	34.0	58.0c	1.0	16.0	27.0c
NA	25	18.0	30.0	34.0b	0.0	0.0	7.0a
NA blank	25	0.0	0.0	4.0a	0.0	0.0	7.0a
Quassin I	25	0.0	0.0	2.0a	0.0	0.0	0.0a
Quassin II	25	1.0	1.0	5.0a	0.0	0.0	2.0a
Quassin III	25	0.0	2.0	11.0a	0.0	1.0	5.0a
Tap water	25	0.0	0.0	1.0a	0.0	0.0	0.0a

Aggarwal *et al.*, 2006

Table 14.10: Effect of Bio-rational Insecticides on the 2nd and 4th Instar Larvae of *S. exigua* Under Laboratory Conditions

Treatments	No. of Larvae Exposed	Mean Percentage Mortality (2nd instar) After			Mean Percentage Mortality (4th instar) After		
		24 h	48 h	72 h	24 h	48 h	72 h
Bta	25	28.0	49.0	58.0d	2.0	5.0	16.0e
Bta+NA	25	38.0	54.0	65.0d	4.0	14.0	26.0f
NA	25	30.0	36.0	43.0c	1.0	8.0	12.0de
NA blank	25	1.0	2.0	7,0ab	0.0	1.0	4.0abc
Quassin I	25	0.0	4.0	6.0ab	0.0	1.0	1.0
Quassin II	25	0.0	5.0	10.0bc	0.0	0.0	6.0
Quassin III	25	1.0	7.0	13.0b	0.0	0.0	9.0*
Tap water	25	0.0	0.0	2.0a	0.0	0.0	0.0

Aggarwal *et al.*, 2006.

The reduction in total mortality over the post application period were recorded in all the treatments under laboratory conditions resulting in significant mortality being recorded 3 days after treatment both in 2nd and 4th instar larvae. However, the rate of mortality differed between the treatments occurring most rapidly in Bta + NA (65 and 26 per cent) and Bta alone (58 and 16 per cent) in the treatments under laboratory conditions in 2nd and 4th instar larvae (Table 14.10).

The data obtained demonstrate that the application of whole cultures as a soil drench of Bti did not significantly improve the growth parameters (plant height, fresh plant weight and fresh root weight). However, Bti significantly reduced final nematode populations (Table 14.11). The percentage control obtained with the application of 2.50 ml dose of Bti per tube was 64. All the four doses of *Bti* significantly (p=0.01) differed from the uninoculated control but these treatments did not differ between themselves.

Table 14.11: Effect of *Bacillus thuringiensis* var. *israelensis* Soil Application on the Control of *Meloidogyne incognita* and Growth of Barley Under Greenhouse Conditions

Dose	*Plant Height*	*Fresh Plant Weight*	*Fresh Root Weight*	*Final Nematode Population*	*Control*
ml/kg	cm	g	g	nc	%
Water check	54.4a	6.54a	10.10a	21076a	0
Bti/1.25	56.6a	6.26a	10.14a	8400b	60
Bti/2,50	59.6a	6.10a	10.58a	7596b	64
Bti/5.00	54.4a	7.34a	12.16a	9964b	53
Bti/7.50	60.6a	732a	10.58a	7995b	62
C.V (%)	11.81	23.88	12.40	41.98	–

Sharma, 1994.

Limitations of Biopesticides

- ☆ Un-availability
- ☆ Limited shelf life
- ☆ Inadequacy of quality
- ☆ Inconsistent field results
- ☆ Slow process and un-predictable stability under field conditions
- ☆ Expensive method of development and production

Feasibility of Biopesticide Acceptance

Economic Incentives

The net gain from the use of a biopesticide must equal or exceed the gain that the grower would receive from conventional pest control tactics (chemicals).

Efficacy

Biopesticides must be as effective as the chemical they would replace. As efficacy of bioinsecticides increase, economic feasibility will increase.

Pest Spectrum

Development of some broad spectrum bioinsectide or mixtures to compete with their synthetic chemical predecessors, can increase the feasibility of those products.

Crop Price

As crop value increase, there is greater interest in using rapid, reliable and effective pest control measuring like the use of bioinsecticides.

Price of Biopesticide

The lower the market price of a biopesticide, the more economically feasible it is to the user.

Variability of Performance

Users prefer consistency and reliability in the pest control methods they choose, therefore economic feasibility will increase as bioinsecticide become more consistent in their field performance.

User Costs

The costs associated with time, labour and management, when a using a new technique or product can increase the overall cost to the user and make the product less economically feasible.

Biopesticides: A Global Projection

- ✰ Biopesticide sale in European market alone reach US $ 167 million by year 2004 (Neale, 2000).
- ✰ Biopesticides will accounts for 15 per cent of the total insecticide market by year 2005 (Koul and Dhaliwal, 2002).

- *Bt* the most sucessfull pest control agent accounts for approx 90-95 per cent of the total sales of biological pest control products world wide amounting to approx an annual sales of US $ 50-55 million (Seema Wahab, 2002).
- In India, present annual demand of Bt based biopesticides in approx 120 tons (Koul and Dhaliwal, 2002).
- Biopesticides represent approx 4.5. per cent of the world insecticide sales (Seema Wahab, 2002).
- Growth rate of biopesticides in next 10 years has been estimated at 10-15 per cent per annum in contrast to 2 per cent for chemical pesticides (Menn, 1996).
- In India, the annual growth rate of biopesticides is estimated to be 2.5 per cent. It is also gathered that all baculoviruses developed so far occupy a share of only 0.2 per cent (Moscardi, 1999).

Potential of Biopesticide in Indian Agriculture

- The concept of biopesticides in farming community is still in infancy. Only 1 per cent of 143 million ha crop area and only 2500 villages out of over 6 lakh villages in the country have been covered so far under IPM (Singhal, 2003).
- Biopesticides represent only 2.89 per cent of the overall pesticide market in India and is expected to exhibit an annual growth rate of about 2.3 per cent in the coming years (Thokore, 2006).
- Consumption of biopesticides has increased from 219 metric tons in 1996-97 to 683 metric tons in 2000-01 and about 85 per cent of the biopesticides used are neem based products (Thokore, 2006).

Conclusions

Biopesticides form the back bone of Integrated Pest Management (IPM), their development, commercialization and use has not yet lived upto the expectations of demand and supply. Biopesticides based on pathogenic organisms specific to their target pests, offer, ecological and effective solution to pest problems and fit well into the desired requirement of sustainable agriculture. Microbial agents seems to provide adequate commercial option to replace conventional chemical control and could overcome the extreme situations of insecticide resistance. Targeted assistance in the form of specialized support, facilities and access to expertise on a multinational and multidisciplinary basis is required to remove constraints and promote development and utilization of biopesticides.

References

Abdul Kareem, 1996. Commercialization of biopesticides a changing scenario. In: *4th National Training Programme on Commercial Production of Biocontrol*. 2-10 TAU, Coimbatore, p. 8.

Aggarwal, N., Holaschke, M. and Basedow, T., 2006. Evalaution of biorational insecticide to control *Helicoverpa armigera* and *Spodoptera exigua* feed on *Vicia faba*. *Mitt. Dtsch. Ges. Allg. Angew. Ent.*, 15: 245-250.

Butter, N.S., Battu, G.S., Kular, G.S., Singh, T.H. and Brar, J.S., 1995. Integrated use of *Bacillus thuringiensis* with some insecticides for the management of bollworms on cotton. *J. Ent. Res.*, 19(3): 255-263.

Graindge, M. and Ahmad, S., 1988. *Handbook of Plant with Pest Control Properties*. John Wiley and Sons Inc. New York, USA, p. 420.

Kalra, A. and Khanuja, S.P.S., 2007. Research and development priorities for biopesticide and biofertilizer products for sustainable agriculture in India. Asian Productivity Organisation, pp. 96-102.

Koul, O. and Dhaliwal, G.S., 2002. *Microbial Biopesticides*. Taylor and Francis, London.

Lowery, D.T. and Isman, M.B., 1994. Insect growth regulating effect of neem extract and Azadirachtin on aphids. *Entomol. Exp. Appl.* 72: 77-84.

Menn, J.J., 1996. Biopesticides: Has their time come? *Journal of Environment, Science and Health*, 31(3): 383-389.

Menn, J.J., 1997. Biopesticides-are they relevant? In: *Focus on Biopesticides*. The Royal Society of Chemistry, pp. 1-2

Moscardi, F., 1999. Assessment of the application of baculoviruses for control of Lepidoptera. *A Review of Entomology*, 44: 257-290.

Neale, M., 2000. The regulation of natural products as crop protection agents. *Pest Management Science*, 56: 677-680.

Pawar, V.M., 1998. Microbial control of *Helicoverpa* sp. on pulse crops. In: *IPM System in Agriculture, Vol. 4: Pulses*, pp. 55-78.

Ramarethinam, S., 1998. Growing importance of biopesticides. *Pestology*, 22: 50-61.

Rao, G.V.R., Rupela, O.P., Rao, V.R. and Reddy, Y.V.R., 2007. Biopesticides status in crop protection. *Indian Journal of Plant Protection*, 35(1).

Seema Wahab, 2002. Biotechnology approaches in plant protection. *Biopesticides in Pest Management*, 1: 113-127.

Shanker, C. and Solanki, K.R., 2000. Botanical insecticides: A Historial Perspective. *Asian Agri-Hist.*, 4(3): 221-232.

Sharma, R.D., 1994. *Bacillus thuringiensis* a biocontrol agent of *Meloidogynae incognita* on barley. *Nematologia Brasileira*, 18: 79-84.

Singal, V., 2003. Biopesticides: Production, utilization and demand. In: *Biopesticides for Sustainable Agriculture: Prospects and Constraints*, pp. 97.

Sinha, B. and Biswas, I., 2008. Potential of biopesticides in Indian agriculture vis-à-vis rural development. *Science and Technology for Rural India and Inclusive Growth.*

Thakore, Y., 2006. The biopesticide market for global agricultural use. *Industrial Biotechnology*, pp. 194-198.

Chapter 15

Light Microscopic as well as Ultrastructural Changes in Adrenal Cortex of *Mus norvegicus* Induced by Sub-lethal Heroin Administration

Kaminidevi K. Bhoir[1], *S.A. Suryawanshi* [1] *and A.K. Pandey*[2*]

[1]*Department of Zoology, Institute of Science, 15 Madam Cama Road, Mumbai – 400 031, India*

[2]*National Bureau of Fish Genetic Resources, Canal Ring Road, Dilkusha, Lucknow – 226 002, U. P., India*

ABSTRACT

Adrenal cortex of *Mus norvegicus* comprised an outer cortex surrounding the inner (central) medulla. Based on cellular and functional characteristics, cortex was divisible into outer zona glomerulosa, middle zona fasciculata and inner zona reticularis. Zona fasciculata was the broadest zone composed of cell cords coursing in a radial direction towards medulla. Each cord was enclosed by sinusoidal capillaries. Parenchymal cells were cuboidal or polyhedral in shape and nuclei appeared more vesicular with less dense chromatin material. These cells were relatively large and their cytoplasm contained more number of lipid droplets. Ultrastructurally, the cells of zona

* Corresponding author: E-mail: akpandey_cifa@yahoo.co.in

fasciculata of control rat were cuboidal or polyhedral in shape, round nucleus with prominent nucleolus and well-distributed chromatin material, large number of mitochondria, lipid droplets, rough endoplasmic reticulum (RER), Golgi complex and lysosomes. Though cells of all the three zones of adrenal cortex of the albino rat were affected by heroin treatment, zona fasciculata cells depicted maximum degenerative changes. Sub-lethal heroin administration for 30 days induced marked deposition of chromatin material in the inner cell membrane, mitochondria with damaged cristae, less secretory granules, scattered free riobosomes and cytoplasm filled with minute vacuoles. Cytoplasm of many cells was devoid of cell organelles and remnants of endoplasmic reticula, mitochondria and granules were also encountered on day 30 of the treatment.

Keywords : *Heroin, Adrenal cortex, Zona fasciculata, Mus norvegicus.*

Introduction

Opiates and cocaine are the main problem drugs of abuse world-over as these are associated with multiple poor health outcomes, reduced quality of life and enhanced criminal behaviour (Sporer, 1999; Cami and Farre, 2003; Brown *et al.*, 2006; Wisniewski *et al.*, 2006). Chronic cocaine and placebo abuse may cause disorders in endocrine function in men and women (Cushman, 1973; Cocores *et al.*, 1986; Al-Gommer *et al.*, 2007). Cocaine administration alters secretion of ACTH of adenohypophysis in the experimental animals and may affect neuroendocrine function in human beings too (Mendelson *et al.*, 1992). ACTH level increased significantly after intravenous cocaine administration while administration of the drug by intranasal inhalation and smoking does not make any significant difference in secretion of adrenal cortex as cortisol and corticosterone remain unchanged (Mendelson *et al.*, 1989). On the other hand, acute and repeated cocaine and amphetamine on intra-peritoneal administration for 8 days elevates the level of corticosterone while amphetamine show similar effect only after 14 days of the treatment. These results indicate that repeated dose of the psychostimulants enhance activity of the hypothalamo-pituitary-adrenal (HPA) axis (Budziszewska *et al.*, 1996).

There exist reports suggesting that narcotic agents may affect the HPA axis of mammals. Both morphine and methadone are concentrated in the hypothalamus. Studies conducted in human have suggested that the HPA axis may be adversely affected by morphine administration (Cushman *et al.*, 1970). Alcohol intake may cause multiple endocrinological changes including stimulation of HPA axis leading to the alcoholic bone diseases (Sarli *et al.*, 1994). In man, ACTH and cortisol increased after two hours of naloxone (an opium alkaloid) dose irrespective of time and day (Martin del Campo *et al.*, 1994). The HPA axis in heroin addicts is affected resulting in significant decrease in cortisol level. As far as effects of opiate are concerned, morphine significantly reduced plasma cortisol level within 60 minutes indicating that chronic opiate abuse leads to a hypoadrenalism, probably because of changes induced by these drugs at the hypothalamic level (Facchinetti *et al.*, 1985).

Physical dependence is an adaptive process to the presence of an exogenous substance and may begin as soon as homeostasis is disrupted (Goldstein *et al.*, 1974). When the exogenous agent such as narcotic is administered, a characteristic addiction syndrome ensued (Goodman and Gilman, 1975). Despite their long history of clinical therapeutic uses and protracted abuse by addicts, little is known regarding possible influences of these drugs on the endocrine system, particularly the HPA axis (El-Daly, 1996; George *et al.*, 2005; Brown *et al.*, 2006; Wisniewski *et al.*, 2006). Since restoration of functional integrity of the HPA axis in man receiving narcotic drugs is of great clinical as well as pharmacological significance, an attempt was made to record the effect of sub-lethal heroin administration on light microscopic as well as ultrastructual alterations in adrenal cortex of *Mus norvegicus*.

Materials and Methods

Healthy male *Mus norvegicus* (Wistar strain) weighing 150-200 gm were purchased from Hoffkin Institute, Parel, Mumbai and housed in specially made plastic cages. They were acclimatized under the ambient laboratory conditions (temparature 28±2^{0}C; photoperiod 14L:10 D) for 10 days, fed *ad libitum* on rat feed (Lipton, Bangalore) and clean water was provided for drinking. 40 male rats were randomly selected and divided into two equal groups - experimental and control. Heroin (85 per cent pure) was initially dissolved in small quantity of alcohol and diluted with physiological saline to prepare the test dose of 0.50 LD_{50} (13.5 mg/kg/day). The drug was administered through subcutaneous (s.c.) route to the experimental rats while the control rats received equal volume (0.2 ml/kg body weight) of physiological saline. The animals were killed on day 30.

Adrenal glands of rats from both the groups were removed and washed in normal saline and fixed immediately in Bouin's solution for light microscopy. After 24 hours, the tissues were dehydrated in ascending series of alcohol, cleared in xylene and embedded in paraffin wax at 60^{0}C. Sections were cut at 5 µm and stained in hematoxylin-eosin (H&E). For electron microscopy, the tissues were removed immediately after the sacrifice and sliced into 1 mm pieces to allow better penetration of the fixative. Tissues were fixed in 3 per cent ice-cold glutaraldehyde for 12 hours followed by 4 hours in 0.1 M cacodylate buffer. They were rinsed in buffer and post-osmicated in 1 per cent osmium tetraoxide (OSO_4) for 1-2 hours. Thereafter, the tissues were dehydrated in ascending series of alcohol followed by propylene oxide and embedded in resin polymerized at 60^{0}C. The blocks were prepared in araldite and 1 µm thin sections were cut with glass knife on LKB-2000 ultramicrotome. The sections were mounted on glass slide and stained with buffered toluidine blue for light microscopic studies. Ultrathin sections of the selected blocks were cut with glass knife, picked up on copper grids and stained with uranyl acetate as well as lead citrate for final observation under ZEIM-EM-109 electron microscope.

Results and Discussion

Adrenal gland of *Mus norvegicus* comprised an outer cortex surrounding the inner (central) medulla. Based on cellular and functional characteristics, the cortex was divisible into three zones - outer zona glomerulosa, middle zona fasciculata and inner zona reticularis. Zona fasciculata was the broadest zone composed of cell cords coursing in a radial direction towards medulla. Each cord was enclosed by sinusoidal capillaries. Parenchymal cells were cuboidal or polyhedral in shape and nuclei appeared more vesicular with less dense chromatin material (Figuers 15.1 and 15.2). These cells were relatively large and their cytoplasm contained more number of lipid droplets. Cytoplasm of zona fasciculata cells of the rat treated with heroin for 30 days showed prominent degenerative changes. Many cells showed vesiculated cytoplasm with eccentric nuclei. There was marked increase in intercellular space suggesting intercellular edema. Treatment of heroin reduced number of lipid droplets in the cells of zona fasciculata. Few cells showed condensation of chromatin material while others showed vesiculated as well as pycnotic nuclei (Figures 15.3 and 15.4).

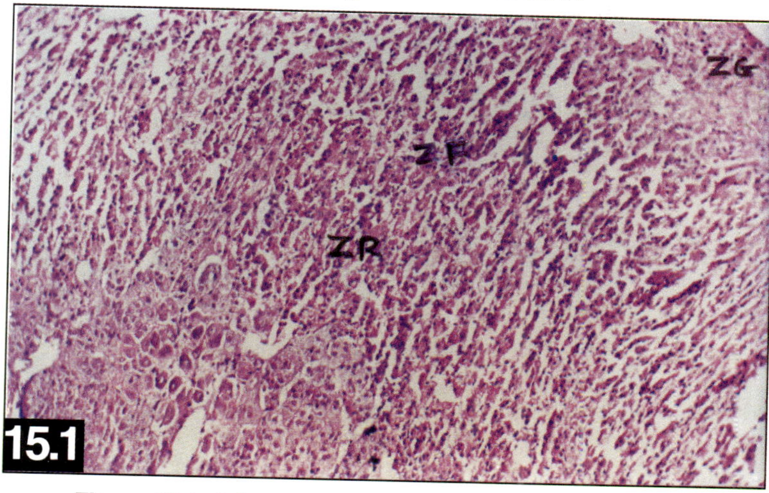

Figure 15.1: Adrenal Cortex of Control *Mus norvegicus* Showing Zona Glomerulosa (ZG), Zona Fasciculata (ZF) and Zona Reticularis (ZR). H&E. x100.

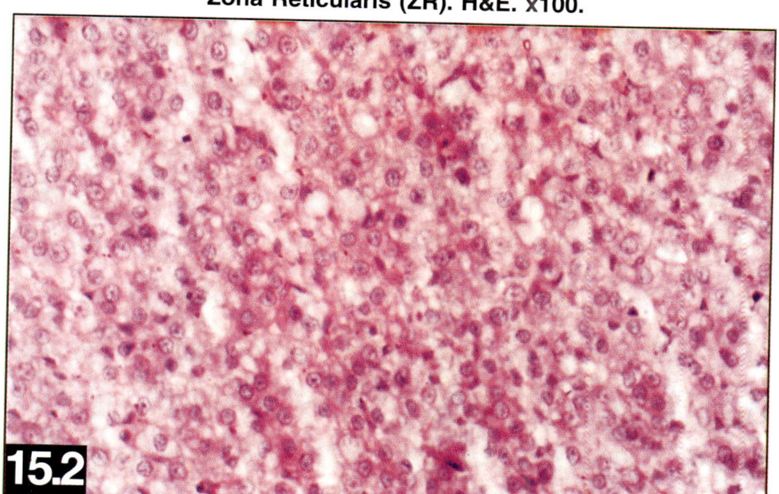

Figure 15.2: Magified View of *Zona fasciculata* of Control Rat Exhibiting Normal Structure of Cells with Round Nuclei. H&E. x 400.

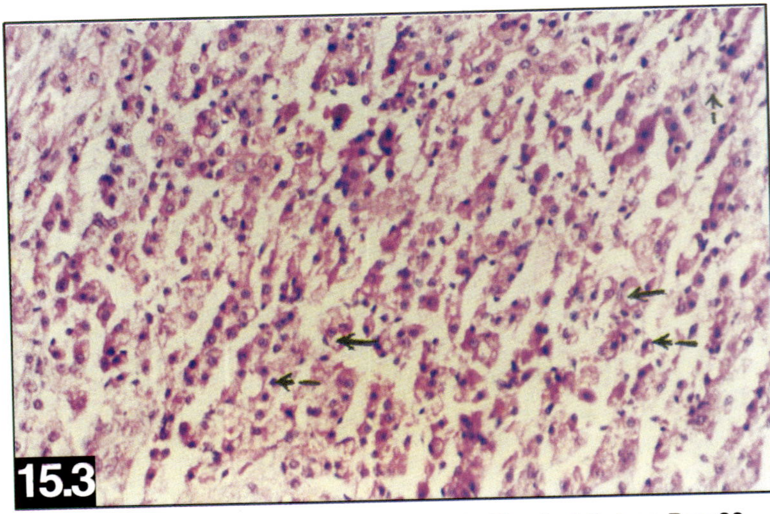

Figure 15.3: *Zona fasciculata* of Heroin Treated Rat on Day 30 Depicting Intercellular Spaces, Marked Vacuolization in Cytoplasm (Arrow) and Pycnotic Nuclei (Broken arrow). H&E. x 250.

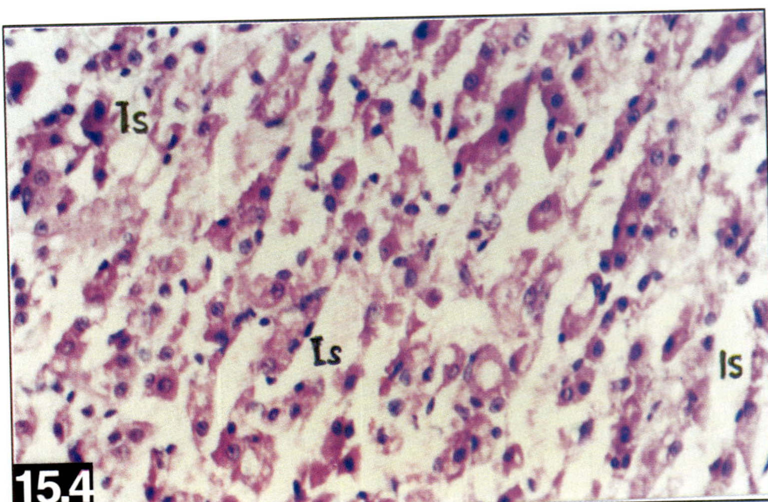

Figure 15.4: Magnified View of *Zona fasciculata* of Heroin Treated *Mus norvegicus* for 30 Days Showing Reduction in Nuclear Size and Prominent Intercellular Spaces (Is). Mark the degeneratice changes in cytoplasm and nucleus. H&E. x 400.

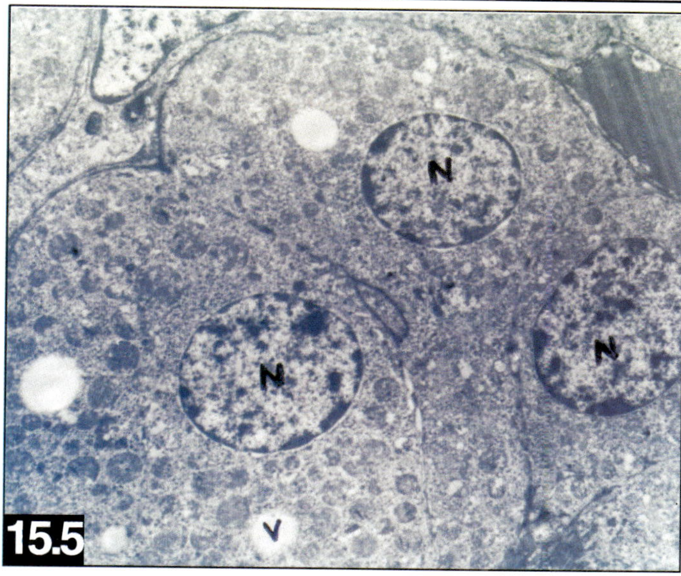

Figure 15.5: ***Zona fasciculata*** **Cells of Control Rat exhibiting Round Nucleus (N), Vacuoles (v) and Mitochondria. x 6,500.**

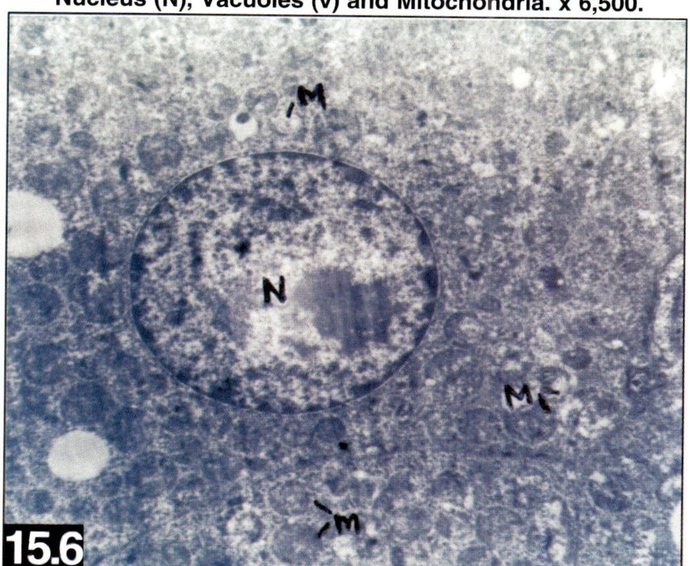

Figure 15.6: ***Zona fasciculata*** **Cells of Control** ***Mus norvegicus*** **Depicting Mitochondria (m) and Nucleus (N). x 10,300.**

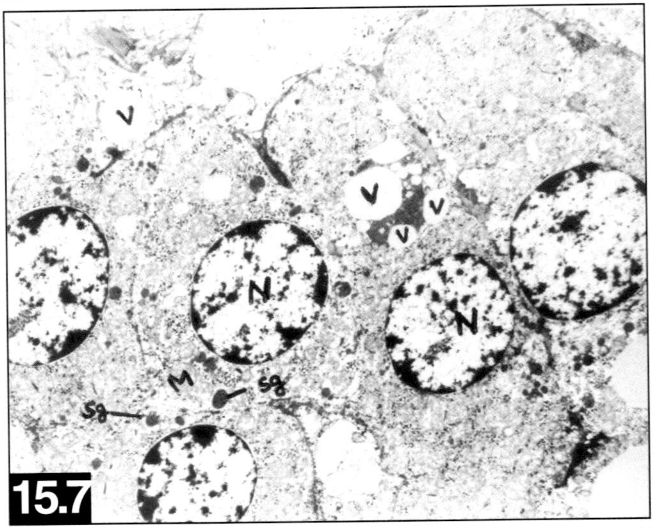

Figure 15.7: ***Zona fasciculata*** **Cells of Heroin Treated Rat on Day 30 Showing Mitochondria (m), Secretory Granules (sg), Nucleus (N) and Vacuoles (v). x 4,300.**

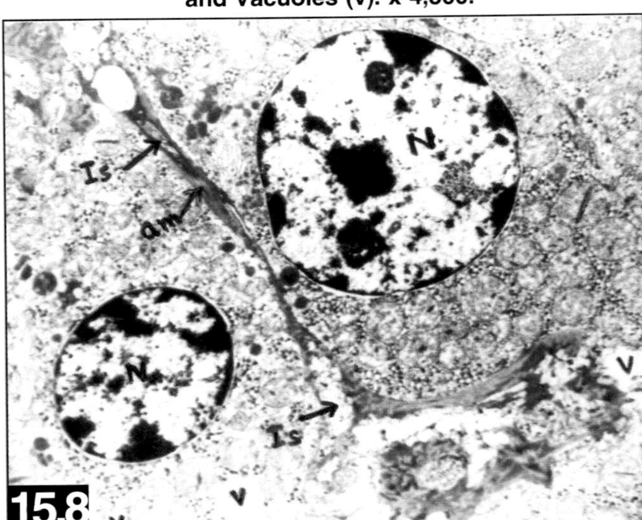

Figure 15.8: ***Zona fasciculata*** **Cells of Heroin Treated Rat for 30 Days Exhibiting Large Number of Vacuoles (v), Amorphous Material (am) in the Intercellular Space (Is) and Deposition of Electron–Dense Material. x 10,100.**

Ultrastructurally, the cells of zona fasciculata of adrenal cortex of control rat exhibited round nucleus with prominent nucleolus and well-distributed chromatin material in nucleoplasm. The cytoplasm contained large number of mitochondria, lipid droplets, rough endoplasmic reticulum (RER) and lysosomes (Figures 15.5 and 15.6). Cells of zonal fascuculata of the rats treated with heroin for 30 days showed large deposition of chromatin material in the inner cell membrane and a number of mitochondria lost their cristae. Some cells showed dense secretory granules along with number of vacuoles. Free riobosomes were seen scattered in the cytoplasm (Figure 15.7). The chromatin-dense nucleus with prominent nucleolus was seen. The cytoplasm was filled with plenty of minute vacuoles. There was deposition electron-dense material in periphery of the plasma membrane together with prominent amorphous material in the intercellular space (Figure 15.8). Exceptionally increased intercellular edema with red blood cells (RBCs) infiltration was visible suggesting that the cell was actively involved in fighting back the adverse effect of heroin. Some cells showed reduced cytoplasm with pycnotic nucleus (Figure 15.9). Furthermore, few cells exhibited deposition of chromatin at periphery of the nuclear membrane while others showed clumps of chromatin material in the nucleolus. Cytoplasm of many cells was devoid of cell organelles and remnants of endoplasmic reticula, mitochondria and granules were seen (Figure 15.10).

Some cells of zona fasciculate also exhibited vacuolated cytoplasm with electron-dense granules. Many of the cell organelles were lost and there was heavy deposition of chromatin expressing pycnotic state of nucleus. The overall picture clearly suggested that the cells were undergoing necrosis (Figure 15.11). The zona fasciculata cells were affected drastically by the drug administration as some region in the cortex exhibited multiple lesions. These cells lost normal architecture and depicted accumulation of amorphous material in the cytoplasm and pycnotic nuclei. Blood infiltration in cell cytoplasm was prominent and intercellular space was seen. Many cells showed hyperactivity exhaustion (Figure 15.12).

The structure of zona fasciculata cells of *Mus norvegicus* resembles to those described for other mammalian species (Chester Jones and Phillips, 1986; Barai *et al.*, 2004). There exist reports indicating that narcotic drugs may affect the HPA axis in mammals

(McDonald *et al.*, 1959; Burdette *et al.*, 1961; Goodman *et al.*, 1967). Acute release of anti-diuretic hormone (ADH) and inhibition of corticotropin-releasing factor (CRF) by the hypothalamus in response to stimuli that usually induce CRF release have been reported (Arimura *et al.*, 1967). In human too, there were suggestions that the HPA axis might be adversely affected by morphine administration (Eisenman *et al.*, 1958, 1961). It is generally agreed that pituitary ACTH is regulated by a neuroendocrine system in which changes in corticotrophin-releasing factor (CRF) determine release of the former. This system is operationally considered in three different interrelated phases *i.e.* stress, feedback and rhythmic periodicity. Suppression of ACTH-dependent cortisol secretion as well as β-endorphin and LDH has been reported following administration of DAMME, a synthetic sedative (Stubbs *et al.*, 1978; Delitala *et al.*, 1981a, b). The fall in serum cortisol level following morphine and nalorphine treatments has been noted in man (McDonald *et al.*, 1959). Delitala *et al.* (1983) observed that DAMME administration resulted in no change in cortisol level in man. High doses of naloxane are able to block the suppression of ACTH by DAMME in patients with Addisson's disease (Gillard *et al.*, 1981) while naloxane alone elevated serum cortisol in man only at relatively high doses (Grossman and Jones, 1983). Non-narcotic drugs also showed similar type of elevation in serum cortisol level. Total intravenous anesthesia in ponies using detomidine, ketamine and guaiphenesin decreased plasma cortisol concentration while plasma 11-deoxycorticoid level increased (Taylor *et al.*, 1995).

Sarli *et al.* (1994) showed that alcohol intake causes stimulation of the hypothalamo-pituitary-adrenal (HPA) axis which leads to alcoholic bone disease because of adverse effect of corticoids on bone. Long-term opioid consumption can induce hyperadrenalism through impairment of the HPA axis. In heroin addicts, saliva cortisol concentration varies according to the amount of heroin consumed and time elapsed since the last self-administered dose (Cami *et al.*, 1992). Hypercortisolism was observed either after abrupt withdrawal of heroin or the last dose of methadone. It is hypothesized that elevated cortisol level may account for untoward effects of adrenergic therapy (Cami *et al.*, 1992).

Facchinetti *et al.* (1985) studied the HPA axis of heroin addicts by evaluating plasma cortisol levels throughout the day in 378 heroin

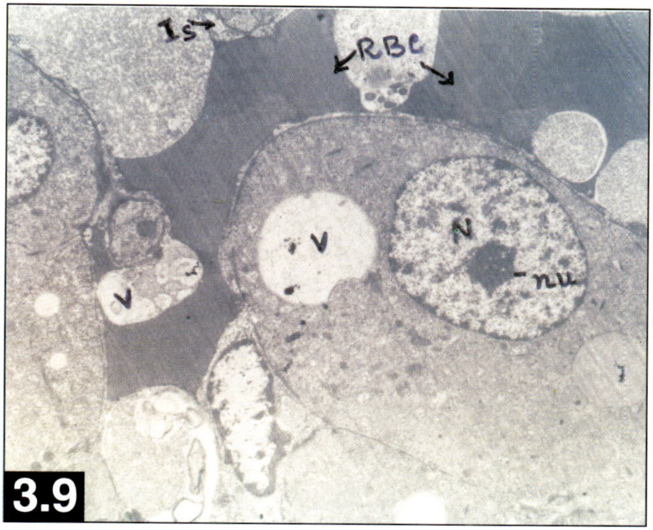

Figure 15.9: ***Zona fasciculata*** **Cells of Heroin Treated** ***Mus norvegicus*** **for 30 Days Depicting Intercellular Space (Is) with Red Blood Cell (RBC) Infiltration and Vacuoles in the Cytoplasm (v) Nucleus (N) and Nucleolus (nu) are also Seen. x 4.400.**

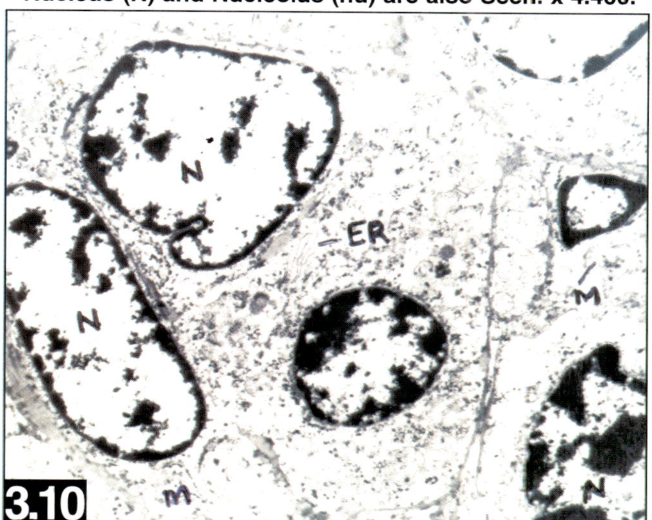

Figure 15.10: ***Zona fasciculata*** **Cells of Heroin Treated Rat on Day 30 Showing Degenerative Changes in Mitochondria (m), Nucleus (N) and Endoplasmic Reticulum (ER). x 6,600.**

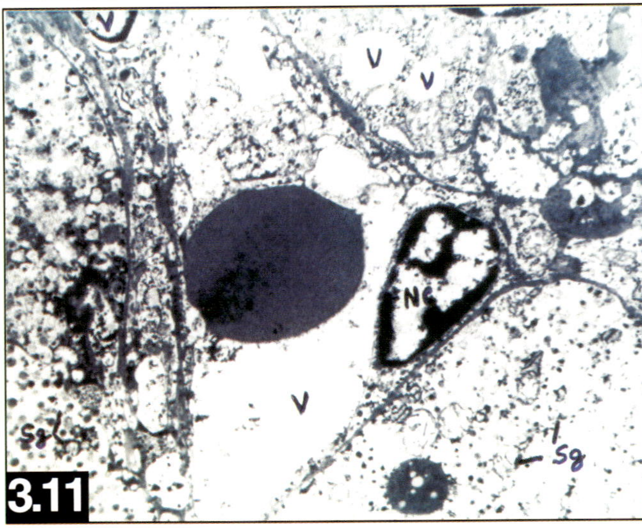

Figure 15.11: ***Zona fasciculata*** **Cells of Heroin Treated Rat for 30 Days Exhibiting Necrotic Cell (Nc) with Pycnotic Nucleus (N), Vacolated Cytoplasm (v) and Secretory Granules (sg). x 6,400.**

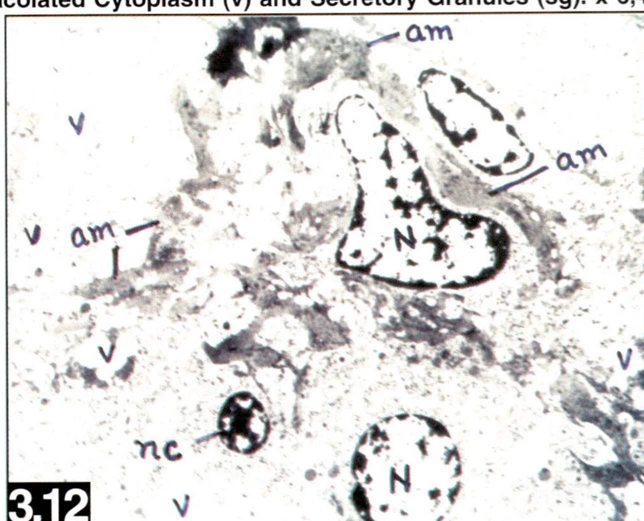

Figure 15.12: ***Zona fasciculata*** **Cells of Heroin Treated** ***Mus norvegicus*** **on Day 30 Depicting Necrotic Cells (Nc) with Electron-Dense Amorphous Material (am) and Pycnotic Nucleus (N). Mark large number of vacuoles in the cytoplasm (v). x 6,400.**

abusers. Morphine significantly reduced plasma cortisol level and produced hypoadrenalism that could be the result of morphine induced changes at the hypothalamic level. In the present investigation, administration of sub-lethal heroin for 30 days produced varying degrees of degenerative changes in zona fasciculata cells of adrenal cortex. These include vacuolization in the cytoplasm, lack of cristae in mitochondria and hypertrophied rough endoplasmic reticulum (RER). These degenerative changes might have resulted owing to the depletion in levels of ACTH and cortisol in heroin treated rat.

Acknowledgements

One of us (KKB) is thankful to N.M. Wadia Trust, Mumbai for partial financial assistance to carry out this work. We are grateful to Hon'ble Justice Mrs. K.K. Baam, the then High Court Judge, Mumbai for permitting us to work on heroin and to Mr. Rahul Rai Sur, the then Deputy Commissioner of Police, Narcotics Cell, Greater Mumbai for the procurement of the drug. Help extended by the staff of Tata Cancer Research Centre, Mumbai in electron microscopy is acknowledged.

References

Al-Gommer, O., George, S. and Haque, S., 2007. Sexual dysfunctions in male opiate users: a comparative study of heroin, methadone and buprenorphine. *Addict. Disord. Their Treat.*, 6: 137-143.

Arimura, A., Sato, T. and Schally, A.V., 1967. Assay for corticotropin-releasing factor (CRF) using rats treated with morphine, chlorpromazine, dexamethasone and nembutal. *Endocrinology*, 81: 235-245.

Barai, S.R., Suryawanshi, S.A. and Pandey, A.K., 2004. Light microscopic and ultrastructural observations on the adrenal cortex of *Rattus norvegicus*. *J. Adv. Zool.*, 25: 12-15.

Brown, T.T., Wisniewski, A.B. and Dobs, A.S. 2006. Gonadal and adrenal abnormalities in drug users: cause of consequence of drug use behaviour and poor health. *Am. J. Infect. Dis.*, 2: 130-135.

Budziszewska, B., Jaworska-Feil, L. and Lason, W., 1996. The effects of repeated amphetamine and cocaine administration on adrenal, gonadal and thyroid hormone levels in rat plasma. *Exp. Clin. Encorinol. Diabet.*, 104: 334-338.

Burdette, B.H., Leeman, S. and Munson, P.L., 1961. The reversal by nalorphine on the inhibitory effect of morphine on the secretion of adrenocorticotropic hormone in stress. *J. Pharmacol. Exp. Ther.*, 132: 323-328.

Cami, J. and Farre, M., 2003. Drug addiction. *N. Eng. J. Med.*, 349: 975-986.

Cami, J., Gilbert, M., San, R. and Torre, R. de la, 1992. Hypercortisolism after opioid discontinuation in rapid detoxification of heroin addicts. *Br. J. Addict.*, 87: 1145-1151.

Chester Jones, I. and Phillips J.G., 1986. The adrenal and interrenal glands. In: *Vertebrate Endocrinology: Fundamental and Biomedical Implications. Vol. 1. Morphological Considerations*, (Eds.) P.K.T. Pang and M.P. Schreibman. Academic Press, San Diego, pp. 319-350.

Cocores, J.A., Dackis, C.A. and Gold, M.S., 1986. Sexual dysfunction: secondary to cocaine abuse in two patients. *J. Clin. Psychiat.*, 47: 384-385.

Cushman, P. Jr., 1973. Plasma testosterone in narcotics addiction. *Am. J. Med.*, 55: 452-458.

Cushman, P. Jr., Bordier, B. and Hilton, J.G., 1970. Hypothalamic-pituitary-adrenal axis in methadone treated heroin addicts. *J. Clin. Endocrinol. Metab.*, 30: 24-29.

Delitala, G., Grossman, A. and Besser, G.M., 1981a. Changes in pituitary hormone levels induced by metenkephalin in man: the role of dopamine. *Life Sci.*, 29: 1537-1544.

Delitala, G., Grossman, A. and Besser, G.M., 1981b. The modulation of opiate induced changes in anterior pituitary function by a dopamine agonist and antagonist. *Neuroendocrinol. Lett.*, 3: 147-152.

Delitala, G., Grossman, A. and Besser, G.M., 1983. Differential effects of opiate peptides and alkaloids on anterior pituitary hormone secretion. *Neuroendocrinology*, 37: 275-279.

Eisenman, A.J., Fraser, H.F., Sloan, J. and Isbell, H., 1958. Urinary 17-ketosteroid excretion during a cycle of addiction to morphine. *J. Pharmacol. Exp. Ther.*, 124: 305-311.

Eisenman, A.J., Fraser, H.F. and Brooks, J.W. ,1961. Urinary excretion and plasma levels of 17-hydroxycorticoids during a cycle of addiction to morphine. *J. Pharmacol. Exp. Ther.*, 132: 226-231.

El-Daly, E.S., 1996. Influence of acute and chronic morphine or stadol on the secretion of adrenocorticotropin and hypothalamic-releasing hormone in the rat. *Life Sci.*, 59: 1881-1890.

Facchinetti, F., Volpe, A., Farci, G., Petraglia, F., Porro, C.A., Barbiri, G., Cioni, A., Bale-Strieri, A. and Genazzani, A.R., 1985. Hypothalamus-pituitary-adrenal axis of heroin addicts. *Drug Alcohol Depend.*, 15: 361-366.

Gaillard, R.C., Grossman, A., Smith, R., Rees, L.H. and Besser, G.M., 1981. The effects of a metenkephalin analogue on ACTH, BLPH, β-endorphin and metenkephalin in patients with adrenocortical disease. *Clin. Endocrinol.*, 14: 471-478.

Goldstein, A., Lowney, L.I. and Pal, B.K., 1974. Opiate receptors. *Life Sci.*, 14: 615-623.

Goodman, L.S. and Gilman, A.G., 1975. *Pharmacological Basis of Therapeutics*. 5th Edn. Macmillan, New York.

Grossman, A. and Jones, A.E., 1983. Opiate receptors: endorphins and enkephalins. *Clin. Endocrinol.Metab.*, 12: 31-56.

Martin del Campo, A.F., Dowson, J.H., Herbert, J. and Paykal, E.S., 1994. Effects of naloxone on diurnal rhythms in mood and endocrine function: a dose-response study in man. *Psychopharmacology*, 114: 583-540.

McDonald, R.K., Evans, F.T., Weise, V.K. and Patrick, R.W., 1959. Effects of morphine and nalorphine on plasma hydrocortisone level in man. *J. Pharmacol. Exp. Ther.*, 125: 241-247.

Mendelson, J.H., Mello, N.K., Toeh, S.K., Ellingboe, J. and Cochin, J., 1989. Cocaine effects on pulsatile secretion of anterior pituitary, gonadal and adrenal hormones. *J. Clin. Endocrinol. Metab.*, 69: 1256-1260.

Mendelson, J.H., Toeh, S.K., Mello, N.K., Ellingboe, J. and Rhodes, E., 1992. Acute effects of cocaine on plasma ACTH, luteinizing hormone and prolactin levels in cocaine-dependent men. *J. Pharmacol. Exp. Ther.*, 263: 505-509.

Sporer, K.A., 1999. Acute heroin overdose. *Ann. Intern. Med.*, 130: 584-590.

Sarli, M., Plotkin, H. and Zanchetta, J., 1994. Alcohol osteopathy. *Medicina*, 54: 363-370

Stubbs, W.A., Delitala, C., Jones, A., Jeffcoate, W.J., Edwards, C.R., Ratter, S.J., Besser, G.M., Bloom, S.R. and Alberti, K.G., 1978. Hormonal and metabolic responses to an enkephalin analogue in normal man. *Lancet*, ii: 1225-1227.

Taylor, P.M., Luna, S.P.L. and Sear, J.W., 1995. Total intravenous anesthesia and guaiphensin pharamacokinetics, cardiopulmonary and endocrine effects. *Res. Vet. Sci.*, 59: 17-23.

Wisniewski, A.B., Brown, T.T., John, M., Cofranceso, J. Jr., Golub, E.T., Ricketts, E.P., Wand, G. and Dobs, A.S., 2006. Cortisol levels and depression in men and women using heroin and cocaine. *Psychoneuroendocrinology*, 31: 250-255.

Chapter 16

Effect of Neem Seed Alkaloid Extract on the Serum Levels of Sex Hormones and Pituitary Gonadotrophins in Male Albino Rats

V. Maruthappan[1], M. Ramesh[1] and K. Sakthi Shree[2]*

[1]Department of Zoology, School of Life Science, Bharathiar University, Coimbatore – 641 046, India

[2]PG and Research Centre, Department of Zoology, Government Arts College (Autonomous), Coimbatore – 641 018, India

ABSTRACT

This study was aimed at determining the activity of alkaloid extract of Neem seed on the serum levels of sex hormones and pituitary gonadotrophins was studied in adult male albino rats. Three tolerated doses obtained from the graph of percentage toxicity (10, 50 and 150 mg/kg) were separately administered orally, daily for seven days to three groups of male rats (n=6) while group of 6 rats received the vehicle (saline) as control. The results showed that 10 mg/kg/d caused increase serum levels of FSH and estrogen but decrease in the serum levels of LH and testosterone compared to control; 50 mg/kg/d

---

* Corresponding author: E-mail: zoomaruthu@yahoo.co.in

elevated the serum levels of FSH, estrogen but inhibited testosterone; while 150 mg/kg/d pretreatments caused a significant decrease ($p<0.01$) in the serum levels of FSH, LH and testosterone. The results permitted the conclusion that Neem seed extract treatment inhibited the serum level of the androgen, testosterone which might result in a male infertility.

Keywords: *Neem extract, Sex hormones, Gonadotrophins, Infertility.*

Introduction

Azadirachta indica (Malvacea, AI) popularly known as Neem, is a medicinal plant that grows freely all over Indian subcontinent. Neem has a role in the treatment of disorders like microbial infections, skin diseases, dental disorders, malaria, syphilis, leprosy and has antiseptic property (Murthy *et al.*, 1978, Pillai and Santha Kumari, 1981, Sen *et al.*, 1992). Anti-inflammatory, immunostimulant and anti-ulcerogenic actions have also been reported in the extracts of *A. indica* (Sen *et al.*, 1992, Ray *et al.*, 1996, Pillai *et al.*, 1978, Balakrishnan *et al.*, 1995). The medicinal and industrial uses of various parts of neem tree and the compounds isolated from it have been reviewed (Schmutterer, 1995). More than 135 compounds of diverse structure have been isolated from various parts of Neem (Kraus, 1995, Devakumar and Sukh Dev, 1996) but few of them have been studied for their biological and pharmacological actions. Alkaloids have been reported to possess anti-infertility activities (Udoh *et al.*, 2009).

The need for fertility regulation in men cannot be overemphasized. While chemical methods for fertility regulation in woman are readily available the 'male pill' remains a distant prospect as effective contraceptive regimens are still toxic and inconvenient (WHO, 1996). Acceptable male contraceptive methods should reduce the burden traditionally placed almost exclusively on the female partner. In Indian system of medicine, plants have been a major source of drugs for the treatment of infertility. World Health Organisation has suggested the evaluation of the potential of plants as effective therapeutic agents, especially in areas where there is lack of safe modern drugs (Eshrat, 2003). Neem has been used in Indian herbal medicine for various diseases. Phytochemistry showed that the Neem seed extract contained alkaloid, glycosides, saponins, flavonoids, coumarin, tannins, aliphatic compounds and tetranortriterpenoids (Chopra *et al.*, 1956). The present paper deals with effect of the seed extract on serum levels of testosterone, LH, estrogen and FSH in male albino rats.

Materials and Methods

Preparation of Plant Extracts

The seeds of *A. indica* were obtained from the University of Bharathiar around the month June and July, 2009. The seeds were washed and oven dried at 80°C for 48 hrs. They were milled into fine powder using electric blender. The powdered material (100 g) was extracted with ethanol by hot continuous percolation method in Soxhlet apparatus. The extract was evaporated to dryness under vacuum and dried in a vacuum desiccator to obtain a residue of 20.65 g. The residue seed extract was preserved in the refrigerator.

Treatment

Twenty four adult male albino rats weighting between 200-250 g were divided into 4 groups (n=6). Group 1 received saline (0.5 ml) daily as control, group 2, 3 and 4 received 10, 50 and 150 mg/kd/d for seven days respectively following the method adopted by Udoh. Seven days after treatment the rats were sacrificed and blood sera were prepared for hormonal assays. Experiments were conducted with the approval of Institutional Animal Ethics Committee.

Hormonal Assays

Serum samples were assayed for the following: follicle stimulating hormones (FSH), luteinizing hormone (LH), testosterone and estrogen (estradiol). The method used was microwell enzyme-linked immuno-sorbent assay (Elisa) using analytical grade reagents (Sigma Chemical Company, USA).

Statistical Analysis

All data for control and experimental groups were subjected to statistical evaluation, using student's 't' test and analysis of variance (ANOVA) for significant differences between the control and experimental groups at $p<0.05$.

Results and Discussion

The study herein presented was instigated by an earlier finding that Neem seed diets, fed for durations lasting 7 days, caused testicular atrophy, reduced relative testis weight, induced spermatogenesis arrest and resulted in degeneration of spermatozoa. These effects were replicated by oral doses of crude alkaloid extracts of the Neem (Sathiyaraj *et al.*, 2010). Table 16.1 shows the effect of Neem seed alkaloid extract on sex hormones and pituitary gonadotrophins in male albino rats. The testosterone level (ng/ml) in control rat was 2.23±0.32. Whereas there was a significant (p<0.05) decreased in testosterone levels of Neem seed alkaloid extract treated rats at 10, 50 and 150 mg/kg/d for 7 days as 1.48±0.56, 1.13±0.14 and 0.76±0.2 respectively. A significant difference (p<0.05) was found on LH by decreasing in its level in treated with Neem seed alkaloid extract treated rat as 0.40±0.01, 0.23±0.01 and 0.13±0.07 (Table 16.1).

Table 16.1: Effect of Neem Seed Alkaloid Extract on Sex Hormones Levels and Pituitary Gonadotrophins in Male Albino Rats

Groups	*Testosterone (ng/ml)*	*LH (μlu/ml)*	*Estrogen (pg/ml)*	*FSH (μlu/ml)*
Control	2.23±0.32	1.07±0.03	16.6±0.10	0.76±0.03
Neem seed extract (10 mg/kg/d)	1.48±0.56	0.40±0.01	61.6±0.02*	1.53±0.03*
Neem seed extract (50 mg/kg/d)	1.13±0.14*	0.23±0.01*	40.0±0.01*	1.80±0.70*
Neem seed extract (150 mg/kg/d)	0.76±0.20*	0.13±0.07*	23.33±0.05*	2.01±0.03*

Values are expressed as mean±SEM.

Number in parenthesis represents number of animals for treatment group, *P<0.05, t-test.

Values are±SD of 6 rats in each group.

The alkaloid extract of (10, 50 and 150 mg/kg/d) caused an increase in the serum level of estrogen in male rats. Doses of 10 and 50 mg/kg/d administered daily for 7 days caused a sharp rise in the serum level of estrogen. Whereas the highest dose of 150 mg/kg/d induced gradual increase (Table 16.1). Pretreatment with the alkaloid extract daily for 7 days caused an increase in the serum level of FSH in males compared to control (Table 16.1). The increase in the serum level of FSH in male rats was statistically significant ($p<0.05$).

Treatment with the extract (dose 10, 50 and 150 mg/kg/d for 7 days) was highly effective in producing reversible functional sterility. The drug treated male rats clearly indicates that the drug caused structural and functional alteration in testes, epididymies and seminal vesicle (Sathiyaraj *et al.*, 2010). The results of the study revealed a decrease in the serum level of testosterone. This observation was similar to the earlier findings of Udoh and Ekpeyong and Udoh *et al.* in their report dietary intake of the seed extract caused reduction in body weight gain compared to control, testicular atrophy, spermatogenesis arrest and degeneration of spermatozoa. The reduction in the serum level of testosterone could probable be due to the decrease of serum levels of LH observed in this investigation. Leydig cells secrete testosterone by the stimulatory effect of LH. In males, reduction of testosterone level might impaire spermatogenesis and cause male infertility (Udoh *et al.*, 2005c).

The above observation may be interpreted variously, depending on the sex of animals involved. In the male rat, following long-term ingestion of Neem seed or oral administration of the alkaloid extract there is marked spermatogenesis arrest (Udoh, 1998). Possible explanations for such observation include a direct action of Neem seed extract on the testis, thereby causing inhibition of gonadotrophic action in that organ. Other possibilities include preventing the release of pituitary gonadotrophins and/or elevation of blood levels of testosterone (*via* inhibition of hepatic metabolism) thereby including negative feedback effect on gonadotrophin release. It is not plausible that prevention of gonadotrophin release is the likely mechanism in operation; because Neem seed extract actually was observed to enhance serum levels of FSH and LH in male rats.

Further, elevation of blood testosterone levels is not a good explanation because Neem seed extract actually decreased serum levels of testosterone in male rats. The most plausible explanation of the observations on male rats in this study is the possibility of Neem seed extract inhibition of gonadotrophic action on the testis. This is in consonance with an earlier study indicating that phenolic compounds are antispermatogenic (Udoh and Patil, 1992, Braide *et al.*, 2003). Any direct damage to the test is likely to impair gonadal response to FSH and LH; such as diminished testosterone production due to lack of gonadal response to LH. Observations in this study indicated that serum levels of testosterone were remarkable low, despite the marked elevation of LH levels in blood. This study further observed a dose dependent increase in the estrogen serum level. This increase might probably be due to the conversion of testosterone to estrogen (Chinoy and Padman, 1996, Udoh *et al.*, 2009).

It is concluded that prolonged high-level exposure to Neem seed alkaloid extract induces profound changes in serum concentrations of gonadotrophins and gonadal hormones in rat; and that the direction of alteration (increase or decrease) depends significantly on the sex of animals under observation. These effects on the levels of gonodal hormones are most likely due to a primary peripheral action of Neem seed alkaloid extract on the male reproductive system, rather than being secondary to alteration by eem seed extract in central gonadotrophin regulation.

References

Balakrishnan, V., Narendranathan, M., Subair, A.S., Raji, E. K., Pillai, N.R. and Santha Kumari, G., 1985. Nimbidin in duodenal ulcer. *Tropical Gastroenterology*, 6: 23-25.

Braide, V.B., Agube, C.A., Essien, G.E. and Udoh, F.V., 2003. Effect of *Garcinia kola* seed alkaloid extract on levels of gonadal hormones and pituitary gonadotrophins in rat serum. *Nig. J. Physiol. Sci.*, 18: 59-63.

Chinoy, R.J. and Padman, P., 1996. Antifertility investigation and benzene extract or *Carica papya* seeds in male albino rats. *J. Med. Aromatic. Plant Sci.*, 18: 489-491.

Chopra, R.N., Nayer, S. and Chopra, I.C., 1956. *Glossary of Indian Medicinal Plants*. CSIR, New Delhi.

Devakumar, C. and Sukh Dev, 1996. Chemistry. In: *Sukh Dev Chemistry Neem*, 2nd edition, (Eds.) N.S. Randhawa and B.S. Parmar, pp. 77-80.

Eshrat, M.H., 2003. Effect of *Coccinia indica* (L.) and *Abroma augusta* (L.) on glycemia, lipid profile and on indicators of end organ damage in streptozotocin induced diabetes rats. *Indian J. Clin. Biochem.*, 18, 54-57.

Kraus, W., 1995. Biologically active ingredients. *In*: *The Neem Tree*, (Ed.) H. Schmutterer. Weinheim, Federal Republic Germany, VCH, p. 35-38.

Murty, K.S., Rao, D.N., Rao, D.K. and Murty, L.B.G., 1978. A preliminary study on hypoglycemic and antihperglycemic effect of *Azadirachta indica*. *Indian J. Pharmacol.*, 10: 247-250.

Pillai, N.R. and Santha Kumari, G., 1981. Hypoglycemic activity of Melia *Azadirachta indica*. *Indian J. Med. Res.*, 74: 931-935.

Pillai, N.R., Suganthan, D., Seshadri, C. and Santha Kumari, G., 1978. Anti-gastric activity of *nimbidin*. *Indian J. Med. Res.*, 68: 169-172.

Ray, A., Banerjee, B.D. and Sen, P., 1996. Modulation of humoral and cell mediated immune response by *Azadirachta indica* (Neem) in mice. *Indian J. Exp. Biol.*, 34: 698-702.

Sathiyaraj, K., Sivaraj, A., Vinoth Kumar, P., Devi, K. and Senthil, Kumar B., 2010. Spermicidal activity of *Azadirachta indica* (Neem) aqueous leaf extract on male albino rats. *Int. J. Pharm. Tech. Res.*, 2: 588-593.

Schmutterer, H., 1995. *In*: *The Neem Tree*, (Ed.) H. Schmutterer. Weinheim, Federal Republic Germany, VCH, p. 1-5.

Sen, P., Mediratta, P.K. and Ray, A., 1992. Effects of *Azadirachta indica* A Juss on some biochemical, immunological and visceral parameters in normal and stressed rats. *Indian J. Exp. Biol.*, 30: 1170-1174.

Udoh, F.V., 1998. Effect of extracts of Garcinia kola seeds and Piper guineense leaves on morphology of reproductive organs of the male rats. *M.Sc. Thesis*, University of Calabar, Calabar, Nigeria, September.

Udoh, F.V., 2007. The effects of *Gnetum africanum* leaf extracts on some biochemical indices and endocrine functions in albino rats. *Ph.D. Thesis*, University of Calabar, Calabar, Nigeria.

Udoh, F.V., Udoh, P.B. and Umoh, E.E., 2005c. Activity of alkaloid extract of *Carical papaya* seeds on reproductive functions in male Wistar rats. *Pharmaceutical Biol.*, 43: 563-567.

Udoh, P. and Ekpeyong, J., 2001. Effects of *Mucuna urens* (Horse eye bean) on the gonads of male guinea pigs. *Phytopher. Res.*, 15: 99-103.

Udoh, P. and Patil, D.R., 1992. Effects of gossypol acetate on pituitary-adrenal axis in male albino rats. *Contraception*, 45: 263-266.

Udoh, P.B., Udoh, F.V., Umoren, E.B., James, U.W., Okeke, C.P. and Agwu, B., 2009. Effect of Caricapryl-99 seed alkaloid extract on the serum levels of sex hormones and pituitary gonadotrophins in male albino rats. *Nig. J. Physiol. Sci.*, 24: 13-17.

WHO, 1996. Task force on methods for the regulation of male contraceptive efficacy of testosterone and oligospermia in normal men, fertility and sterility. *Int. J. Androl.*, 65: 821-823.

Section II

Animal Reproduction

Chapter 17

Trypterygium wilfordii: A New Hope for Male Contraception

Mukesh Kumar[1]* and N.K. Lohiya[2]

[1]*Department Zoology, M.S.J. (Government P.G.) College, Bharatpur, Rajasthan, India*

[2]*Department Zoology, University of Rajasthan, Jaipur, Rajasthan, India*

ABSTRACT

Present study summarizes the findings of the major experiment with dose level (6mg/animal/day, oral of GTW) (total glycosides of *Trypterygium wilfordii*) being tested in male langur monkeys for 120 days to assess its ability to suppress fertility, mechanism of action, reversibility and toxic effects, if any. Semen analysis, semen and blood biochemical parameters were done fortnightly. GTW treatment caused gradual reduction in sperm density and motility from 45-days of dosing in all the treated animals when compared with control group without affecting accessory sex glands functioning and circulating level of testosterone. But 6-mg dose level could not suppress the spermatogenesis completely during treatment period.

No noticeable changes were observed in clinical chemistry during the course of investigation. This treatment effects

* Corresponding author: E-mail: prof.mukeshkumar@rediffmail.com

gradually disappeared during recovery period. In conclusion, GTW affects spermatogenesis without affecting accessory sex glands functioning and circulating level of testosterone. It does not cause damage to Leydig and Sertoli cells at the dose level being used and treatment effects were reversible. GTW may have potentiality for male contraceptive in future.

Keywords: *GTW, Male contraception, Langur monkey, Toxicity and Reversibility.*

Introduction

Trypterygium wilfordii Hook F., a perennial twinning vine belonging to the family celastraceae is cultivated widely in Southern China. Since late 1970s active constituent *i.e.* so called multiglycosides of *Trypterygium wilfordii* Hook F. (hereafter GTW) are being used for the treatment of renal, liver, skin, collagenous diseases and arthritis and in few patients (male) this treatment caused necrospermia/ azoospermia and suppression of fertility incidentally (Li, *et al.*, 1982; Qin *et al.*, 1982; Jia, 1985). Visualizing the possible effect on male fertility, Chinese researchers have done some studies with GTW in rat, mice and human volunteers (some) suffering from above cited diseases and these investigations have shown reduction/ suppression of male fertility (Qin *et al.*, 1986; Qian *et al.*, 1986). These preliminary studies on GTW seem to be encouraging but its ability to suppress male fertility properly, precise mechanism of action safety and reversibility are yet to be investigated. Present study was designed aiming at all those uninvestigated aspects of GTW in male langur monkey because this non-human primate animal model is very close to human being in its endocrine and exocrine profile and lack of seasonality provides opportunity to conduct long term experiment (Lohiya *et al.*, 1985) and findings could be extrapolated for further studies in human.

Materials and Methods

Experimental Animal

Adult male langur monkeys (*Presbytis entellus entellus* Dufresne) were caught from the jungle around Jaipur, India and recruited for this study. The selection of adult male langur monkeys was based on following characters:

- ☆ The animal should have well developed musculature with pinkish oedomatous band on rump and large erupted canines.
- ☆ The animal should have good general health and should have the normal range of clinical laboratory tests in blood, urine and semen.

Housing and Feeding

Animals were housed in metallic cages under semi-natural conditions in our Primate Research Facility (PRF). Wheat chapaties, green leaves, seasonal fruits and roasted/soaked grams were given with free access to drinking water. Animals were quarantined for 3-4 months before commencing the experiment. Reproductive status of the animal was examined by semen analysis.

Experimental Design

One long term experiment with 6 mg. dose level was done. Experiment composed of two groups and each group consisted of five animals.

Experiment Protocol

Group – A: Animal of this group received vehicle (banana) alone during treatment phase to serve as a control.

Group – B: Animals of this group received 6 mg GTW/day/oral during treatment phase.

This study was divided into three phases

- ☆ Pre-treatment phase: 30 days
- ☆ Treatment phase: 120 days
- ☆ Recovery phase: 90 days

Body Weight

Body weight of the animals was recorded once a month during all the phases of study.

Semen Analysis

Semen samples were collected fortnightly by penile electro ejaculation (Mastroianni and Manson, 1963) and analysed for:

(a) Seminal Characteristic

Semen weight, volume, colour, pH, sperm motility, density and sperm morphology (WHO, 1980).

(b) Semen Biochemistry

Biochemical analysis of seminal plasma fructose (Man, 1964), acid phosphates (Gutman and Gutman, 1940) lactic de-hydrogenase (Cabaud and Wroblewski, 1958), glycerylphosphorylcholene (White, 1959), Magnesium (Neill and Neely, 1956) and citric acid (Lindner and Mann, 1960).

Circulating Level of Testosterone

To estimate the serum testosterone level (WHO, 1950) three blood sample at 15 minute intervals (08.00, 08.15, 08.30 am) were collected monthly. Animals were introduced to receptive female one every month for observing mounting and copulating behaviour (Lohiya and Sharma, 1983).

Clinical Investigation

Following laboratory clinical investigations were done during the entire course of study.

(a) Haematology

Haemoglobin (Crosby *et al.*, 1954), haematocrit. (Natelson, 1951), RBC and WBC (Lynch *et al.*, 1969).

(b) Serum Biochemistry

SGOT and SGPT (Reitman and Frankel, 1957), LDH (Cabaud and Wrobelewski, 1958), CPK (Hughes, 1962) and blood glucose (Asatoor and King 1954).

(c) Electrolyte Metabolism

Na (John, 1960), K (John, 1960) Cl (Schales and Schales, 1941) PO_4 (Gomorri, 1942) and Mg (Neil and Neely 1956).

Statistical Analysis

Data were expressed as mean ± S.E. and analysed for statistical difference using student "t" test.

Results

Body Weight

No appreciable changes were recorded in the body weight in

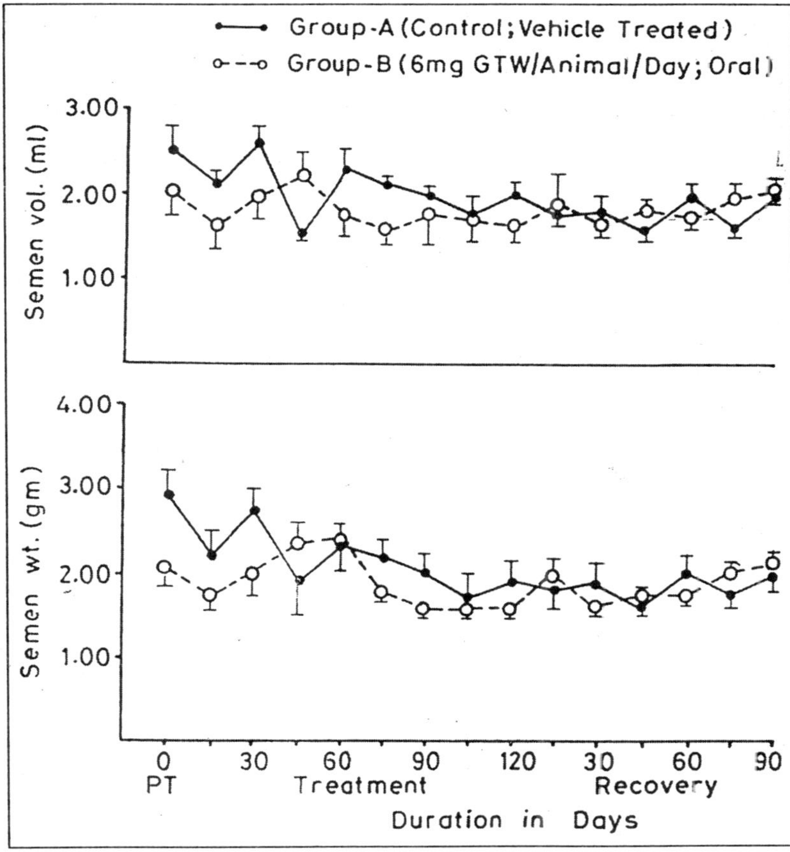

Figure 17.1: Showing Normal Semen Weight and Volume of Group-A (Control; vehicle treated) and Group-B (6 mg GTW/animal/day; oral) During Pretreatment, Treatment and Recovery Phases. Each value represents mean ± S.E. (Vertical bars)

all the treated animals when compared with control group during the course of study.

Seminology

Macroscopic evaluation of semen revealed no drug-related change in semen weight, volume, seminal fluid volume, colour and pH during experimentation. The ejaculatory responses were found normal.

Treatment of GTW caused gradual decline in sperm density but semen volume of all the animal possessed adequate numbers of spermatozoa (ranged 20 – 40 million/ml) at the end of treatment (Figure 17.2). Sperm motility also showed gradual decline

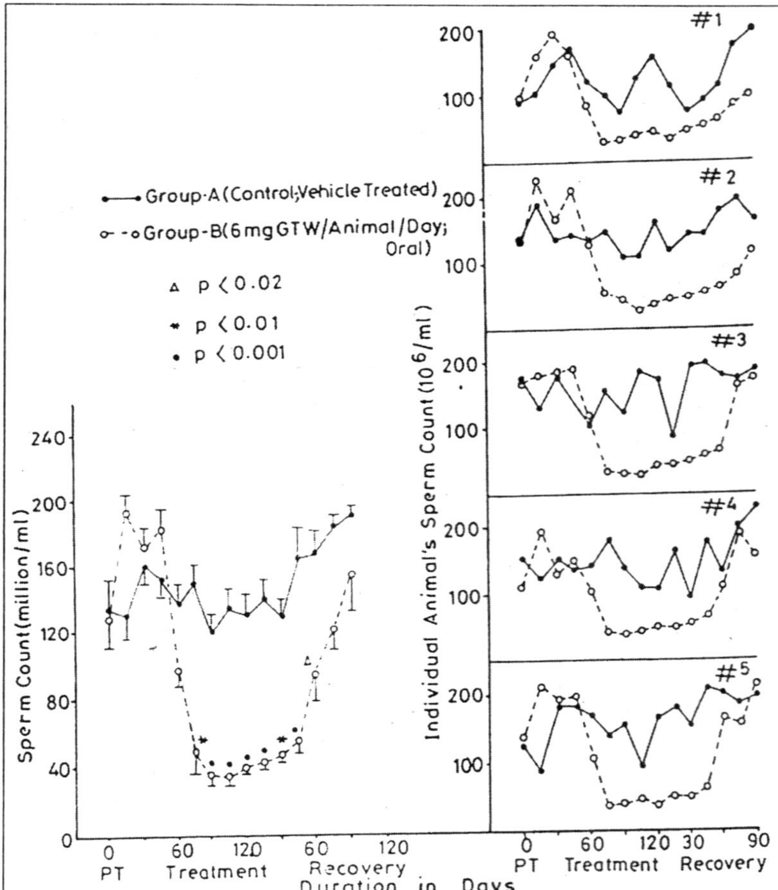

Figure 17.2: Showing the Sperm Count (million/ml) of Group-A and Group-B (6 mg/animal/day; oral) Animals. Gradual decline is evident in sperm count from 45-60 days of the GTW treatment. It was significant at the end of the treatment (ranged 20-40 million/ml). Gradual recovery was observed during 90 days of the termination of the treatment.

Figure # 1–5: Revealing individual animal's sperm count (million/ml) of both the groups during experimentation.

(qualitatively and quantitatively) (Figure 17.3) with increased production of deformed spermatozoa. Complete restoration of sperm density and motility was evident during the end of the recovery period.

Seminal Plasma Biochemistry

Treatment of GTW did not reveal any significant change in fructose, acid phosphates, glycerylphosphorylcholine, lactic dehydrogenase, citric acid and magnesium during the course of experimentation.

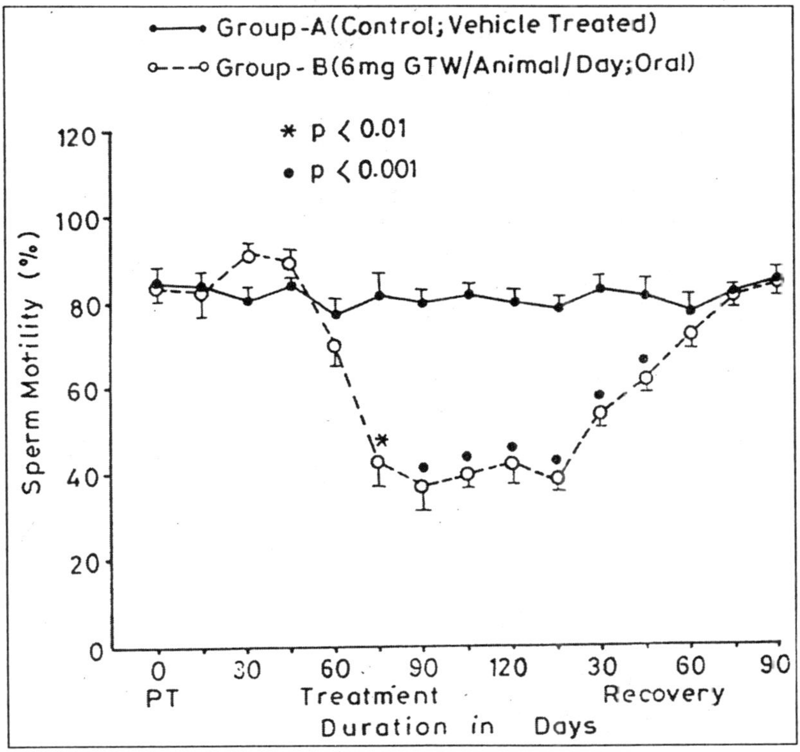

Figure 17.3: Showing the Decrease in Sperm Motility of GTW Received Animals During 45-60 Days of Treatment and it is Significant at the End of the Treatment. Each value represents mean ± S.E. (Vertical bars)

Libido

No remarkable changes were observed in ejaculatory responses latencies. Animals showed normal mounting and copulating behaviour throughout the study period.

Haematology

Haematelogical variables: haemoglobin, RBC, WBC and haematocrit remained within normal range during the entire period of investigation.

Clinical Chemistry

Activity of serum transaminases (GOT and GPT) CPK, LDH was observed within control range. Rate of critinine clearance and

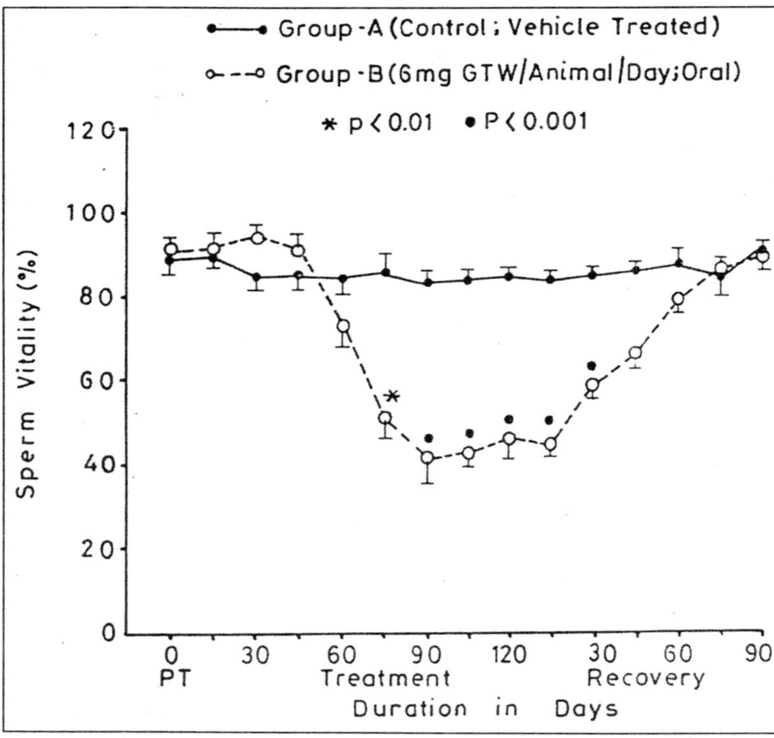

Figure 17.4: Alive Sperm Percentage of GTW Treated and Control Animals during the Experimentation. Each value represents the mean ± S.E. (Vertical bars).

level of blood glucose fluctuated within normal range during the course of investigation.

Electrolytes

Treatment of GTW didn't affect the metabolism of serum electrolytes: Na, K, Mg, PO_4 and Cl during the study period.

Circulating Level of Testosterone

No significant change were observed in the circulating levels of testosterone in treated animals when compared with control group.

Discussion

In present study, treatment of GTW caused gradual reduction in sperm production and motility with increased number of deformed spermatozoa which reflects that GTW primarily affects spermatozoa and spermatogenesis. Earlier studies done in mice and rat have shown similar findings but these researchers didn't propose the mechanism of action of GTW in suppressing the spermatogenesis precisely (Qian *et al.*, 1986).

Results of the present study show normal circulating level of testosterone which reflects that GTW does not affect testosterone metabolism. Qian *et al.* (1984) also reported that GTW does not affect testosterone level and morphology of Leydig cells.

Presence of normal concentration of seminal plasma contents; fructose, magnesium, zinc, alkalinephosphatase, lacticdehydrogenase, glycerylphophorylcholine during the course of investigation shows that GTW does not affect the accessory sex glands functioning.

Haematological and biochemical parameters being done during entire course of investigation fell/fluctuated within normal range which indicates that GTW does not cause any untoward effect in treated animals. Changes noticed during course of treatment gradually returned to normalcy which reflects the reversibility of this approach. In conclusion, GTW impaired/suppresses spermatogenesis without affecting the functioning of accessory sex glands and circulating level of testosterone. All effects were reversible. These findings in langur monkeys seem to be encouraging and suggest further studies on this plant products, which may explore the possibility for a male contraceptive.

Acknowledgements

This study was sponsored by Indian Council of Medical Research (ICMR), New Delhi and financial assistance to Dr. Mukesh Kumar in the form of Senior Research Fellowship (SRF) and Research Associateship (RA) from ICMR is gratefully acknowledged.

References

Asatoor, A.M. and King, E.J., 1954. Simplified colorimetric blood sugar method. *Biochem. T. J.* 56: XLIV.

Cabaud, P.G. and Wroblewski, F., 1958. Colorimetric measurement of lactic dehydrogenase activity of body fluids. *Am. J. Clin. Pathol.*, 30: 234–236.

Crosby, W.H., Mann, J.I. and Furth, F.W., 1954. Standardizing a method for clinical hemo-globinometry. *U.S. Armed Forces. Med. J.*, 5: 693–703.

Gomorri, C.J., 1942. Colorimetric determination of Phosphate. *Lab. Clin. Med.*, 27: 955.

Gutman, E.B. and Gutman, A.B., 1940. Estimation of acid phosphates activity of blood serum *J. Biol. Chem.*, 136: 201–209.

Hughes, B.P., 1962. Colorimetric determination creatinine phosphokinase. *Clin. Chem. Acta.*, 7: 597.

Jia, L., 1985. *Chin. Pharm. Bull.*, 20: 101-105.

Jonh, A.D., 1960. *Flame Photometry*. McGraw-Hill Book Company Inc., p. 295.

Lindner, H.R. and Mann, T., 1960. Relationship between the content of androgenic steroids in the testes and the secretary activity of the seminal vesicles in the bull. *J. Endocr.*, 21: 341–360.

Lohiya, N.K. and Sharma, O.P., 1983. Effect of cyproterone acetate with combination of testosterone enanthate on seminal characteristic, andragenecity and clinical chemistry in langur monkey. *Contraception*, 28: 575–56.

Lohiya, N.K., David, G.F.X. and Anand Kumar, T.C., 1983. The langur monkeys as an experiment model for research in reproduction. *Contracept. Deliv. Syst.*, 4: 89.

Li, L.S., Zhang, Chen, H.P. Li, Y., Ji, D.X., Zhan, J. H., How, F.F. and Chen, P.D., 1982. Effect of *Trypterygium wilfordii* in the treatment of nephritis. *Natl. Med. J. China*, 62: 581–585.

Lynch, M.J., Raphael, S.S., Mellore, L.D., Spare, P.D. and Inwood, M.J.H., 1969. *Medical Laboratory: Technology and Clinical Pathology*. W.B. Saunders Company, Philadelphia.

Mann, T. (Ed.) 1964. *The Biochemistry of Semen and of the Male Reproductive Tract*. Methuen, London.

Mastroianni, L., Jr. and Manson, W.A. Jr., 1963. Collection of monkey semen by electro ejaculation. *Proc. Soc. Exp. Biol. Med.*, p. 1025–1027.

Natelson, S., 1951. Routine use of ultramicro methods in the clinical laboratory. *Am. J. Clin. Pathol.*, 21: 1153–1172.

Neill, D.W. and Neely, R.A., 1959. Estimation of magnesium in serum using titan yellow. *J. Clin. Pathol.*, 9: 162–163.

Qin, G.W., Yang, X.M., Gu, W.H., Wang, B.D., Chen, Z.X., Guo, R.X. and Shao, K.W., 1982. The structure of two new diterpene lactones from *Trypterygium wilfordii, wilforlide* A and B. *Acta Chimica Sinica.*, 40: 637-647.

Qian, S.Z., Zhang, C.Q. and Xu, Y., 1986. Effect of *Trypterygium Wilfordii* on the fertility of rats. *Contraception*, 33: 105–110.

Qian, S.Z., Zhang, C.Q., Xu, N. and Xu, Y., 1986. Anti-fertility effect of *Trypterygium wilfordii* in men. *Adv. Contracept.*, 2: 253–254.

Reitman, S. and Frankel, S., 1957. A colorimetric method for determination of serum glutomic oxalo acetic and glutamic pyruvic transaminases. *Am. J. Clin. Pathol.*, 28: 56–63.

Schales, O. and Schales, S., 1941. A simplified and accurate method for determination of chloride in biological fluids. *J. Biol. Chem.*, 140: 879-884.

W.H.O., 1980. Laboratory manual for the examination of Human Semen and Semen – Cervical Mucus interaction. WHO special programme of Research, Development and Research Training in Human Reproduction. World Health Organization, Geneva, Switzerland.

White, I.G., 1959. Studies on the estimation of glycerol, fructose and lactic acid with particular reference to semen. *Aust. J. Exp. Biol.*, 37: 441–450.

Chapter 18

Mating Behaviour of Commercially Important Portunid Crab *Portunus pelagicus* (Linnaeus, 1758)

Anand, T. and P. Soundarapandian*

CAS in Marine Biology, Faculty of Marine Science, Parangipettai, Tamil Nadu, India

ABSTRACT

The blue swimming crab *Portunus pelagicus* is one of the commercially important crab along Parangipettai coast. Berried females are important to start a commercial hatchery. The berried females are not available throughout the year from natural resources. So the production of berried females in controlled condition is essential. Hence on mating behaviour of the blue swimming crab *P. pelagicus* was studied under the controlled conditions in the laboratory. The mating was took place in three phases, that are Contact, Cradle- Carry position and mating after the female entered premating moult. The male was attracted by the moulted female by releasing sex pheromones through their urine in the water and sensing the pheromones by males and contacts the particular female by stretching the chelate in front of the female, then embraces the female using his walking legs and hold her beneath him in what is termed the cradle-carry position and carried the female

* Corresponding author: E-mail: soundsuma@yahoo.com

to suitable position for mating. Then the male mate the female and transfers the spermatophores into the female's spermatheca. The sperms from the spermatophores fertilize the egg at the time of spawning. The fertilized eggs are extruded through the gonophores and get attached to pleopods of the abdominal flab to form a egg mass is called berry. Those females are also called as berried or ovigerous females.

Keywords: *Mating behaviour, Blue swimming crab, Portunus pelagicus.*

Introduction

The crab fishery in India is fast developing and there is a vast scope for the crab meat both national and international markets (Dinakaran and Soundarapandian, 2009). Crabs rank third next to the shrimps and lobsters for their esteemed seafood delicacy and also value of fishery they support (Mohammed Saved and Rajeev Rahavan, 2001). The economically important portunid crabs found along east coast of India are *Scylla serrata, S. tranquebarica, Portunus pelagicus, P. sanguinolentus, Charybdis feriata, C. lucifera* and *C. truncate* (John Samuel *et al.,* 2004). The blue swimming crab *P. pelagicus* inhabits coastal marine and estuarine waters throughout the Indo-west pacific (Stephenson, 1962; Kailola *et al.,* 1993) is the basis of important commercial and recreational fisheries. In recent times the blue swimming crabs are fished in large quantities from all the seas in India and finally sold as a processed food (Dinakaran and Soundarapandian, 2009). So the demand of these crabs is increasing day by day. Hatchery technology and forming activities are available here and there for bigger sized crabs (*S. serrata, S. tranquebarica*) but economically viable mass seed production technology is lacking for swimming crabs in general and *P. pelagicus* in particular (Soundarapandian *et al.,* 2007). Berried females are important to start a commercial hatchery. The berried females are not available throughout the year from the natural resources. So the production of berried females in a controlled condition is essential for this one should know the mating behaviour of any aquaculture organism. Hence in the present study mating behaviour of the blue swimming crab *P. pelagicus* was studied under controlled condition in the laboratory.

Materials and Methods

The crab for the present study was collected from the Parangipettai (Lat 11°29'N; Long 79°49°E) landing center. The live hard shelled male crabs at the size of 105–110 mm carapace width and females at the size of 98 – 104mm carapace width were selected and kept in a plastic container with sea water and brought to the laboratory. In the laboratory, the crabs were immediately acclimatized with sterilized and filtered sea water (salinity 30-32ppt; temperature 26-33°C; pH – 7.6 to 8.3 and dissolved oxygen 5ppm). At the beginning the water level was maintained at 20cm depth and it was observed that the male struggle to carry the female and eventually turn over for mating. In order to avoid the above problem the water depth was increased upto 35cm. So the males were carried the females very easily for mating. Optimum environmental parameters were maintained during the experimental period (salinity 30-32ppt; temperature 26-31°C; pH 7.5 – 8.5 and dissolved oxygen 5ppm). During acclimatization and experimental periods the crabs were fed with mixture of clam, squid and prawns at 10 per cent of the body weight (daily morning and evening) twice a day. The water quality was maintained by partial exchange of 50 per cent water daily. The uneaten and excretory wastes from the tanks were removed while water exchange.

Results

Observation of Mating Behaviour

For convenient, the mating behaviour of *P. pelagicus* divided into three phases as follows:

Contact

The hard shell male crab introduced into the experimental tank along with soft shell female crab. The male was attracted by the female by releasing sex pheromones. These pheromones triggered the males and guide them towards the female (Glesson, 1980). In turn the female was able to utilize chemical cues (possibly a male pheromone) to locate males which are an important mechanism for optimizing reproduction success. This chemicals released by the female was to attract the male for the selective capture and contact.

Cradle – Carrying position

The male after making contact with the soft shell female

ultimately move towards her extending his bigger chelate, then embraces the female in a short while using his walking legs hold her beneath him to form a position called cradle-carrying position. During this position both animals are facing in the same direction. In general the male is active and aggressive but the female is defunct. The male crabs only extend his chelates in an attacking position vigorously and try to attack whenever disturbed but no reactions were observed from the female's side. Sometimes the pair is broken at the time of disturbing but afterward's the pair is reformed in the same position. Both animals were eating during this period and also locomotion was observed.

Mating

At the time of mating, the male crab carried the female to a suitable position for mating in a cradle-carrying position. Once the male became active eventually rotate the female using his waking legs and chelate turned over her. The assistance rendered by the male crab, she positioned herself upside down beneath him and extends her abdomen exposing gonophores allowing the male to insert his paired coupulatory appendages called gonopods into her genital pores. By this time male and female crabs facing in the opposite direction. The female is in reverse position, her lower side is directed towards the males ventral side and the abdomen of both are flung backwards. During copulation the male often walked around with the female attached to its ventral surface, holding her with third and fourth walking legs. After copulation the cradle carrying position is continued for only few hrs. The female is inactive until she attains normal hardness of her exoskeleton.

Extrusion of Eggs

The male crabs deposited spermatophores in the female's spermatheca during mating will be stored until the female is ready for extrusion. During the process of spawning or extrusion, the eggs are liberated from the ovaries passing through the seminal receptacles. In seminal receptacles the stored sperms are liberated from the spermatophores to fertilize the eggs and fertilized eggs are extruded through the gonophores present in the sternites of the sixth thoracic segments of third pair of legs and these eggs become attached to the smooth setae present in the endopodites of the four pair of pleopods in the abdominal flab. The egg mass seggregated and carried on the abdominal flab is called as berry or sponge. The females carrying eggs is also called as berried crabs. The freshly extruded eggs are initially orange in colour and become black before hatched into zoeae.

Discussion

In decapods sex pheromones induce mate search and courtship behaviour of con-specifics (Atema and Engstrom, 1971; Dunham, 1978). Many crustaceans use pheromones to find mates and induce mating behaviours (Anna-Sarakrang and Mattiasekerlolm, 2006). Pupertal females attract males with a urinary born pheromone that is released for several days before mating, and they actively participate in courtship behaviour with males (Teytand, 1971; Glesson, 1980) and these pheromones are detected by chemoreceptor's located on the aesthetasis of the antennules (Glesson, 1982). According to Glesson (1980) the pheromone signal is of primary important for initiating the male's courtship behaviour and that visual cues are secondarily used to orient this behaviour towards any crab in the immediate vicinity. In the present investigation it is not sure whether the male *P.pelagicus* was attracted by pheromone or visual cues as reported in *P. sanguinolentus* (Dinakaran and Soundarapandian, 2009). Teytaud (1971) noted that pubertal *C. sapidus* female exhibit significant changes in particular behaviours like rocking and chelate waving when presented with a visual image of a crab and simultaneously exposed to water containing male odour. These type of movements were not observed in *P. sanguinolentus* (Dinakaran and Soundarapandian, 2009) and in the present study too. Male blue crabs *C. sapidus*, has shown a courtship display in which they elevate their body by standing high on their legs, open their chelate and paddle their swimming legs. Jaroensatasinee and Jaroensatasine (2003) studied the courtship in *U. paradussumieri*. They have observed male display in the form of claw waving to attract the females to the burrows of males for mating. Lucas (1980) suggested that the conspicuous colouring of some male Hymenosomatids might be evidence for visual displays. The portunid crabs, *Ovalipes punctatus* from South Africa, after pairing, the male would bury himself and the female in the sand with only their eyes protruding (Du Preez and McLachlan, 1984).This type of behaviours had never been observed in the present study.

Cradle carrying is a pre-coupulatory mate guarding behaviour which is required to guarantee a successful mating and to ensure paternity and is therefore of great ecological importance. Male mate-guarding is energetically expensive and considered a measure of male fitness (Adams *et al.*, 1984; Elwood *et al.*, 1987). In *C. sapidus* pupertal females are frequently initiate the cradle carrying position themselves by approaching and repeatedly bumping against non displaying males (Glesson, 1982). This type of approach by pupertal female was not observed in *P. sanquinolentus* in laboratory conditions (Dinakaran and Soundarapandian, 2009). In the present study the males only initiate the cradle-carry position by approaching the pupertal females and the pupertal females has not shown any sort of approach towards the male. The female is protected by a male before and after her pubertal moult by being grasped by the males first pair of walking legs and hold right side up in a cradle carry position under the male. The same behaviour has been reported previously by Van Engel (1958), Glesson (1980) and Johnson (1980).

The mating of *P.pelagicus* is basically corresponding with the pattern of brachyuran crabs (Hartnoll and smith, 1979), generally occurred between hard shelled males and soft shelled females (Hartnoll and Smith, 1979). Previously soft-female mating had been reported in crabs belongs to Portunidae (Hard, 1942; Cheung, 1996; Ryan, 1966; Heasman *et al.*, 1985; Norman and Jones, 1993; Haddon, 1994). Alternatively some species where multiparous females can mate in a hard-shell condition, there is often little pre-coupulatory guarding, but the male may guard the female for some time following copulation. As females of these species are not especially vulnerable to predation, post-coupulatory mate guarding is likely to result from male-male competition. This type of post coupulatory guarding is not seen in *P. sanguinolentus* (Dinakaran and Soundarapandian, 2009). In the present study also such behaviour is not observed. Mating was reported when the females were in hard shelled condition in *Pugettia product* (Boolotian *et al.*, 1959), in goldan crab, *Geryon fenneri* (Hines, 1988), in *Cyclograpsus lavauxi*, *Helice crassa*, *Hemigrapsus crenulatus*, *H. sexdentatus* (Brockrohoff and Melay, 2005) and in portunid species *Thalamita prymna*, *T. sima* (Norman, 1996). In other crabs, such as *Cancer pagurus* and *S. serrata*, pair formation takes place just before the female undergo moulting (Hill, 1975).

During coupulation the male positions the ventral parts of its body facing upwards and the female places herself on top of the male with the ventral side facing that of the male (Hartnoll, 1969; Brosnan, 1981). Similar type of position has not been observed in the present study. The first pair of pleopods of the male is the functional intromittent organs, each receiving spermatophores and semen from the respective penis. The second pair of pleopods are inserted into the posterior foramen of the first pleopods, forcing the spermatophores and semen through the tube like, first pleopods. During copulation semen and spermatophores are passed from the first pleopods of the male into the paired oviducts and eventually the seminal receptacles (spermathecae) of the female (Cronin, 1947). At the time of mating the brachyuran males transfer their spermatophores to the female spermatheca. The female store the spermatophores until fertilization (Pinheiro and Fransozo, 2002). The eggs are subsequently fertilized at the time of extrusion (Smith, 1982). Van Engel (1958) found that sperm in a female *C. Sapidus* spermathecum can remain viable for at least 12 months. This is likely to also be the case of *P. pelagicus*. Eggs are fertilized when passing from the ovaries to the seminal receptacles before being extruded onto the female's pleopods. Egg extrusion onto endopodites of the female's pleopods may be complete within 2 hrs (Van Engel, 1958).

Many species, including mammals, may mate each time the female ovalutes, others must rely stored sperm for atleast some fertilization events. Females of *Inachus phalangium* the spider crab commonly extrude a brood shortly after mating (Jones and hortnoll, 1997), but may store sperm for over six months and fertilize as many as six broods before mating again (Diesel, 1989). Females usually extrude a clutch of eggs within 1-5 days of moulting, whether mated or not (Paul and Adams, 1984; Sainte-Marie and Lovrich, 1994). Both fertilized and unfertilized eggs attached to the pleopods; those fertilized are incubated for upto 2 years; those not fertilized are lost within 5-6 months of attachment (Sainte-Marie, 1993; Sainte-Marie and Carriere, 1995; Moriyasu and Lanteigne, 1998). The number of eggs extruded in each brood was defined as the reproductive success of females because egg loss through the breeding period is quite small (Henmi, 1989) and almost all eggs extruded are fertiled under natural conditions (Koga *et al.*, 1993; Koga, 1994). Laboratory rearing of sand crabs has shown that female sand crabs have to maturity moults and each of these moults can extrude upto four batches of eggs (Campbell, 1984).

Acknowledgement

The financial support provided by the UGC is greatly acknowledged.

References

Adams, J., Greenwood, P., Pollitt, R. and Yonow, T., 1984. Loading constraints and sexual size dimorphism in *Asellus aquaticus*. *Behaviour*, 92: 277–287.

Anna-Sara, Krang and Ekerholm, Mattias, 2006. Copper reduced Mating behaviour in male shoe crabs [*Carcinus Maenas* (L.)]. *Aquatic Toxicology*, 80(2006): 60-69.

Atema, J. and Engstrom, D.G., 1971. Sex pheromone in the Lobster, *Homarus americanus*. *Nature*, 232: 261–263.

Boolootian, R.A., Giese, A.C., Farnan, A. and Tucker, J., 1959. The reproductive cycles of five west coast crabs. *Physiol. Zool.*, 32: 213–220.

Brockrehoff, A.M. and McLay, C.L., 2005. Mating behaviour female receptivity and male- male competition in the intertidal crab *Hemigrapsus sexdentatus* (Brachyura: Grapsidae). *Marine Ecol. Prog. Series*, 290: 179-197.

Brosnan, D.M., 1981. Studies on the biology, ecology and fishery of the spider crab *Maia squinado* Herbst (1768) off the west coast of Ireland. *M.Sc. Thesis*, Department of Zoology, University College Galway, Ireland, 133 pp.

Campbell, G.R., 1984. A comparative study of adult sexual behaviour and larval ecology of three commercially important portunid crabs from the Moreton Bay region of Queensland, Australia. *Ph.D. Thesis*. The University of Queensland, 253 pp.

Cheung, T.S., 1966. An observed act of coupulation in the shore crab, *Carcinus maenas* (L.). *Crustaceana*, 11: 107-108.

Cronin, L.E., 1947. Anatomy and histology of the male reproductive system of *Callinectes sapidus* Rathbun. *J. Morphol.*, 81: 209-219.

Diesel, R., 1989. Structure and function of the reproductive system of the symbiotic spider crab, *Inachus phalangium* (Decapoda:

Majidae): Observations on sperm transfer, sperm storage, and spawning. *J. Crustac. Biol.*, 9: 266-277.

Dinakaran G.K. and Soundarapandian, P., 2009. Mating behaviour and broodstock development of commercially important blue swimming crab, *Portunus sanguinolentus* (Herbst). *Indian Journal of Science and Technology*, Vol. 2 No. 4.

Du Preez, H.H. and Mc Lachlan, A., 1984. Biology of the three-spot swimming crab, *Ovalipes punctatus* (De Haan) II. Growth and moulting. *Crustaceana*, 47(2): 1984, E.J.Brill. Leiden.

Dunham, P.J., 1978. Sex pheromones in crustaceans. *Biological Reviews*, 53: 555–583.

Elwood, R., Gibson, J. and Neil, S., 1987. The amourous Gammarus: size assortative mating in *G. pulex*. *Anim. Behav.*, 35: 1–6.

Glesson, R.A., 1980. Pheromone communication in the reproductive behaviour of the blue crab, *Callinectes sapidus*. *Mar. Behav. Physiol.*, 7: 119-134.

Glesson, R.A., 1982. Morphological and behavioural identification of the sensory structures mediating pheromone reception in the blue crab, *Callinectes sapidus*. *Biol. Bull. (Woods Hole)*, 163: 162-171.

Haddon, M., 1994. Size-fecundity relationships, mating behaviour, and larval release in the New Zealand paddle crab, *Ovalipes catharus* (White 1843) (Brachyura : Portunidae), N.Z.J. *Mar. Freshw. Res.*, 28: 329-334.

Hard, W.L., 1942. Ovarian growth and ovulation in the mature blue crab, *Callinectes sapidus* Rathbun. *Chesapeake Biol. Lab. Publ.*, 46: 1 –17.

Hartnoll, R.G. and Smith, S.M., 1979. Pair formation in the edible crab, *Cancer pagurus*, Decapoda, Brachyura. *Crustaceana*, 36: 23–28

Hartnoll, R.G., 1969. Mating in Branchyura. *Crustaceana*, 16: 161-181.

Heasman, M.P., Fielder, D. R. and Shepherd, R.K., 1985. Mating and spawning in the mud crab, *Scylla serrata* (Forskal) (Decapoda: Portunidae), in Moreton Bay, Queensland. *Australian Journal of Marine and Freshwater Research*, 36:773-783.

Henmi, Y., 1989. Reproductive ecology of three ocypodid crabs. II. Incubation sites and egg mortality. *Ecol. Res.*, 4: 261–269.

Hill, B. J., 1974. Salinity and temperature tolerance of Zoeae of the portunid crab *Scylla serrata*. *Mar. Biol.*, 25: 21–24.

Hines, A.H., 1988. Fecundity and reproductive output in two species of deep sea crabs, *Geryon fenneri* and *G. quinquedens* (Decapoda, Brachyura). *J. Crustac. Biol.*, 8: 557– 562.

Jaroensatasinee, M. and Jaroensatasinee, K., 2003. Male body size influence female choice and male-male competition in the fiddler crab *Uca paradussumieri* Bott, 1973 (Decapoda, Brachyura, Ocypodidae). *Crustaceana*, 76(2): 177-186.

John Samuel, N., Thirunavukkarasu, N., Soundarapandian, P., Shanmugam, A. and Kannupandi, T., 2004. Fishery potential of commercially important portunid crabs along Parangipettai coast. In: *Proc. of Ocean Life Food and Medicine Expo.*, pp. 165-173.

Johnson, P.T., 1980. Histology of the Blue Crab, *Callinectes sapidus*: A Model for the Decapoda. Praeger Scientific Publishing Company, New York, NY, pp. 1–440.

Jones, D.R. and Hartnoll, R.G., 1997. Mate selection and mating behaviour in spider crabs. *Estuar. Coast. Shelf Sci.*, 44: 185–193.

Kailola, P.J., Williams, M.J, Stewart, P.C., Riechelt, R.E., McNee, A. and Grieve, C., 1993. Editors, *Australian Fisheries Resources*, Bureau of Resource Sciences, *Canberra*, p. 422.

Koga, T., 1994. Alternative mating behaviours in the sand-bubbler crab *Scopimera globosa* (De Haan) (Decapoda : Ocypodidae). *Ph.D. Thesis*, Kyushu University, Fukuoka, p. 71.

Koga, T., Henmi, Y. and Murai, M., 1993. Sperm competition and the assurance of underground copulation in the sand-bubbler crab, *Scopiemera globosa* (Brachyura: Ocypodidae). *J. Crustac. Biol.*, 13: 1.

Lucas, J.S., 1980. Spider crab of the familyHymenosomatidae (Crustacea : Brachyura) with particular reference to Australian species: Systematics and biology. *Records of the Australian Museum*, 33(4): 148-247.

Mohammed Saved, A. and Rahavan, P. Rajeev, 2001. Mud crab-culture and fattening techniques, status and prospects. *Sea. Exp. Journal*, 32(1): 25-29.

Moriyasu, M. and Lanteigne, C., 1998. Embryo development and reproductive cycle in the snow crab, *Chionoecetes opilio* (Crustacea: Majidae), in the southern Gulf of St.Lawrence, *Canada. Can. J. Zool.*, 76: 2040-2048.

Norman, C.P. and Jones, M.B., 1993. Reproduction ecology of the velvet swimming crab, *Necora puber* (Brachyura: Portunidae), at Plymouth.*J. Mar. Biol. Assoc. U.K.*, 73: 379–389.

Norman, C.P., 1996. Reproductive biology and evidence for hard-female mating in the branchyuran crab *Thalamita sima* (Portunidae). *Journal of Crustac. Biology*, 16(4): 656-662.

Paul, A.J. and Adams, A.E., 1984. Breeding and fertile period for female *Chionoecetes bair* (Decapoda, Majidae). *J. Crustac. Biol.*, 4: 589-594.

Pinheiro, M.A.A. and Fransozo, A., 2002. Reproductive dynamics of the speckled swimming crab *Arenaeus cribrarius* (Lamarck, 1818) (Branchyura, Portunidae), on the north coast of Ssao Paulo State, Brazil. *Journal of Crustac. Biology*, 22(2): 416-428.

Ryan, E.P., 1966. Pheramone: evidence in a decapods crustacean. *Science*, 151:340-341.

Sainte-Marie, B., 1993. Reproductive cycle and fecundity of primiparous and multiparous female snow crab, *Chionoecetes opilio*, in the northwest Gulf of Saint Lawrence. *Can. J. Fish. Aquat. Sci.*, 50: 2147– 2156.

Sainte-Marie, B., and C. Carrie're, 1995. Fertilisation of the second clutch of eggs of snow crab, *Chionoecetes opilio* from females mated once or twice after their moult to maturity. *Fish. Bull.*, 93: 759–764.

Sainte-Marie, B., and Lovrich, G.A., 1994. Delivery and storage of sperm at first mating of female *Chionoecetes opilio* (Brachyura: Majidae) in relation to size and morphometric maturity of male parent. *J. Crustac. Biol.*, 14: 508– 521.

Smith, H., 1982. Blue crabs in South Australia: Their status potential and biology. *South Australian Fishing Industry Council* (*Adelaide, Australia*), 6: 6-9.

Soundarapandian, P., Thamizhazhagan, E. and Samuel, N. John, 2007. Seed production of commercially important blue swimming crab *Portunus pelagicus* (Linnaeus). *J. Fish. Aqua. Sci.*, 2 (4): 302-309.

Stephenson, W., 1962. Evalution and ecology of portunid crabs, with special reference to Australian species. In: *The Evolution of Living Organisms*, (Ed.) G.W. Leeper. Melbourne University Press, Melbourne, p. 311-327.

Teytaud, A.R., 1971. The laboratory studies of Sex Recognition in the Blue Crab. *Callinectes sapidus* Rathbun. *Sea Grant Tech. Bull.* No. 15, University of Miami Sea Grant Program.

Van Engel, W.A., 1958. The blue crab and its fishery in Chesapeake Bay. Part I: reproduction, early development, growth, and migration. *Commer. Fish. Rev.*, 20: 6–17.

Chapter 19

Leydig Cell Differentiation in Adult Amphibian (*Euphlyctis cyanophlyctis*) Testis

Katti Pancharatna

Department of Zoology, Karnatak University, Dharwad – 580 003, Karnataka, India

ABSTRACT

Leydig cells or interstitial cells are the main steroidogenic components of the testis in vertebrates. In the testis of the Indian skipper frog, *Euphlyctis cyanophlyctis* morphological diversity in the populations of these intertubular interstitial cells was observed. Three types of Leydig cells were distinguishable depending on the size, shape and details of the nucleus *i.e.* fibroblastic, vesicular and pycnotic cells. There was a seasonal variation in the number of these three types of Leydig cells. Hypophysectomy resulted in a decrease in the number of vesicular type with a corresponding increase in that of pycnotic ones. Administration of human chorionic gonadotropin (hCG) to 3 month hypophysectomized animals caused an increase in vesicular cells while injections of testosterone to operated animals enhanced fibroblastic and pycnotic cells with a corresponding decrease in vesicular cells. Unilateral castration (ULC) resulted in an increase in vesicular cells in the remaining testis. Injections of testosterone propionate (TP) or estradiol

* Corresponding author: E-mail: pancharatnak@gmail.com

17β (E_2) to ULC animals caused a reduction in the total count and number of vesicular cells with an increase in the number of fibroblastic and pycnotic cells. These findings suggest that fibroblastic cells form precursors for hormone synthesizing vesicular ones and pycnotic cells are those undergoing degeneration; further hypophyseal gonadotropins stimulate the differentiation of fibroblastic to vesicular cells and steroid hormones, testosterone and estradiol-17β interfere with the process in the testis of *E. cyanophlyctis*.

Keywords: *Leydig cells, Amphibian, Euphlyctis cyanophlyctis, Seasonal variation, Hypophysectomy .*

Introduction

The large body of the literature existing on the reproduction of amphibians reveals that environmental cues greatly influence the gametogenesis and steroidogenesis in these animals (Lofts, 1968, 1974, 1984, 1987; Saidapur, 1989; Denver *et al.*, 2002; Pierantoni *et al.*, 2002; Cobellis *et al.*, 2003; Royere *et al.*, 2004). Annual testicular cycles, patterns of spermatogenesis, factors controlling spermatogenesis are well documented for amphibians (Lofts, 1974, 1984, 1987; Saidapur, 1989; Denver *et al.*, 2002). Comparatively, studies on Leydig cells/interstitial cells are limited and are confined to only annual variation in the nuclear diameter and steroid synthesizing ability in different species of amphibians (Lofts, 1974, 1984, 1987' Saidapur, 1989). Morphological variations in the Leydig cell populations and the possible renewal mechanism in the production of new Leydig cells are studied in a few temperate amphibian species (Pudney *et al.*, 1983; Pudney and Callard, 1984; Minucci *et al.*, 1990, 1994; Hardy *et al.*, 1992; Kao *et al.*, 1993; Huang *et al.*, 1996). Corresponding studies on tropical amphibians are virtually lacking.

The present work was initiated in the tropical frog *Euphlyctis cyanophlyctis* to examine (1) the morphological distinctions if any, in the Leydig cell populations of testicular interstitium, (2) seasonal numerical variation if any, in Leydig cells and (3) role of gonadotropins (human chorionic gonadotropin) and steroid hormones (testosterone propionate and estradiol-17β) on the production and maintenance of populations of Leydig cells in adult testis using unilaterally castrated or hypophysectomized frogs.

Materials and Methods

Adult male *E. cyanophlyctis* (Schn.) collected from the vicinity of Dharwad (15°7′N 75°3E) in the first week of every month (n = 6) for a period of one year (September 1994 – August 1995) were used. Body weight (g), body length (snout-vent length –cm) and testicular weight (mg) of each animal were recorded. Testes were excised and fixed in Bouin's fluid and embedded in paraffin wax. Sections of 4 μm thick were cut on a rotary microtome, stained with haematoxylin-eosin and observed under a binocular compound microscope. Leydig/interstitial cells were counted from the intertubular regions of 10 randomly chosen testicular sections per animal. Careful observations revealed that in the cross sections of the testis of *E. cyanophlyctis* Leydig cells could be differentiated into three (fibroblastic, vesicular and pycnotic) types. The differential count (per cent distribution of fibroblastic, vesicular and pycnotic cell types) was also made. Data were analyzed using analysis of variance (ANOVA) followed by Duncan's multiple range test. The results were judged significant at 5 per cent level of significance (Steel and Torrie, 1980).

Effects of Hypophysectomy and Hypophysectomy Plus Exogenous hCG or Testosterone Propionate on Leydig Cell Populations (Experiment–I)

Adult male *E. cyanophlyctis* procured in the month of March 1997 were hypophysectomized. Following the surgery, frogs received injections of 100 IU benzyl penicillin (antibiotic) for three days. In addition, hypophysectomized frogs received 0.2 ml of saline twice a week until autopsy in order to compensate salt balance. Corresponding sham operated controls were maintained. Operated frogs were housed in glass aquarium (size 30 X37 X 22.5 cm). The room temperature ranged between 22 – 28° C and photophase from 11.10 – 13.5 hours. Frogs were fed on live guppies (*Gambusia affinis*) *ad libitum* on every alternate day. A group of 5 operated and 5 sham operated frogs were autopsied at a regular interval of 3 months each, from the date of operation *i.e.* in the month of June (3 month), September (6 month) and December (9 month).

After 3 months of the operation remaining operated frogs were divided into 5 groups and received the following treatment:

Group 1: Intact/sham operated controls (0.2 ml saline)

Group 2: Operated initial controls at the beginning of the hormone treatment.

Group 3: Hypophysectomized controls (0.2 ml saline)

Group 4: Hypophysectomy + 20 IU hCG (Gonadotrophin LH, Amsa Laboratori. Chimico Farmaceutic, Rome, Italy) in 0.2 ml saline

Group 5: Hypophysectomy + 10 μg TP (testosterone propionate) in 0.2 ml saline

Injections (ip) were given daily for 30 days. Frogs were autopsied 24 hours after the last injection.

Effects of Unilateral Castration (ULC) and Exogenous Testosterone and Estradiol-17β on the Compensatory Hypertrophy Response of Residual Testis in ULC Frogs (Experiment–II)

Male *E. cyanophlyctis* procured in May 1997 were used in the present study. Five frogs were autopsied at the beginning of the experiment that served as initial controls. Remaining frogs were unilaterally castrated (ULC). Sham operated controls were maintained. All operated frogs received injections of 100 IU benzyl penicillin for 3 days following the surgery and were maintained under the laboratory conditions mentioned above. This experiment comprised the following groups:

Group I: Initial controls

Group II: Sham operated controls

Group III: ULC controls (0.2 ml distilled water)

Group IV: ULC+10 μg testosterone propionate (TP) in 0.2 ml distilled water

Group V: ULC + 5 μg estradiol-17β (Sigma) in 0.2 ml distilled water

Injections were given on alternate day for 45 days starting from the third day of the operation. Testosterone and estradiol suspensions were prepared by dissolving a known quantity of hormone in 0.5 ml of acetone and then diluting the solution with distilled water to the required concentration. Frogs belonging to group II-IV were autopsied 24 hours after the last injection on 46th day.

At the end of both the experiments (Experiment I and II) body weights and lengths of animals were recorded. Testes were excised and fixed in Bouin's fluid; embedded in paraffin wax, sectioned at 4 μm thickness and stained with haematoxylin-eosin. Leydig cell (total and differential) counts were made from 10 testicular sections per frog chosen randomly. The data were analyzed using analysis of variance (ANOVA) followed by Duncan's new multiple range test (Steel and Torrie, 1980). The results were judged significant at 5 per cent level of significance.

Results

Seasonal Variation in the Total Number and Differential Counts of Leydig Cells

Leydig cells were observed in the intertubular region of seminiferous tubules in the testis of *E. cyanophlyctis* (Figures 19.1 and 19.2). Morphologically they were distinguishable into three distinct types *i.e.* (*i*) fibroblastic cells with spindle shaped nucleus (Figure 19.1a), (*ii*) vesicular cells with spherical nucleus and granular nuclear material, and one or two nuclei (Figure 19.1b) and (*iii*) cells with pycnotic nuclei containing highly condensed chromatin material (Figure 19.1c). The differential counts indicated that vesicular cells were more in number (30-90 per cent) during all the months of the year (Figure 19.2). Fibroblastic cells formed 1 – 2 per cent and pycnotic cells formed 5-30 per cent of total cell number during annual cycle. Pycnotic Leydig cells were highest in number in April (Figure 19.2).

Effects of Hypophysectomy

In the testis of initial control frogs, Leydig cells were conspicuous, ranged from 120 –130 per cross section of testis. Fibroblastic cells formed 2.5 per cent, vesicular 87.2 per cent and pycnotic 10.3 per cent (Figure 19.2). After three and six months of hypophysectomy, the total number of vesicular Leydig cells decreased and pycnotic cells increased (Figure 19.3). In nine month hypophysectomized frogs total Leydig cell number and the percentage of pycnotic cells were significantly higher compared to six months operated and corresponding sham operated.

Effects of Hypophysectomy+ (hCG) or TP

In initial control frogs, Leydig cell number ranged between 361 and 387, of which fibroblastic cells formed 2.3 per cent, 88 per cent

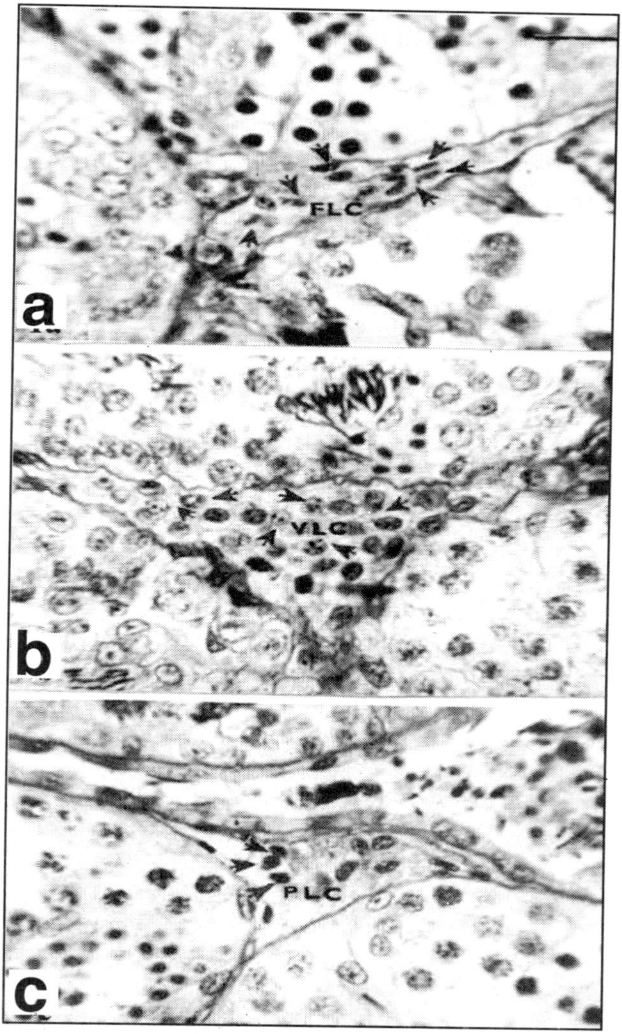

Figures 19.1a–c: Cross Sections of Testis of *E. cyanophlyctis* (Haematoxylin-eosin)

a: Cross section of testis showing fibroblastic cells (arrows) in the intertubular region; b: Cross section of testis showing vesicular Leydig/interstitial cells (arrows) in the intertubular region; c: Cross section of testis showing pycnotic Leydig/interstitial cells (arrows) in the intertubular region. Scale line = 30 μm.

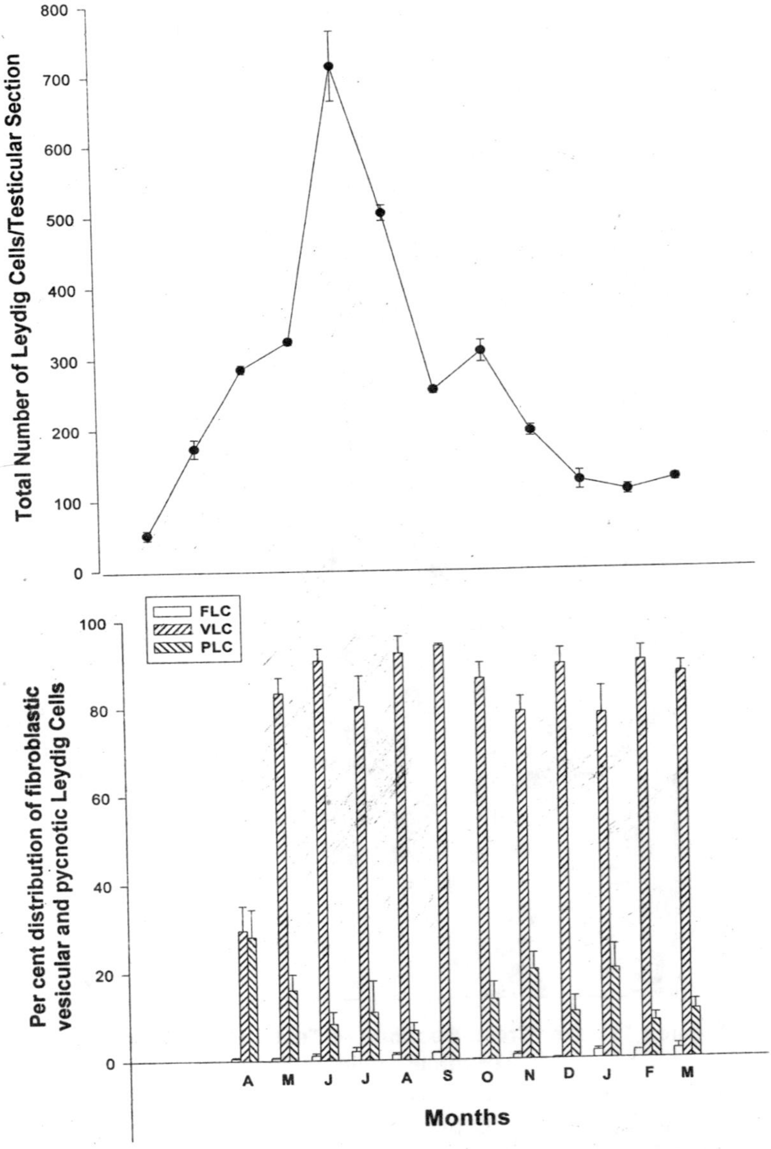

Figure 19.2: Monthly Variations in the Number of Leydig Cell and per cent Distribution of Fibroblastic, Vesicular and Pycnotic Type of Leydig Cell in *E. cyanophlyctis*

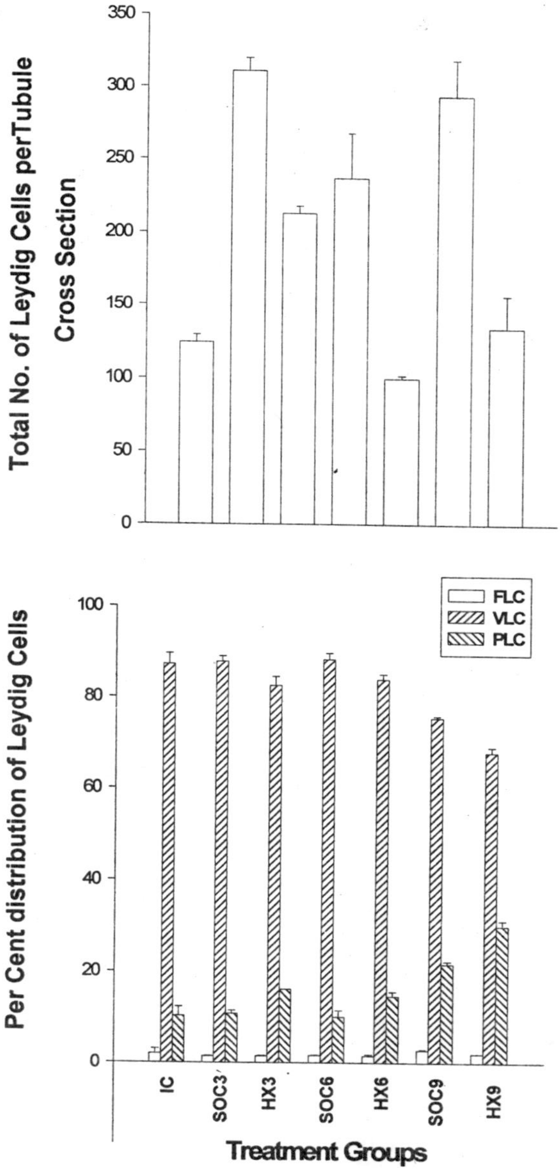

Figure 19.3: Effects of 3, 6 and 9 Months of Hypophysectomy on the Total Number and per cent Distribution of Leydig Cells in *E. cyanophlyctis* Testis

were vesicular and 9.5 per cent were pycnotic (Figure 19.4). In sham operated control frogs, the total number of Leydig cells was lower compared to the initial controls (Figure 19.4). After 3 months of hypophysectomy, the total number of Leydig cells and vesicular cells decreased, while pycnotic cells doubled in number (Figure 19.4). In operated animals treated with distilled water (hypophysectomized controls) the total number of Leydig cells, fibroblastic and vesicular cells were significantly lower, but the pycnotic cells increased, compared to that of sham operated controls. In hCG treated hypophysectomized frogs, the total number of Leydig cells was higher by four folds, while the percentage of pycnotic cells decreased (Figure 19.4). In operated animals treated with testosterone propionate the percentage of fibroblastic and pycnotic cells was higher and that of vesicular cells was lower when compared to hypophysectomized controls and hCG treated frogs (Figure 19.4).

Effects of Unilateral Castration (ULC), ULC + TP and ULC + E_2 on Leydig Cells

In initial control frogs, the Leydig cell number varied from 336 to 342, of which, fibroblastic cells formed 4.56 per cent, Vesicular 77.44 per cent and pycnotic 17.3 per cent (Figure 19.5) After 3 months, in the testis of sham operated controls Leydig cells increased significantly over initial controls (Figure 19.5). ULC caused an increase in the number of vesicular Leydig cells, while the number of fibroblastic and pycnotic cells decreased ($P < 0.05$) compared to sham operated controls. Injections of Testosterone propionate caused a decrease in the number of Leydig cells, particularly vesicular cells, while fibroblastic and pycnotic cells were significantly higher in number (Figure 19.6). In E2 treated ULC frogs, total Leydig cell and vesicular interstitial cell numbers decreased, while fibroblastic and pycnotic cell number was significantly higher in these frogs (Figure 19.6).

Discussion

Seasonal numerical variation, morphological and functional heterogenity in the population of Leydig interstitial cells and possible mechanisms controlling the production of new Leydig cells are now reported for a few amphibian species (Callard *et al.*, 1980; Pudney *et al.*, 1983; Pudney and Callard, 1984; Minucci *et al.*, 1990, 1994; Hardy *et al.*, 1992; Kao *et al.*, 1993; Huang *et al.*, 1996). However, the data is

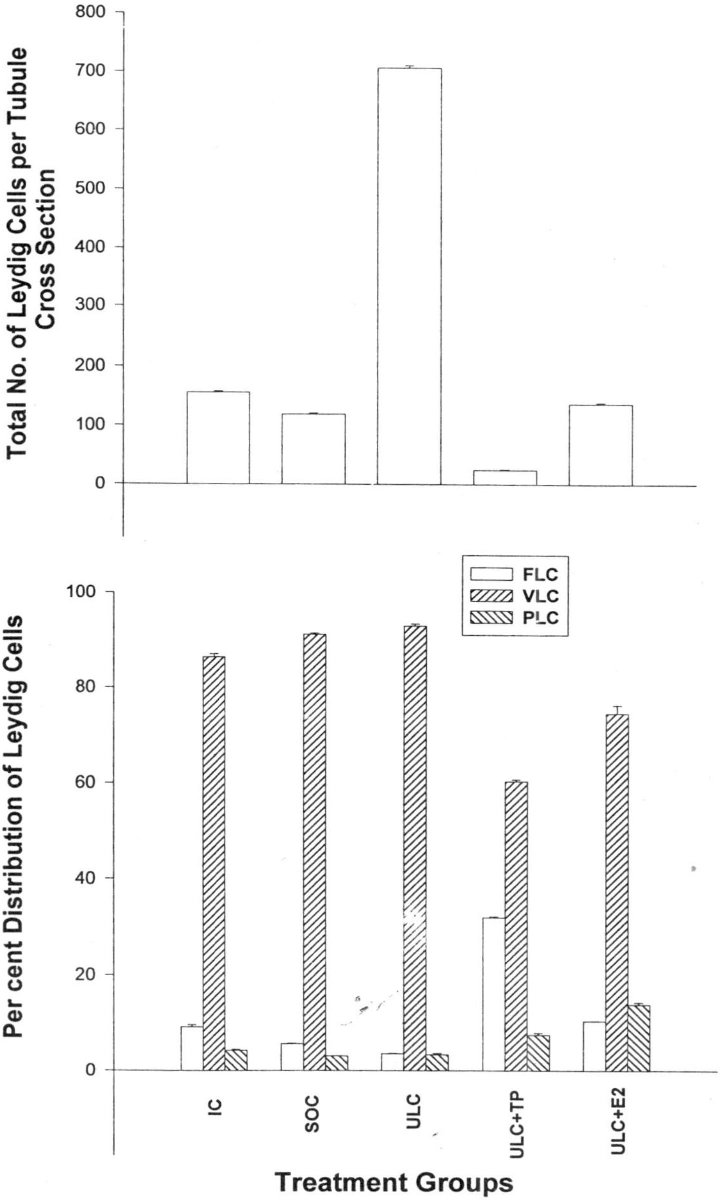

Figure 19.4: Effects of Hypophysectomy and Treatment with hCG and Testosterone on the Leydig Cells in *E. cyanophlyctis*

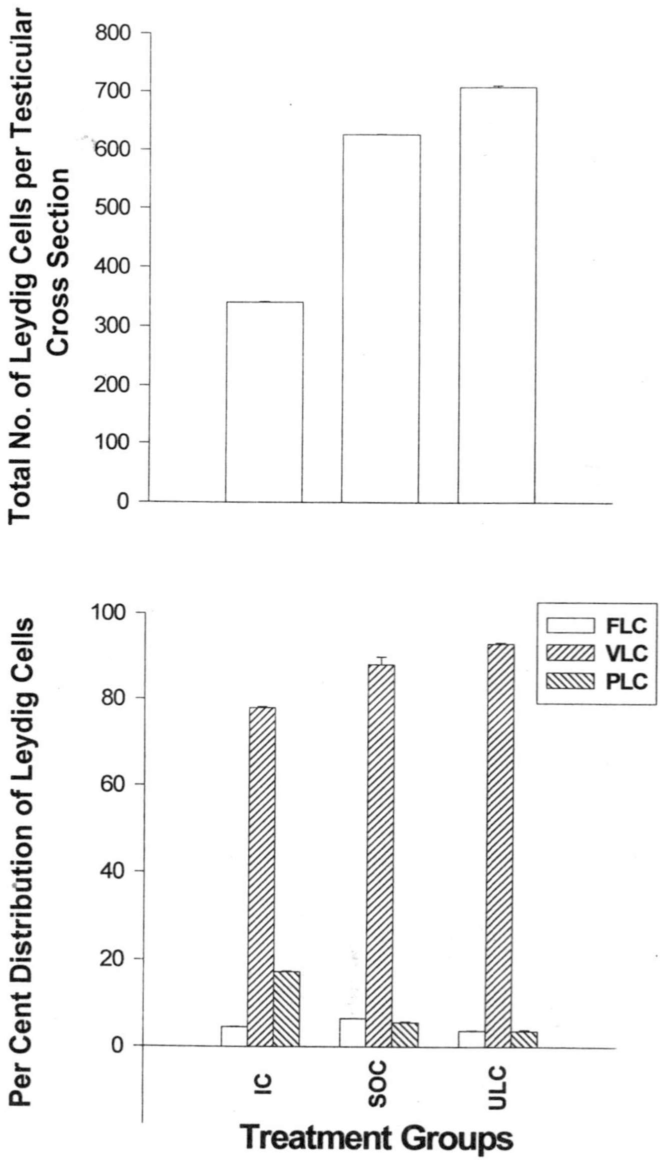

Figure 19.5. Effects of Unilateral Castration (ULC) on the Total Number and per cent Distribution of Leydig Cells in the Remaining Testis in *E. cyanophlyctis*

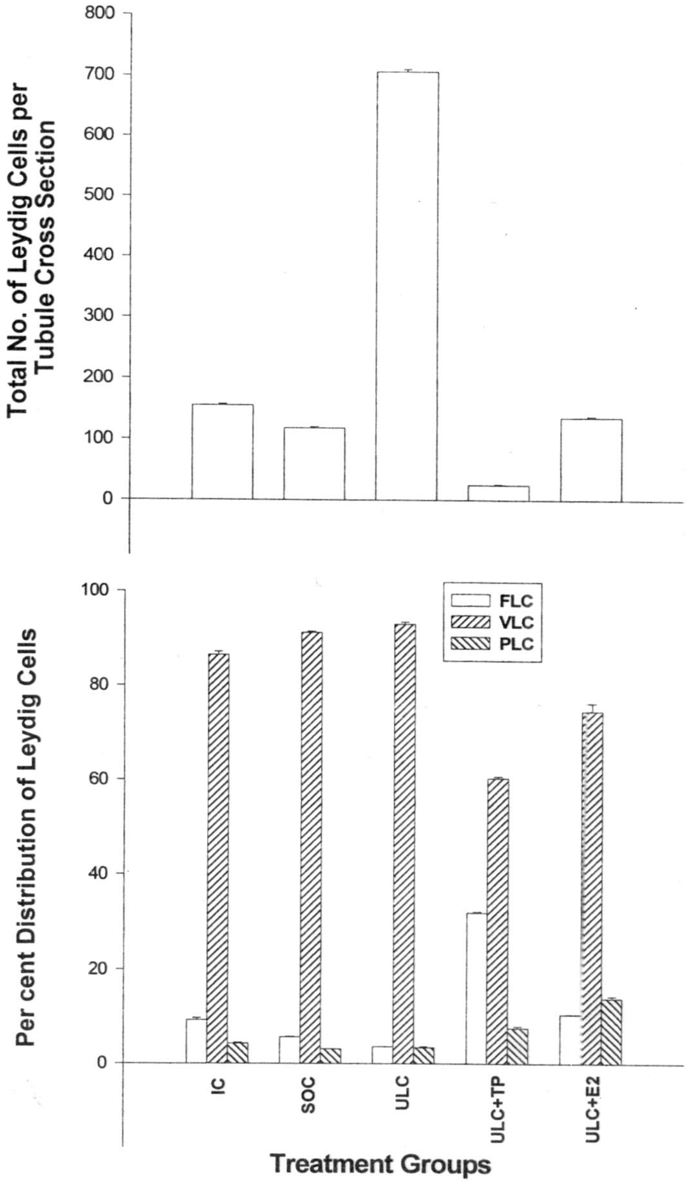

Figure 19.6: Effects of ULC and Treatment with hCG and Testosterone on the Leydig Cells in the Remaining Testis in *E. cyanophlyctis*

still insufficient to resolve any generalization for amphibians as a whole. The present study is first of its kind on an Indian anuran amphibian.

In *E. cyanophlyctis* morphologically 3 distinct types of cells were found in the intertubular region (Figure 19.1a–c); (i) fibroblastic cells with spindle shaped nucleus (ii) vesicular cells with spherical nucleus, and granular chromatin material and one or two nucleoli and (iii) pycnotic cells with a nucleus containing highly condensed chromatin. The differential counts indicated that vesicular cells were more in number (30–90 per cent) during all the months of the year. Fibroblastic cells formed 1–2 per cent and pycnotic cells formed 5–30 per cent of total cell number during annual cycle. Pycnotic Leydig cells were maximal in number in April.

Interstitial cells/Leydig cells are known to make androgenic and also estrogenic steroids (Callard *et al.*, 1978; Callard *et al.*, 1980; Lofts, 1987). The seasonal changes in the nuclear diameter and 3β HSDH activity are reported for a number of amphibians (Callard *et al.*, 1978; Lofts, 1984; Saidapur, 1989). But recent studies report that annual variation in Leydig cell number occur in some urodelan amphibian species such as *Necturus maculosus* (Pudney *et al.*, 1983), red spotted newt (Hardy *et al.*, 1992) and anurans, *Rana rugulosa*, (Kao *et al.*, 1993), *Rana esculenta* (Minucci *et al.*, 1990, 1994) and *Bufo bankorensis* (Huang *et al.*, 1996).

Further, Leydig cells undergoing division were never noticed suggesting that production of new Leydig cells may be by the process of differentiation of stromal fibroblast cells. There seems to be a species variation with regard to the factors affecting Leydig cell population in amphibians, for example in *Rana pipiens*, Leydig cell number increased with the increase in number of pituitary implants (Wada *et al.*, 1976). In *Bufo japonicus*, it is reported that development of interstitium is under the control of pituitary gonadotrophins (Moriguchi and Iwasawa, 1987). In *B. bufo*, hypophysectomy caused depletion in the interstitial cells (Guha and Jorgensen, 1978). However, in *Rana esculenta* it is reported that Leydig cell differentiation from fibroblastic cells may not require pituitary hormones (Minucci *et al.*, 1990, 1994). In the present study it was noticed that hypophyseal gonadotropins are essential for the differentiation of fibroblastic cells into vesicular hormone secreting cells and to maintain the pool of the latter; therefore removal of hypophysis resulted in degeneration of vesicular cells leading to the increase in pycnotic cells. While steroid hormones, testosterone and estradiol caused decrease in the total number of Leydig cells and percentage of vesicular cells indicating that steroid hormones interfere with the process of differentiation which was also evident by the increase in fibroblastic and pycnotic cells in steroid hormone treated ULO frogs compared to ULO controls.

In conclusion, the present study suggests that there is morphological variation in the populations of Leydig cells, seasonal changes occur in the differential counts of Leydig cells, gonadotropins stimulate the differentiation of fibroblastic cells into hormone secreting vesicular cells while steroid hormones testosterone and estradiol interfere with the differentiation in the testis of *E. cyanophlyctis*.

Acknowledgements

Dr. KP thanks Ms. Sapna Chandran for assisting in carrying out the experiments.

References

Callard, I. P., Callard, V. G., Lance, V., Bolaffi, J. L. and Rosset, S. J., 1978. Testicular regulation in nonmammalian vertebrates. *Biol. Reprod.*, 18: 16-43.

Callard, G. V., Canick, J. A. and Pudney, J., 1980. Estrogen Synthesis in Leydig Cells: Structural-Functional Correlations in Necturus Testis. *Biology of Reproduction*, 23: 461-479.

Cobellis, G., Meccariello, R. and Fasano, S., 2003. Intratesticular signals for progression of germ cell stages in vertebrates. *Gen. Comp. Endocrinol.*, 134(3): 220-228.

Denver, R. J., Glennemeier, K. A. and Boorse, G. C., 2002. Endocrinology of complex life cycles: Amphibians. In: *Hormones, Brain and Behaviour, Vol. 2*, (Eds.) D. Pfaff; A Arnoild, A. Etgin, S. Fahrbach, R. Moss and R. Rubin. Academic Press Inc, San Diego, pp. 469-513.

Guha, K. and Jorgensen, C. B., 1978. Effects of hypophysectomy on structure and function of testis in adult toads *Bufo bufo bufo* (L.). *Gen. Comp. Endocrinol.*, 34: 201-210.

Hardy, M. P., Sprando, R.L. and Ewing, L. L., 1992. Leydig Cell Renewal in the testes of seasonally breeding animals. *J. Exp. Zool.*, 261: 161-172.

Huang, L., Jun-Yi, L. and Yu-Lin, J. N., 1996. The male reproductive cycle of the toad, *Bufo bankorensis* in Taiwan. *Zool. Studies*, 35(2):128-137.

Kao, Y., Alexander, P. S., Cheng Yang, V. V. and Yu Yuh-Lin., 1993. Annual patterns of testicular development and activity in the Chinese bull frog (*Rana rugulosa* Weigmann). *Zool. Sci.*, 10: 337-351.

Lofts, B., 1968. Patterns of testicular activity. In: *Perspectives in Endocrinology Hormones in the Lives of Lower Vertebrates*, (Eds.) E.J.W. Barrington and C.B. Jorgensen. Academic Press Inc, New York and London, p. 239-404.

Lofts, B., 1974. Reproduction. In: *Physiology of Amphibia*, (Ed.) B. Lofts. Academic Press, New York, pp. 107-218.

Lofts, B., 1984. Reproductive cycles of vertebrates: Amphibians. In: *Marshall's Physiology of Reproduction*, (Ed.) G.E. Lamming. Churchill Livingstone, London, pp. 127-205.

Lofts, B., 1987. Testicular function. In: *Hormones and Reproduction in Fishes, Amphibians and Reptiles*, (Eds.) D.O. Norris and R.E. Jones. Plenum Press, New York, pp. 283-314.

Minucci, S., Fasano, S., DiMatteo, L., Chieffi, G.B. and Pierantoni, R., 1990. Morphological and Hormonal Changes in the frog, *Rana esculenta*, testis after administration of ethane dimethane sulfonate. *Gen. Comp. Endocrinol.*, 79: 335-345.

Minucci, S., DiMatteo, L., Fasano, S., Baccari, G. C. and Pierantoni, R., 1994. Regeneration of the testicular interstitial compartment after ethane dimethane sulfonate treatment in the hypophysectomized frog, *Rana esculenta*: Independence of pituitary control. *Gen. Comp. Endocrinol.*, 95: 84-91.

Moriguchi, Y. and Iwasawa, H., 1987. Annual changes in male reproductive organs in *Bufo japonicus formosus*: Histological observation. *Gen. Endocrinol.* (Life Sci. Adv)., 6: 115-120.

Pierantoni, R., Cobellis, G., Meccariello, R., Palmiero, C., Fienga, G. Minucci, S. and Fasano, S., 2002. The amphibian testis as model to study germ cell progression during spermatogenesis. *Comparative Biochemistry and Physiology Part B: Biochemistry and Molecular Biology*, 132(1): 131-139.

Pudney, J. and Callard, G. V., 1984. Organization of interstitial tissue in the testis of the salamander *Necturus maculosus* (Caudata: Proteidae). *J. Morphol.*, 181(1): 87-95.

Pudney, J., Canick, J. A., Mak, P. and Callard, G. V., 1983. The differentiation of Leydig Cells, Steroidogenesis and the spermatogenetic wave in the testis of *Necturus maculosus. Gen. Comp. Endocrinol.*, 50: 43-66.

Royere, D., Guerif, F., Laurent-Cadoret, V. and Hocherea, M., 2004. Apoptosis in testicular germ cells. *International Congress Series*, 1266: 170-176.

Saidapur, S.K., 1989. Reproductive Cycles of amphibians. In: *Reproductive cycles of Indian Vertebrates*, (Ed.) S.K. Saidapur. Allied Press, New Delhi, pp. 166-224.

Steel, R.G.D. and Torrie, J.N., 1980. *Principles and procedures of Statistics*. McGraw Hill, London.

Wada, M., Wingfield, J. C. and Gorbman, A., 1976. Correlation between blood level of androgens and sexual behaviour in the male leopard frogs, *Rana pipiens*. *Gen. Comp. Endocrinol.*, 29: 72-77.

Chapter 20

Biochemical Changes in Ovary and Uterus of Mice After Exposure to Indoxacarb

T.Y. Mudaraddi and B.B. Kaliwal*

P.G. Department of Studies in Biotechnology and Microbiology, Karnatak University, Dharwad – 580 003, Karnataka, India

ABSTRACT

Indoxacarb: (S)-methyl 7-chloro-2,5-dihydro-2-[[(methoxycarbonyl) [4-(trifluoromethoxy)phenyl]amino] carbonyl]indeno[1,2-e][1,3,4]oxadiazine-4a(3H) carboxylate, is a pyrazoline broad spectrum insecticide. The indoxacarb containing technical formulation was evaluated for its effects on the ovary and uterus biochemical contents in mice. Normal 90 days old Swiss albino mice, weighing about 25-30g were used in the experiment. The mice were administered with 6, 12, 18, and 24 mg/kg body wt indoxacarb for 30 days. The mice administered with distilled water served as control and mice were sacrificed on day 31st or 24 hours after the terminal exposure. Ovary and uterus were dissected out, freed from adherent tissue and weighed to the nearest milligram, estimations of biochemical contents and enzyme activities were carried out. Ovary and uterus biochemical contents showed that the levels of DNA, RNA, protein and glycogen were

* Corresponding author: E-mail: b_kaliwal@yahoo.com

decreased but there was an increase in the level of cholesterol in the mice treated with 18 and 24 mg/kg/day indoxacarb. The mice treated with 18 and 24 mg/kg/day of indoxacarb caused a decrease in the enzyme activities of SDH (Succinate dehydrogenase), Na^+-K^+ ATPase, Mg^{++}ATPase, Ca^{++}ATPase, ACP (Acid phosphatase) 3-βhydroxysteroid dehydrogenase (3-βHSD), 17-βhydroxysteroid dehydrogenase (17-βHSD) and increase in LDH (Lactate dehydrogenase) and AKP (Alkaline phosphatase). These observed effects of indoxacarb biochemical constituents may be due to imbalance in the hormone or toxic effect.

Keywords: *Indoxacarb, Ovary and uterus, Biochemical contents, Toxicity, Mice.*

Introduction

Pesticides are used in agriculture and public health to control insects, weeds, animals, and vectors of disease. Pesticides may cause reproductive toxicity through several different mechanisms: direct damage to the structure of cells, interference with biochemical processes necessary for normal cell function, and biotransformation resulting in toxic metabolites (Henderson 1995; Schettler *et al.*, 2003).

The decrease in the protein content in the ovaries of rats after long term treatment with low doses of dimethoate, methyl parathion and monocrotophos indicates degenerative changes (Gopal and Ahuja, 1979). The decrease in the level of ovarian glycogen and protein and increase in cholesterol content in higher doses of pesticides treated rats and mice (Mahadevswami *et al.*, 2000; Baligar and Kaliwal, 2001; Ksheerasagar and Kaliwal, 2005; Parimala and Kaliwal, 2005; Shreelakshmi and Kaliwal, 2006). Chemicals affect the metabolism by imbalancing homeostasis of the organism. It has been reported that, carbamate and organophosphorus pesticides play important role in chronic poisoning and take part in number of process, as a pathophysiological and on biochemical constituents of ovary and other vital organs (Ksheerasagar, 2005; Manawadi, 2006; Shreelakshmi, 2008). Oxidative stress occurs when formation of reactive oxygen species (ROS) exceeds the ability of the cells to defend themselves from increased ROS. When oxidized molecules overwhelm the cell system, a cascade of detrimental effects ensures affecting the whole organ at biochemical and molecular levels (lipids, proteins, DNA and RNA) (Pelicano *et al.*, 2003). Recently it has been reported that indoxacarb induces oxidative stress in testes, kidney and induces changes in biochemical constituents of liver and also induces effects on estrous cycle and ovarian follicles in albino mice (Mudaraddi and Kaliwal, 2009).

It has been reported that organophosphate pesticide quinolphos, carbamate pesticides thiram and mancozeb are known to cause decreased activity of SDH and increased LDH activity in testis of rats (Kackar *et al.*, 1997; Mishra *et al.*, 1998; Pant and Srivastava, 2003). Reactive oxygen induced injury is lipid peroxidation, and peroxidation of membrane phospholipids which not only alters lipid milieu and structural and functional integrity of cell membrane but also affects the activities of various membrane bound enzymes including total ATPase, Na^+- K^+-ATPase and Mg-ATPase (Shao *et al.*, 1995; Fritz *et al.*, 1999). It has been reported that carbamate pesticides such as thiram and mancozeb exposure causes decrease in ACP and increase in AKP activity in gonads of the rats (Kackar *et al.*, 1997; Mishra *et al.*, 1998).

Indoxacarb is a recently introduced oxadiazine insecticide derived from pyrazoline with activity against a wide range of pests (Harder *et al.*, 1996). In insects, indoxacarb appears to be decarbomethoxylated to DCJW by an esterase/amidase (Wing *et al.*, 2000). Several studies have demonstrated that DCJW is effective at blocking sodium channels at this target site (Tsurubuchi and Kono, 2003; Tsurubuchi *et al.*, 2001; Narahashi, 2002; Zhao *et al.*, 1999). However, indoxacarb and DCJW have also been shown to affect mammalian nicotinic acetylcholine receptors and have a weak effect on mammalian GABA receptors (Tsurubuchi *et al.*, 2001). Therefore present investigation was carried out to evaluate toxicity of indoxacarb in ovary and uterus of mice.

Materials and Methods

Insecticide

The sample of indoxacarb (indoxacarb 14.5 per cent) used in experiments was commercial insecticide supplied by E.I DuPont India Pvt., Ltd., Haryana obtained from the local company's market containing indoxacarb (a.i) 14.5 (w/w) in active enantiomer 6 per cent (w/w) amorphous silicon dioxide 7 per cent (w/w) polyethoxylated polyalyl phenol 9 per cent (w/w) polyethoxylated polyalyl phenol phosphate 6 per cent (w/w) distilled methyl soyate 57.5 per cent (w/w).

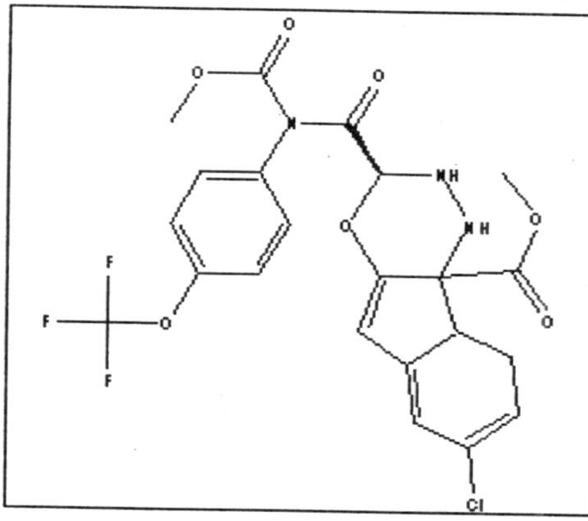

Structural Formula of Indoxacarb $C_{22}H_{17}ClF_3N_3O_7$
Indoxacarb: (S)-methyl 7-chloro-2,5-dihydro-2-[[(methoxycarbonyl) [4-(trifluoromethoxy) phenyl]amino] carbonyl]indeno [1,2-e][1,3,4]oxadiazine-4a(3H) carboxylate

Animals and Treatments

Laboratory bred adult virgin female Swiss albino mice were used in the experiments. Mice aged 90 days old weighing between 25-30g were used. The mice were maintained in the P.G. Department of Studies in Zoology, Karnatak University, Dharwad. Mice breed quite normally, almost throughout the year. They were housed in separate polypropylene cages containing sterile paddy husk as bedding material. The mice were provided with standard mice pellet diet "Gold Mohar" (Hindustan Liver Company, Mumbai) and water *ad libitum*. The mice were maintained under normal day/night schedule (12 L: 12 D) at room temperature 25 ± 2°C.

The doses were given orally in distilled water, below their acute level of intoxication according to their weight. The mice were divided in to 5 groups, 1st group was used as control and remaining 4 groups were used for graded dose study. Each group consists of 10 mice. The mice were given 6, 12, 18 and 24 mg/kg body weight indoxacarb for 30 days. Control mice were provided distilled water. All mice were autopsied by cervical dislocation on 31st day or 24 hrs after the terminal exposure. The ovary and uterus of all mice were dissected out and in each group mice were processed for biochemical study.

Biochemical Studies

The biochemical study such as estimation of DNA and RNA carried out as per the method described by Schneider (1957), protein by Lowry *et al.* (1951), glycogen by Carrol *et al.* (1956), cholesterol by Abell *et al.* (1952), activities of enzymes such as SDH by Nachlas *et al.* (1960), LDH by King (1965), 3-βHSD by Shivanandappa and Venkatesh, 17-βHSD by Jarabak *et al.*, Na^+-K^+ ATPase, Ca^{++} ATPase, Mg^{++} ATPase were assayed according to the method described by Jinna *et al.* (1989), ACP and AKP by method of Bergmeyer and Bernt (1963).

Statistical Analysis

Statistical significance between the control and experimental data were subjected to analysis of variance (ANOVA) together with Dunnett's test ($P<0.05$).

Results and Discussion

Biochemical Studies

In graded dose study the mice treated with 18 and 24 mg/kg/day indoxacarb for 30 days showed decrease in DNA, RNA, Protein, Glycogen and increase in the level of cholesterol. There was no change in the biochemical contents of the mice group treated with 6 mg and 12 mg/kg/day indoxacarb for 30 days. (Tables 20.1 and 20.2)

In the present investigation the decreased levels of biochemical contents in ovary and uterus of mice are found with higher dosage. It has been revealed that pesticides cause chromosomal breaks by breaking phosphodiester backbone of DNA and induce decreased mitotic index (Adhikari and Grover, 1988; Zefesco *et al.*, 1990; Cid *et al.*, 1990; Georgellis *et al.*, 1989; Barale *et al.*, 1993; Topktas *et al.*, 1996). Flessel *et al.* (1993) have reported that malathion an organophosphate insecticide affects the activity of estrogens and other enzymes and possibly causes a disturbance in cell division machinery. The enzyme DNA polymerase-alpha (pol-alpha) is one of the enzymes essential in nuclear DNA replication. Gorski *et al.* (1971) have reported that uterine RNA synthesis is influenced by ovarian estrogens. Estrogen administration accelerated ribosomal RNA synthesis representing the transcriptional activity is increased to provide more ribosomes for increased protein synthesis, which appears to control glucose metabolism, lipid synthesis and other

Table 20.1: Effect on Biochemical Contents of the Ovary in Mice After Exposure to Indoxacarb

Group	Treatment (mg/kg/day)	Biochemical Contents (mg/mg wet weight of tissue)				
		DNA	RNA	Protein	Glycogen	Cholesterol
I	Control	2.31± 0.30	3.95± 0.24	190.05± 5.76	4.81± 0.28	5.85 ± 0.38
II	6	2.26± 0.28	3.72± 0.36	185.05± 4.72	4.76 ± 0.32	6.0 ± 0.30
III	12	2.29± 0.20	3.51± 0.45	177.33± 8.72	4.30 ± 0.25	6.15 ± 0.34
IV	18	2.02± 0.10*	3.20± 0.25*	170.33± 6.72*	3.93 ± 0.32*	6.73 ± 0.29*
V	24	1.86± 0.15*	2.66± 0.21*	159.6± 6.72*	3.43± 0.30*	7.30 ± 0.38*

Values are mean ± SEM of 10 animals.

* Significant $P \leq 0.05$ compared to control.

Table 20.2: Effect on Biochemical Contents of the Uterus in Mice After Exposure to Indoxacarb

Group	*Treatment (mg/kg/day)*	*Biochemical Contents (mg/mg wet weight of tissue)*				
		DNA	*RNA*	*Protein*	*Glycogen*	*Cholesterol*
I	Control	2.03± 0.15	4.78± 0.24	195.09± 8.30	3.84± 0.42	8.18 ± 0.84
II	6	1.98± 0.09	4.45± 0.40	185.86± 6.40	3.44 ± 0.50	8.44 ± 0.82
III	12	1.90± 0.05	4.05± 0.30	176.25± 6.46	3.05± 0.35	9.20 ± 0.40
IV	18	1.67± 0.20*	3.65± 0.30*	170.23± 8.20*	2.90± 0.22*	10.49 ± 0.50*
V	24	1.27± 0.30*	2.52± 0.25*	161.72± 5.38*	2.64 ± 0.24*	12.87 ± 0.51*

Values are mean ± SEM of 10 animals.

* Significant $P \leq 0.05$ compared to control.

activities. This stimulation culminates in cellular growth, cell division and hyperplasia at uterine cells (Gorski *et al.*, 1985). In the present study, the observed results in the levels of nucleic acids in ovary and uterus under the influence of indoxacarb treatment in mice might have caused decrease in mitotic index and disturbed cell division (Walter *et al.*, 1980; Flessel *et al.*, 1993; Topktas *et al.*, 1996), which may be due to inhibition of DβH (Dopamine-β-hydroxylase) and release of GnRH gonadotropins and thereby affecting the production of gonadal steroids (Maj *et al.*, 1969; Prezewlock *et al.*, 1975).

In the present study it was found that indoxacarb caused decrease in the level of total protein and glycogen in the ovary and uterus of mice after exposure to indoxacarb. Similar observations have been made in rats and mice exposed to other pesticides like monocrotophos, dimethoate, methoxychlor, methyl parathion (Janardhan *et al.*, 1990; Mahadevaswami and Kaliwal, 2002; Gupta *et al.*, 2006; Radhika and Kaliwal, 2006; Shreelakshmi and Kaliwal, 2007). It has been reported that the decrease in the proteins, lipids, phospholipids and cholesterol (cytoplasmic and membrane bound) in the ovaries of rats after long term treatment with low doses of dimethoate, methyl parathion and monocrotophos indicates degenerative changes (Sukhdeep and Dhanju, 2005).The changes in the levels of protein, glycogen and lipids with mancozeb treatment indicated either an increased catabolism of the biomolecules to compensate the energy demand under stress or their reduced synthesis due to impaired tissue function (Ivanova-Chemishanska, 1962). The decreased tissue glycogen levels with indoxacarb exposure signifies their utilization for energy requirements to face the toxic stress or this may be due to pesticide effect on ovarian hormone production, as the ovarian hormones are known to regulate glycogen metabolism in ovary and uterus or may be due to leakage of glucose from the tissue into blood due to tissue damage on indoxacarb exposure thereby affecting ovarian function, follicular dynamics and estrous cycle in albino mice (Sukhdeep and Dhanju, 2005).

In the present study higher dose of indoxacarb caused increase in the level of cholesterol in the ovary and uterus of mice. Similar observations have been made in rats and mice exposed to other pesticides like monocrotophos, dimethoate, methoxychlor, methyl parathion (Janardhan *et al.*, 1990; Mahadevaswami and Kaliwal, 2002; Gupta *et al.*, 2006; Radhika and Kaliwal, 2006; Shreelakshmi and Kaliwal, 2007). It has been reported that the decrease in the proteins, lipids, phospholipids and cholesterol (cytoplasmic and membrane bound) in the ovaries of rats after long term treatment with low doses of dimethoate, methyl parathion and monocrotophos indicates degenerative changes (Sukhdeep and Dhanju, 2005). Increased cholesterol level in the testes and adrenals found as indicator of steroidogenesis inhibition in rats exposed to BHC (Shivanandappa and Krishnakumari, 1981). The organophosphate pesticide (monocrotophos) and carbamate pesticide (Diethyl dithiocarbamates) are known to inhibit cyt P450 Inhibition in the activity of enzyme causes deposition of cholesterol in the cell (Siddiqui *et al.*, 1987; Stott *et al.*, 1997). The results indicate that increase in dose of indoxacarb caused increase in the cholesterol level of the ovary and uterus. The increased cholesterol levels are also suggestive of the inhibition of steroidogenesis in testis and adrenal (Shivanandappa and Krishnakumari, 1981; Chitra *et al.*, 1987; Sujatha *et al.*, 2001) or inhibition of P450 enzymes (Sidiqui *et al.*, 1987; Stott *et al.*, 1997) which are essential for cholesterol break up, thus causing deposition of cholesterol in the cell. Thus, this may cause reduced steroidogenesis (Eik-Nes and Hall, 1962; Dorfman *et al.*, 1963).

Effect on Enzyme Activities

In graded dose study the mice dosed with 18 and 24 mg/kg/day for 30 days indoxacarb showed decrease in the SDH, Na^{+}-k^{+} ATPase, Mg^{++} ATPase, Ca^{++} ATPase, ACP 3-βhydroxysteroid dehydrogenase (3-βHSD), 17-βhydroxysteroid dehydrogenase (17-βHSD) and increase in the activity of LDH and AKP. There was no change in the levels of enzyme activities in the mice group treated with 6 mg and 12 mg/kg/day indoxacarb for 30 days. (Tables 20.3 and 20.4)

The present findings revealed that, increase in dose exposure of indoxacarb showed increase in LDH and decrease in the activity of SDH in the ovary and uterus of albino mice, similar observations have been made in rats and mice exposed to carbofuran (Ksheerasagar, 2005), methomyl and organophosphate pesticide phosphomidon (Manawadi, 2006; Shreelakshmi, 2008). In the present investigation, the observed decrease in the SDH activity under

Table 20.3: Effect on Dehydrogenase and Phosphatase Enzyme Activity of the Ovary in Mice After Exposure to Indoxacarb

Group	Treatment (mg/kg/day)	Enzyme Activity μmoles/min/g tissue								
		LDH[a]	SDH[b]	3βHSD[c]	17βHSD[d]	Na^+-K^+ ATPase[e]	Mg^{++} ATPase[e]	Ca^{++} ATPase[e]	ACP[f]	AKP[f]
I	Control	18.81±0.24	12.56±0.30	0.50±0.002	0.90±0.05	10.20±0.29	12.30±0.16	9.40±0.34	13.10±0.30	14.50±0.62
II	6	19.00±0.34	12.40±0.34	0.48±0.002	0.85±0.06	10.01±0.25	12.40±0.23	9.10±0.27	12.90±0.45	14.91±0.45
III	12	19.49±0.45	12.08±0.27	0.45±0.003	0.81±0.03	9.41±0.20	11.34±0.45	8.80±0.27	12.40±0.40	15.54±0.40
IV	18	21.21±0.48*	11.43±0.20*	0.42±0.001*	0.72±0.05*	8.54±0.19*	10.02±0.34*	8.50±0.35*	11.40±0.35*	16.47±0.51*
V	24	23.01±0.34*	11.10±0.29*	0.40±0.001*	0.60±0.05*	8.30±0.23*	9.48±0.33*	8.28±0.25*	10.50±0.50*	18.09±0.47*

Table 20.4: Effect on Dehydrogenase and Phosphatase Enzyme Activity of the Uterus in Mice After Exposure to Indoxacarb

Group	Treatment (mg/kg/day)	Enzyme Activity μmoles/min/g tissue						
		LDH[a]	SDH[b]	Na^+-K^+ ATPase[c]	Mg^{++} ATPase[c]	Ca^{++} ATPase[c]	ACP[d]	AKP[d]
I	Control	10.67±0.58	11.45±0.66	10.09±0.45	9.89±0.42	9.96±0.44	15.49±0.54	17.47±0.52
II	6	11.41±0.64	10.91±0.56	9.66±0.58	9.52±0.43	9.21±0.43	13.96±0.53	17.99±0.47
III	12	12.97±0.53	10.30±0.45	8.86±0.60	9.01±0.44	8.36±0.56	13.12±0.63	18.84±0.43
IV	18	13.89±0.55*	9.26±0.55*	7.98±0.43*	8.23±0.35*	7.54±0.51*	12.09±0.49*	19.57±0.46*
V	24	14.80±0.48*	8.15±0.53*	6.93±0.53*	7.34±0.45*	6.36±0.53*	13.12±0.59*	20.56±0.42*

a: μmoles of pyruvate formed/min/g tissue; b: μmoles of formazon formed/min/g tissue; c μmoles of NAD converted to NADH/min/g tissue;

d: μmoles of NADPH converted to NADP/min/g tissue; e: μmoles of inorganic phosphorus formed/min/g tissue

f: μmoles of p-nitrophenyl formed/min/g tissue.

Values are mean±SEM of 10 animals.

* Significant $P \leq 0.05$ compared to control.

high-dose treatment with indoxacarb may be attributed to, effect on carbohydrate metabolism of the tissues, increased follicular atresia as indicated by decrease in SDH activity (Preidkatns and Weber, 1968), as this enzyme is related with high metabolic activity such as absorption and secretion (Padykula, 1952). The rise of LDH activity in tissue suggests high turnover of pyruvate to lactate or vice-versa to yield required energy to over come pesticide induced metabolic stress (Kacker *et al.*, 1997; Mishra *et al.*, 1988; Pant and Shrivastava, 2003). Ovarian hormones are known to regulate the activity of LDH in the uterus. Therefore, synthesis of LDH subunits can be stimulated by ovarian hormones (Richards, 1980). Thus enhanced activity of LDH in the present findings with indoxacarb treatment may be due to metabolic stress by affecting the ovary and uterine metabolism or decreased production of ovarian steroid hormones in albino mice.

The present findings revealed that, increase in dose exposure of indoxacarb showed a decrease in 3-βhydroxysteroid dehydrogenase (3-βHSD), 17-βhydroxysteroid dehydrogenase (17-βHSD). It has been found that the increase in the duration of exposure to carbosulfan caused an increase in the cholesterol level in the ovary and uterus and decrease in the 3 βHSD activity in the ovary of albino mice, suggesting its effect on steroidogenesis in the ovary (Shivanandappa Krishnakumari, 1981) and further causing effect on follicular dynamics and estrous cycle in albino mice exposed to carbosulfan. It has been reported that the fungicide azole affects the steroidogenesis and there by disturbs the physiological balance of androgens and estrogens (Zarh *et al.*, 2002). Similar results have been reported by the intoxication of carbosulfan (Ksheerasagar, 2005), methomyl and organophosphate pesticide phosphomidon (Sudheer, 2006; Shreelakshmi, 2008). The present study imply that the toxic action of indoxacarb was exerted by impaired steroidogenesis in the granulosa- thecal cells in the ovary or may be due to inhibition of certain pathways of steroidogenesis (Shivanandappa *et al.*, 1981; Chitra *et al.*, 1999; Sujatha *et al.*, 2001) by affecting cytochrome P450 and G-6PD (Siddiqui *et al.*, 1987; Stott *et al.*, 1997; Reddy *et al.*, 1988) or might be due to high affinity binding of pesticide (Zarh *et al.*, 2002) causing ovarian toxicity either by its direct action on reproductive system.

The present findings revealed that, increase in dose exposure of indoxacarb showed a decrease in Na^{+}-K^{+}ATPase, Ca^{++}ATPase and Mg^{++}ATPase. One of the targets of reactive oxygen induced injury is lipid peroxidation and peroxidation of membrane phospholipids not only alters lipid milieu and structural and functional integrity of cell membrane but also affects the activities of various membrane bound enzymes including total ATPase, Na^{+}-K^{+}ATPase and Mg^{++}ATPase (Shao *et al.*, 1995; Rauchova *et al.*, 1995). In the present study, it has been found that increase in dose exposure of indoxacarb caused significant decrease in the activity of ATPases in the ovary and uterus. This may be due to (a) pesticide induced effect on cell membrane because of their strong affinity for interaction with member of lipids (Antuner-Maderia and Maderia, 1987) causing inhibition of membrane bound ATPase enzymes by affecting enzyme complex (Kinter *et al.*, 1972; Basha and Nayeemunnisa, 1993; Shao *et al.*, 1995; Rauchova *et al.*, 1995; Blaisak, 1995; Mishra *et al.*, 1998). (b) Mitochondrial disorganization as reported during pesticide toxicities (Pardini *et al.*, 1980) might have caused inhibition of Na^{+}-K^{+}ATPase, Mg^{++}ATPase and Ca^{++}ATPases activities in ovary and uterus with respect to increase in the dose and duration of indoxacarb exposure.

The present findings revealed that, increase in dose and exposure of indoxacarb caused a decrease in ACP and increase in AKP activity in ovary and uterus of mice. Similar changes in the activities of AKP have been reported in carbon tetrachloride treated rats (Berman *et al.*, 1992) and HCH and gamma HCH treated mice (Ravinder *et al.*, 1989). Decrease and increase in liver, testis and serum AKP activity were also reported by HCH, methyl parathion, diazinon and monocrotophos treated rats (Dikshith *et al.*, 1975; Janardhan and Sisodia, 1990; Dikshith *et al.*, 1991), which may be indicative of an adaptive rise in enzyme activity to the persistent stress (Murphy and Porter, 1966). On the other hand the level of acid phosphatase decreased significantly. This enzyme is known to be associated with the lysosomes, which participate in the intra and extra cellular digestive processes (Novikoff, 1961). Riar *et al.* (1973) have also suggested that it is associated with scavenging activity. In the present study, the decrease in ACP activity may be due to an altered transport of phosphate (Engstrom, 1964) and inhibitory effect on the cell growth and proliferation (Goldfisher *et al.*, 1964). The elevated AKP activity in kidney which is suggestive of an increase in tissue synthesis of these enzymes as an adaptive mechanism to chemical stress (Kackar *et al.*, 1997; Mishra *et al.*, 1998)

Acknowledgements

The authors are grateful to the Post-Graduate Department of Studies in Microbiology and Biotechnology, Karnatak University, Dharwad for providing the necessary facilities.

References

Abell, L.L., Levy, B.B., Brodie, B.P. and Kendal, F.E., 1952. Simplified method for estimation of total cholesterol in serum and demonstration of its specificity. *J. Biol. Chem.*, 195: 357-361.

Adhikari, N. and Grover, I.S., 1988. Genotoxic effects of some systemic pesticides: in vivo chromosomal aberrations in bone marrow cells in rats. *Environ. Mol. Mutagen.*, 12: 235-242.

Akbarsha, M.A. and Averal, H.I., 1998. Male reproductive toxicity of vincristine: Ultrastructural changes in the epididymal principal cell. *Biomedical Letters.* 57: 159-169.

Antunes-Mudeira, M.C., Madeira, V.M.C., 1987. Partition of malathion in synthetic and native membranes, *Biochem. Biophys Acta.*, 901: 61.

Baligar, P.N. and Kaliwal, B.B., 2001. Induction of gonadal toxicity to female rats after chronic exposure to mancozeb. *Ind. Health.* 39: 235-243.

Barale, R.C., Seapoli, C., Meli, D., Casini, M., Minunni, A., Marrazzini, N., Loprieno and Barrai, I., 1993. Cytogenetic effects of benzimidazoles in mouse bone marrow. *Mutation Res.*, 300: 15-28.

Basha, P.M. and Nayeemunnisa, 1993. Effect of methyl parathion on Na^+-K^+ and Mg^{2+} adenosine triphosphatase activity in developing central nervous system in rats. *Ind. J. Exptl. Biol.*, 31: 785.

Bergemeyer, H.V. and Bernt, E., 1963. In: *Methods of Enzymatic Analysis,* (Ed.) H.V. Bergmeyer. Academic Press, Weinheim, N.Y. and London, 837.

Berman, E., House, D.F, Allis, J.W. and Simmons, J.L., 1989. Hepatotoxicity interaction of ethanol with ethyl alcohol or carbon tetrachloride in rats. *J. Toxicol. Environ. Hlth.*, 37(1): 161-176.

Blasiak, J., 1995. Inhibition of erythrocyte membrane (Ca^{2+}+Mg^{2+}) ATPase by organophosphorus insecticides parathion and methyl parathion, *Comp. Biochem. Physiol. Pharmacol. Toxicol. Endocrinol.*, 110C: 119.

Carrol, N.V., Langely R.W. and Row R.H., 1956. Glycogen determination in liver and mode by use of anthrone reagent. *J. Biol. Chem.*, 20: 583-593.

Chitra, K.C., Latchoumycandane, C. and Mathur, P.P., 1999. Chronic effects of endosulfan on the testicular function of rat. *Asian J. Androl.*, 1(4): 203-206.

Dikshith, T.S., Behari, J.R., Datta, K.K and Mathur, A.K., 1975. Effect of diazinon in male rats, Histopathological and biochemical studies, *Environ. Physiol. Biochem.*, 5: 239-299.

Dikshith, T.S.S., Raizada, R.B., Singh, V., Pandey, M. and Srivastava, M.K., 1991. Repeated dermal toxicity of tech.HCH and methyl parathion (50 EC) to female rats (*Rattus norvegicus*). *Ind. J. Exptl. Biol.*, 29(2): 149-155.

Engstrom, L., 1964. Phosphate incorporation. *Biochem. Biophys. Acta.*, 92: 71.

Flessel, P., Quintana, P.J.E. and Hooper, K., 1993. Genetic toxicity of malathion: a review. *Environ. Mol. Mutagen.*, 22: 7-17.

Fritz, K.I., Groenendaal, F., Andersen, C., Ohnishi, S.T. and Mishra, O.P. 1999. Deleterious brain cell membrane effects after NMDA receptor antagonist administration to new born piglets. *Brain Res.*, 816: 438.

Georgellis, A, Purvinen, M. and Rydstrom, J., 1989. Inhibition of stage-specific DNA, synthesis in rat spermatogenic cells by polycyclic aromatic hydrocarbons. *Chem. Biol. Interact.*, 72: 79-92.

Goldfisher, S., Essner, E. and Novikoff, A.B., 1964. The localization of phosphatase activities at level of ultrastructure. *J. Histochem. Cytochem.*, 12: 72-95.

Gorski, J., De Angelo, A.B. and Barnea, A., 1971. Control of gene expression: An early response to estrogen. In: V.H.T. James and C. Martini, (Eds.) *Proc. 3rd Internat. Congr. Hormonal Steroids, Excerpta Medica*, Amsterdam, p. 426.

Gupta, R.K., Schuh, R., Fiskum, G. and Flaws, J.A., 2006. Methoxychlor caused mitochondrial dysfunction and oxidative damage in the mouse ovary. *Toxicol. and Appl. Pharmacol.* (In Press).

Harder, H.H., Riley, S.L., McCann, S.F. and Irving, S.N., DPXMP062, 1996. A novel broad-spectrum, environmentally soft, insect control compound. *Proc. Brighton Crop. Prot. Conf.*, p. 449.

Henderson, P.T., Borm, P.J.A., Kant, I.J., 1995. Basisboek Arbeidstoxicologie risicoinventarisatie en-evaluatie Zeist: Uitgeverij Kerckebosch bv.

Hore, S. K., Maitis, S. K., Chauhan, H. V., Neelu, Gupta, S. and Koley K.M., 1997. Effect of longterm exposure of mancozeb on clinico-haemato-biochemical and pathological changes in rats. *Indian Vet. J.*, 74: 26–8.

Ivanova-Chemishanska, L., 1962. Dithiocarbamates. In: Toxicity of pesticides, health aspects of chemical safety WHO Copenhagen, Interim Document. 9: 158-169.

Janardhan, A., and Sisodia, P., 1990. Monocrotophos: short term toxicity in rats. *Bull. Environ. Contam. Toxicol.*, 44: 230-239.

Jinna, R.R., Ozodinma, J.E. and Desaiah, D., 1989. Age related changes in rat brain ATPases during treatment with chlordecone. *J Toxicol Environ Hlth.*, 27: 199-208

Kackar, R., Srivastava, M. K. and Raizada, R.B., 1997. Induction of gonadial toxicity to male rats after chronic exposure to mancozeb. *Indus Health*, 35: 104-11.

King J., 1965. In: *Practical Clinical Enzymology*, Edn. Van Z., Norstrand D., Co. London, p. 83.

Kinter, W.B., Merkens, L.S., Janiki, R.H. and Guarino, A.M., 1972. Studies on the mechanism of toxicity of DDT and PCBS; Disruption of osmoregulation in marine fish. *Environ. Hlth. Persps.*, 8: 169-173.

Ksheerasagar R.L., 2005. Application of biotechnology in the evaluation of gonadal, hepatic and renal toxicity of A carbamate insecticide carbofuran in a albino mice. *Ph.D. Thesis*, Karnatak University, Dharwad, India

Lowry, H., Rosebrough, N.I., Far, A.L. and Randall, R.J., 1951. Protein measurement with Folin phenol reagent. *J. Biol. Chem.*,193: 265-275.

Mahadevaswami, M.P. and Kaliwal, B.B., 2002. Effect of dimethoate administration schedules on compensatory ovarian hypertrophy, follicular dynamics and estrous cycle in hemicastrated mice. *Jour. Basic. Clinic. Phys. Pharmacol.*, 13(3): 225-248.

Maitra and Sarkar, 1996. Morphological study of the testes in relation to the brain and testicular acetyl cholinesterase activity in an organophosphate pesticide ingester wild passerine bird (*Lonchura malabarica*). *Folia Biologica*, 43: 143-149.

Maitra, S.K. and Sarkar, R., 1996. Influence of methyl parathion on gametogenic and acetyl cholinesterase activity in the testis of white throated munia (*Bonchura malabarica*). *Arch. Environ. Contam. Toxicol.*, 30: 384-389.

Maj, J. and Vetulani, J., 1969. Effect of some N, N-disubstituted dithiocarbamates on catecholamines level in rat brain. *Biochem. Pharmacol.*, 18: 2045-2047.

Manawadi, S.I., 2006. Evaluation of toxicity by a carbamate pesticide methomyl in female albino mice. *M. Phil Thesis*, K. U. Dharwad India.

Mishra, V.K., Shrivastava, M.K. and Raizada, R.B., 1998. Testicular toxicity in rat to repeated oral administration of tetramethyl thiuram disulfide (Thiram). *Ind. J. Exptl. Biol.*, 36: 390-394.

Mudaraddi, T.Y. and Kaliwal, B.B., 2009. Indoxacarb induces testes oxidative stress in swiss albino mice. *International J. Biotechnology Research*, 2: 40-48

Mudaraddi, T.Y. and Kaliwal, B.B., 2009. Indoxacarb induces kidney oxidative stress in swiss albino mice. *Ind. J. of Comparative Animal Physiology*, 27(2): 106-112.

Mudaraddi, T. Y. and Kaliwal, B.B., 2009. Indoxacarb induces effects on estrous cycle and ovarian follicles in albino mice. In: *97th Session of Indian Science Congress* (Accepted).

Mudaraddi, T.Y. and Kaliwal, B.B., 2009. Indoxacarb induces hepatic toxicity in Swiss albino mice. *Research J. Chemistry and Environment* (Accepted).

Nachles, M.M., Margulius, S.I. and Sellirgman, A.M., 1960. Site of electron transfer to tetrazolium salts in the succinoxidase. *J. Biol. Chem.*, 235: 27–39.

Narahashi, T., 2002. Nerve membrane ion channels as the target site of insecticides. *Mini Rev. Medic. Chem.*, 2: 419.

Novikoff, A.B., 1961. Lysosomes and related particles in the cell: Biochemistry, physiology, morphology, (Eds.) J. Brachet and A.E. Mirskey. Academic Press, New York, pp. 423-488.

Pant, N. and Srivastava, S.P., 2003. Testicular and spermatotoxic effects of quinolphos in rats. *J. Appl. Toxicol.*, 23: 271-274.

Pardini, R.S., Heidken, J.C., Baker, T.A., Payme, B., 1980. Toxicology of various pesticides and their decomposition products on mitochondrial electron transport. *Arch. Environ. Contam. Toxicol.*, 9: 87-97.

Parimala, M.D. and Kaliwal, B.B., 2005. Dose-dependent estrous cycle, ovarian follicles and biochemical contents reversal in albino mice after exposure to mancozeb. *Caspian J. Env. Sci.*, 3(2): 118-131.

Preidkalns, J. and Weber, A.F., 1968. The succinic dehydrogenase and lipid content of follicular and luteal cells of the bovine ovary. *Acta. Anat.*, 71: 542-564.

Przewlocka, B., Sarnek, J., Szmielski, A. and Niewiakomsha, A., 1975. The effect of some dithiocarbamic acids on dopamine-β-hydroxylase and catecholamines level in rats brain. *Pol. J. Pharmacol. Pharm.*, 27: 555-559.

Radhika, P. and Kaliwal, B.B., 2002. Monocrotophos induced dysfunction on estrous cycle and follicular development in mice. *Indust. Health*, 40: 237-244.

Rathnasooriya, W.D., Peiries, L.D.C. and Jayatunga, Y.N.A., 1995. Analgesic and sedative action of monocrotophos following oral administration in rats. *Med. Sci. Res.*, 23: 401-402.

Rauchova, H., Ledvinkova, J., Kalous, M. and Drahota, Z. 1995. The effect of lipid peroxidation on the activity of various membrane-bound ATPases in rat kidney. *Int. J. Biochem. Cell Biol.*, 27: 251–261.

Rauchova, H., Ledvinkova, J., Kalous, M. and Drahota, Z., 1995. The effect of lipid peroxidation on the activity of various membrane-bound ATPases in rat kidney. *Int. J. Biochem. Cell Biol.*, 27: 251.

Reddy, A.N., Venugopal, N.B.R.K. and Reddy, S.L.N., 1992. Effect of endosulfan 35EC on ATPases in the tissues of a freshwater field crab *B. querini. Bull. Environ. Contam. Toxicol.*, 48: 216-222.

Riar, S.S., Setty, B.S. and Kar, A.B., 1973. Studies on the physiology and biochemistry of mammalian epididymis: Biochemical composition of epididymis. A comparative study. *Fertil. Steril.*, 24: 355.

Richards, J.S., 1980. Maturation of ovarian follicles: Actions and interactions of pituitary and ovarian harmones of follicle cell differentiation. *Physiol., Rev.*, 60: 51-89.

Schettler, T., Solomon, G., Kaplan, J. and Valenti, M., 2003. Generations at risk: How environmental toxicants may affect reproductive health in California Brisbane, CA: George Lithograph.

Schneider, W.C., 1957. Determination of nucleic acids in tissues by pentose analysis. In: *Methods in Enzymology*, (Eds.) S.P. Colowick and N.D. Kaplan. Academic Press, New York, p. 680-684.

Shao, Q., Matsubara, T., Blott, S.K. and Dhalla, N.S., 1995. Inhibition of cardiac sarcolemma Na^+-K^+-ATPase by oxyradical generating systems. *Mol.Cell Biochem.*, 147: 139.

Shivanandappa, T. and Krishnakumari, M.K., 1983. Hexachlorecyclohaxane induced testicular dysfunction in rats. *Acta. Pharmacol. Toxicol.*, 52: 12-17.

Shivanandappa, T. and Krishnakumari, M.K., 1981. Histochemical and biochemical change sin rats fed dietary benzene hexachloride. *Indian J. Exp. Biol.*, 19: 1163–1168.

Shreelakshmi T.S., 2008. Studies on possible mechanism of phosphamidon induced intoxication on reproductive and neurobehavioural changes in swiss albino mice. *Ph.D. Thesis*, Karnatak University, Dharwad, India.

Shreelakshmi, T.S. and Kaliwal, B.B., 2006. Phoaphamidon induced effects on estrous cycle, ovarian, uterine biochemical parameters in swiss albino mice. *Pesticide Biochemistry and Physiology*, 87: 204-210.

Siddiqui, M.K.J., Rahman, M.F, Anjum, F. and Quadri, S.S.H., 1987. Effect of oral administration of endosulfan on some haematological parameters and serum enzymes in rats. *Pesticides*, 21: 25-27.

Stott, Ian, Anupam, M., Alex, R., Norman, W.T. and Jeffrey, R.F., 1997. Low dose dithiocarbamate attenuates the hepatotoxicity of 1,3-dichloro-2-propanol and selectivity inhibits CYP2E1 activity in the rat. *Human Expt. Toxicol.*, 16: 262-266.

Sujatha, R., Chitra, K.C., Latchoumycandave, C. and Mathur, P.P., 2001. Effect of lindane on testicular anti oxidant system and stroidogenic enzymes in adult rats. *Asian J. Androl.*, 3: 135-138.

Sukhdeep, K. and Dhanju, C.K., 2005. Biochemical effects of some organophosphorus pesticides on the ovaries of albino rats, *Indian J. of Physiol. Pharmacol.*, 49(2): 148–152.

Topaktas, M., Rencizogullari, E. and Ila, H.B., 1996. *In vivo* chromosomal aberrations in bone marrow cells of rats with marshal. *Mut. Res.*, 371: 259-264.

Tsurubuchi, Y. and Kono, Y., 2003. Modulation of sodium channels by the oxadiazine insecticide indoxacarb and its N-decarbomethoxylated metabolite in rat dorsal root ganglion neurons. *Pest. Manag. Sci.*, 59: 999.

Tsurubuchi, Y., Karasawa A., Nagata K., Shono T. and Kono Y., 2001. Insecticidal activity of oxadiazine insecticide indoxacarb and its N-decarbomethoxylated metabolite and their modulations of voltage-gated sodium channels. *Appl. Entomol. Zool.*, 36: 381.

Walter, Z., Czakowska, A. and Lipecka, K., 1980. Effect of malathion on the genetic material of human lymphocytes stimulated by phytohemagglutinin (PHA). *Human Genet.*, 53: 375-381.

Wing, K.D., Sacher M., Kagaya Y., Tsurubuchi Y., Mulderig L., Connair M. and Schnee M., 2000. Bioactivation and mode of action of the oxadiazine indoxacarb in insects. *Crop. Prot.*, 19: 537

Zarh, J.A., Bruschweiler, B.J. and Schlatler, J.R., 2002. Azole fungicides affect mammalian steroidogenesis by inhibiting sterol 14α-demethylase and aromatase. *Environ Health Perspect.*, 111: 255–61.

Zefesco, P.A., Barbieri, I. and Graves, J.A.M., 1990. Use of a cell hybrid test system to demonstrate that Benomyl induces aneuploidy and polyploidy. *Mut. Res.*, 242: 329-335.

Zhao, X., Nagata, K., Marszalec, W., Yeh J.Z. and Narahashi T., 1999. Effects of the oxadiazine insecticide indoxacarb, DPXMP062, on neuronal nicotinic acetylcholine receptors in mammalian neurons. *Neuro Toxicology*, 20: 561.

Chapter 21

Ethno-Medicinal Use of Herbal Drugs for Enhancing Male Fertility

Pallavi Gupta[1]*, *Amita Kanaujia*[1] *and Poonam Singh*[2]

[1]*Department of Zoology, University of Lucknow, Lucknow – 226 007, U.P., India*

[2]*Divison of Toxicology, C.D.R.I., Lucknow – 226 001, U.P., India*

ABSTRACT

It is surprising to know the presence of male infertility in an over populated country like India. Infertility in males is the inability to conceive after at least one year of unprotected intercourse. In men, hormonal disorders, illness, reproductive anatomy trauma and obstruction, and sexual dysfunction can temporarily or permanently affect sperm count and prevent conception. Men's sperm counts have dropped dramatically and some experts fear an even greater decline in fertility in the future. The most common male infertility factors include azoospermia (no sperm cells are produced) and oligospermia (few sperm cells are produced). Sometimes, the quality of sperm cells is very poor, resulting in poor fertility. The healthcare system in India is characterized by multiple systems of medicine, mixed ownership patterns and different kinds of delivery structures. Ayurveda is basically the knowledge of wellbeing living dealing with the normal as well as abnormal pathological

* Corresponding author: E-mail: pallavi.gupta.2007@gmail.com

condition. It has a galaxy of medicines with special properties. Herbal remedies have long been used to address problems with fertility. In fact, evidence of the use of herbal remedies for male fertility dates all the way back to 200 A.D. These fertility herbal remedies are made out of special plants and plant extracts believed to have a positive effect on the reproductive organs, hormonal system, and sex drive. *Allium sativum, Ceropegia bulbosa, Setaria italica, Tribulus terrestris, Ficus bengalensis,* Ashwagandha, Shatavari are used for fertility enhancing properties. Recently, several important developments have been reported in scientific literature that may help to improve male fertility. Thus importance should be given to the potentiality of ethno-medicinal studies as these can provide a very effective strategy for the discovery of useful medicinally active identity. A detailed and systematic study is required for identification, cataloguing and documentation of herbal medicinal plants for enhancing male fertility.

Keywords: *Male fertility, Herbal remedies, Ayurveda, Sperms, Medicines.*

Introduction

It is surprising to know the presence of male infertility in an over populated country like India. Human infertility is a major worldwide health problem for individuals and their partners because over the past twenty years, fertility problems have increased dramatically. At least 25 per cent or more of couples will have trouble in conceiving, and more couples are turning to fertility treatments to help themselves to have a family. Infertility is a complex disorder with significant medical, psycho-social and economic aspects. Human infertility is an inability of a couple to achieve pregnancy after at least one year of trying to do so without using any means of birth control. Infertility can be caused by a wide variety of factors. One-third of problem lies with the male, one-third lies with the female, and one-third infertility is caused by problems with both the male and the female. Like all complex organ systems the human reproductive system is also affected by many diseases.

In men, hormonal disorders, illness, reproductive anatomy trauma and obstruction, and sexual dysfunction can temporarily or permanently affect sperm count and prevent conception. Men's sperm counts have dropped dramatically and some experts fear an even greater decline in fertility in the future. There are two types of infertility; Primary infertility, which is infertility without any previous pregnancy; and secondary infertility, when there has been a previous pregnancy. Common causes of infertility are ovulation problems, tubal causes, sperm causes, unexplained infertility and age-related problems whether some less common causes are uterine problems, endometriosis, previous tubal ligation, previous vasectomy and cervical factors.

The healthcare system in India is characterized by multiple systems of medicine, mixed ownership patterns and different kinds of delivery structures. Ayurveda is basically the knowledge of wellbeing living dealing with the normal as well as abnormal pathological condition. It has a galaxy of medicines with special properties. Herbal remedies have long been used to address problems with fertility. Medicinal herbs are among the oldest medicines and their increasing use in recent years is evidence of alternatives to conventional medicine. Yet the conventional approach of the drugs tends to focus on suppressing symptoms without looking at the bigger picture and finding the root cause of the problem. Herbal remedies have long been used to address problems with fertility.

In fact, evidence of the use of herbal remedies for male fertility dates all the way back to 200 A.D. Herbal remedies have been used successfully for thousands of years in traditional medicine in order to increase fertility and improve the functioning of the male reproductive systems. Phytotherapy (herbal therapy) has helped many couples to conceive the children. These fertility herbal remedies are made out of special plants and plant extracts believed to have a positive effect on the reproductive organs, hormonal system, and sex drive. When treating infertility using herbal fertility tonics, the remedies should be taken by both male and female for maximum results. The natural approach to increase fertility is and has been enormously successful, largely because fertility is multi-factorial, meaning that there are many elements that can be at the root of the fertility problems. Hence one has to turn to indigenous drugs to treat these maladies. The present article reviews the role of some such remedies in various male sexual disorders.

Disorders Related to Male Reproductive System

Traditionally the definition of male infertility is based on one or more abnormalities within semen analysis. As we all know there are several causes of infertility where the semen analysis can be, at least on superficial examination, perfectly normal (Anne M. Jequier, 1999). Male infertility is involved in a sexually paired couple's inability to conceive in a significant number of cases, with estimates ranging from 40-50 per cent. In the past it was considered necessary to address the reproductive function of a man only if sperm count is found to be low (Male Fertility Supplement Proceptin, 2009). However, it is now known that sperm count is not the only factor in impaired fertility. Male infertility increases with age, but fertility does not decline in men as sharply as it does in women. About six per cent of males between the ages of fifteen and fifty are struggling with infertility. The presence of anatomical defects or scar tissue formation, in the recovery process of the reproductive tract from infection is responsible for infertility in some men. Oxidative stress is a common pathology seen in approximately half of all infertile men (Tremellen, 2008).

Male infertility can be caused by a range of problems. Some common disorders are listed below:

- *Azoospermia*: It occurs when no sperm is produced.
- *Oligospermia*: It is diagnosed when few sperm are produced.
- *Abnormal sperm production*: It occurs when shape and structure of sperm is hampered, sperm may not be able to reach the egg.
- *Undescended testicle or testes*: It occurs when one or both testicles fail to descend from the abdomen into the scrotum during fetal development.
- *Varicocele*: A varicose vein around one of the two spermatic cords can cause blood to pool in the testes.
- *Ductal Obstruction*: Blockage or damage to the spermatic tubes.
- *Ejaculatory Dysfunction*: These disorders are characterized by the failure to deliver sperm to the vagina.
- *Cystic fibrosis*: This is a condition associated with both an absence and or blockage of the vas deferens.
- *Testicular cancer*: This condition may cause obstructions or dysfunctions or problems related to chemotherapy used to treat the disease.

Table 21.1: Herbs for Male Reproductive System

Sl.No.	*Plant Name*	*Botanical Name*	*Part Used*	*Picture*	*Effective in*
1.	Banyan	*Ficus bengalensis*	Latex	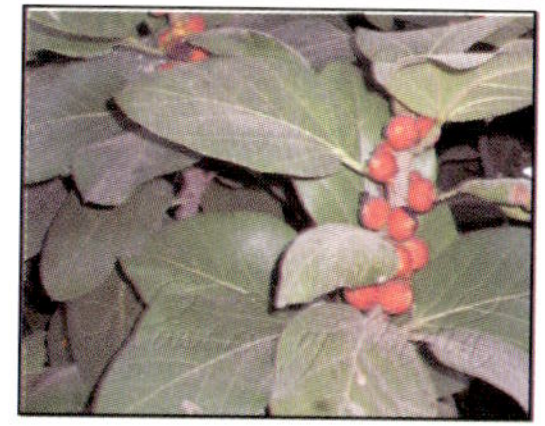	Make semen thick and regain sexual potentiality
2.	*Garlic*	*Allium sativum*	Bulb	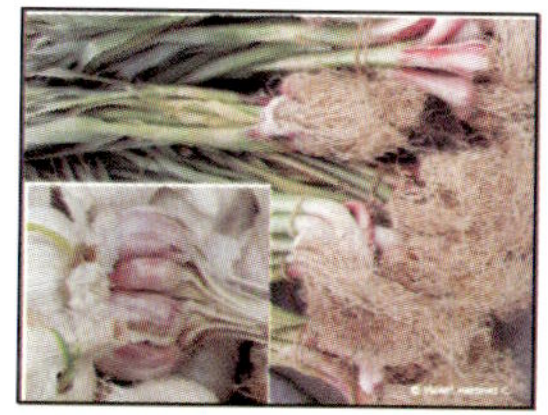	Increase sexual potency
3.	Gangl angoor	*Vitis vitiginea*	Tuber	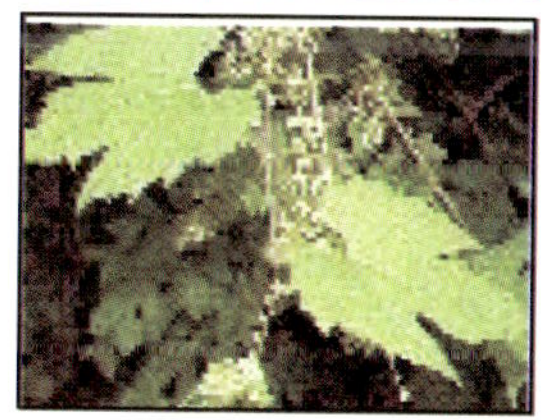	Enhance sexual potency

Contd...

Table 21.1–Contd...

Sl.No.	*Plant Name*	*Botanical Name*	*Part Used*	*Picture*	*Effective in*
4.	Bakhara	*Tribulus terrestris*	Mucilaginous infusion	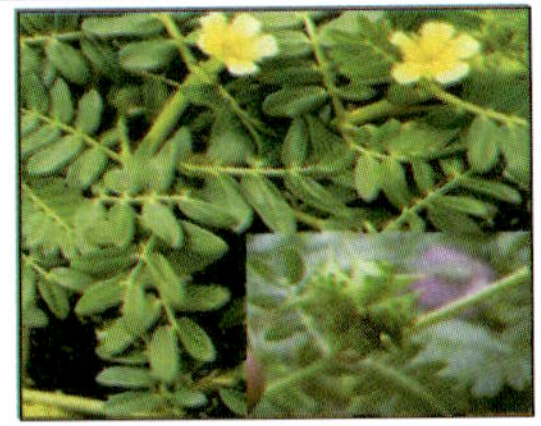	Enhance sexual potency
5.	Milk-vetch, locoweed	*Astragalus* spp.	Roots	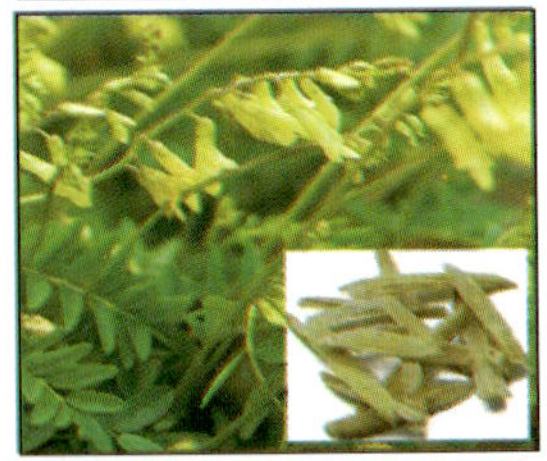	Increase motility of sperms
6.	Pumpkin	*Cucurbita maxima*	Seed	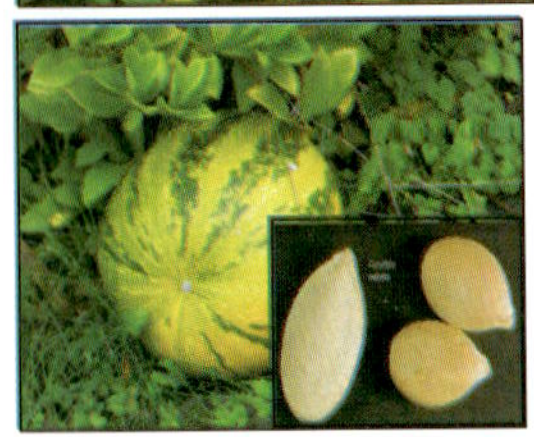	Increase functioning of male reproductive system

Contd...

Table 21.1–Contd...

Sl.No.	*Plant Name*	*Botanical Name*	*Part Used*	*Picture*	*Effective in*
7.	Ashwagandha	*Withania somnifera* (L.) *Dunal*	Root	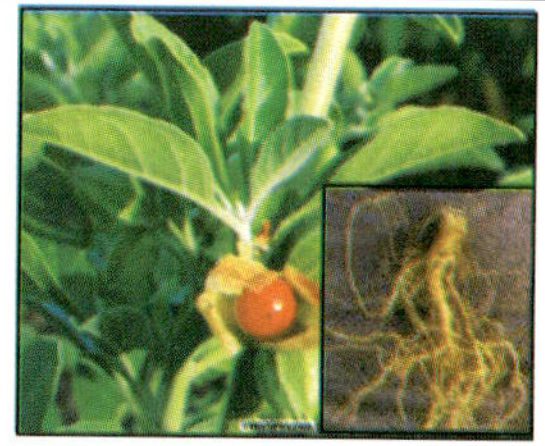	Increase sexual potency
8.	Giloy	*Tinospora cordifolia*	Stem	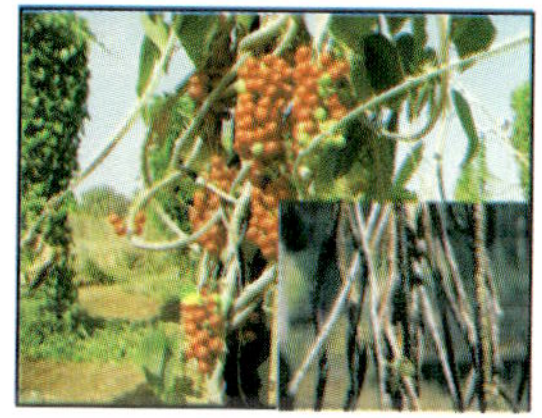	Increase sexual potency
9.	Flax	*Linum usitatissimum*	Seed	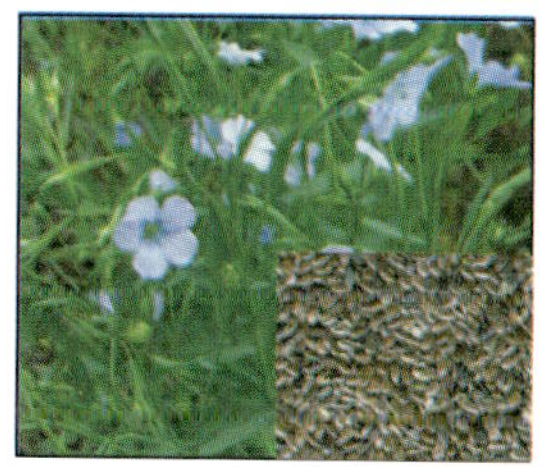	Increase sperm count and boost testosteron product

Contd...

Table 21.1–Contd...

Sl.No.	Plant Name	Botanical Name	Part Used	Picture	Effective in
10.	Kwao Krua Dang	*Butea superba*	Tuberous root	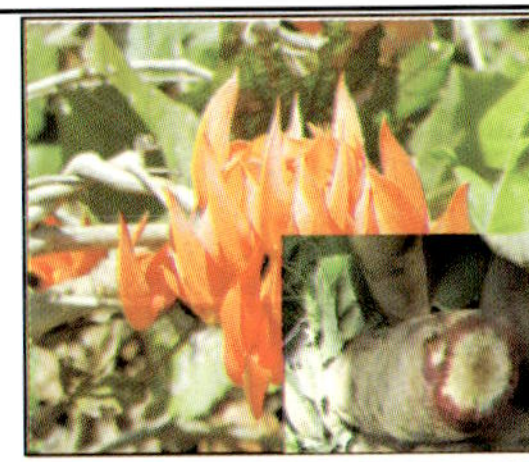	Aphrodisiac and for erectile dysfunction
11.	Bala	*Sida cordifolia*	Root	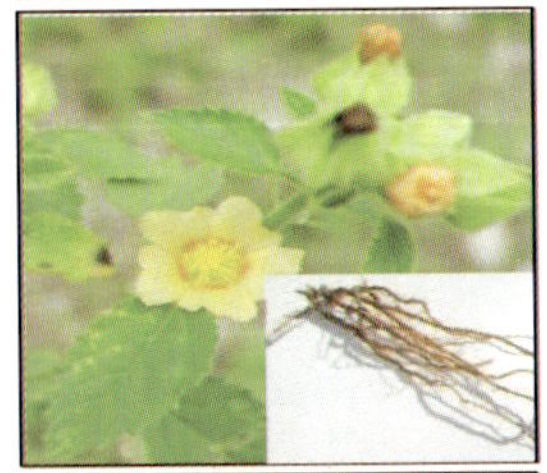	Promote spermatogenesis and fertility
12.	Safed Musli	*Cholorophytum* spp.	Root	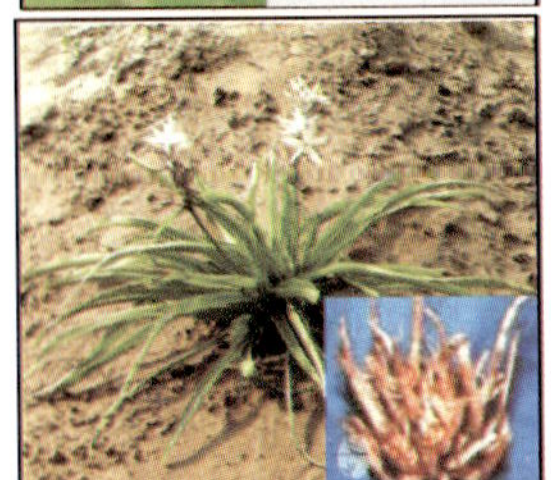	Aphrodisiac

- *Testicular trauma*: This condition causes damage to testes, impairing their ability to function.
- *Hemochromatosis*: It is a metabolic disorder that causes iron deposition in the testes.
- *Retrograde ejaculation*: It is an anatomical defect that involves the muscles and nerves of the bladder neck.
- *Systemic diseases*: In this condition high fever, infections, kidney diseases, or metabolic disorders can impair spermatogenesis.

The presence of anatomical defects or scar tissue formation, in the recovery process of the reproductive tract from infection is responsible for infertility in some men.

Effectivity of Herbs

There are a number of treatment options such as drug therapy, surgery and assisted reproductive therapy. While these treatments can be effective they are often costly and may have some serious side effects. For centuries, natural and holistic treatments have been used to cure infertility as well as overall male reproductive health. Herbal treatments are gentle enough to use, without the harsh side effects of allopathic medicine. Ayurveda can certainly help to get a deeper understanding of these complex issues and deal with them in a holistic manner with the use of herbs along with diet and lifestyle guidelines (Vishnu Das, 2007). Herbs that are most effective in treating male infertility generally help to raise testosterone levels, increase sexual desire, maintain erections longer and increase sperm count. Action of herbal remedies may vary from human to human and care should be observed in using it.

Nutritional Supplements that Helps to Improve Male Fertility

Optimizing fertility is one of the delicious arts of Ayurveda. There are certain foods like almonds, walnuts, pumpkin seeds milk, cream, ghee, seaweeds, roses, saffron, jasmine, flower pollen, dates, grapes and pomegranates etc. that have an affinity for the male reproductive system that anyone wanting to enhance their fertility should include in their diet. These are usually foods that have qualities of sweetness, nourishing and building.

The following supplements can help increase sperm count and mobility.

- *Arginine*: This non essential amino acid and is needed to produce healthy sperm. Natural production of arginine declines with age and a supplement here may help older patients. This is an amino acid that may affect both sperm count and motility. The heads of sperm contain large amounts and abnormal sperm counts often indicate a deficiency of arginine in the semen.
- *Coenzyme Q10*: Helps increase sperm count and motility. Co-enzyme Q10 is a vital catalyst in the conversion of food to energy within cells. In sperm cells it is concentrated in the mid piece where it is an energy promoter and antioxidant. Research is showing that it may be effective in improving fertilization rates.
- *Zinc*: Required for a healthy male reproductive system and sperm production. Zinc is a trace mineral, and perhaps one of the most well known nutrients important in male fertility. Zinc deficiency decreases both testosterone and sperm counts. It is highly concentrated in the seminal fluid and seminal plasma zinc concentration is significantly correlated with sperm density, motility and viability. However zinc supplementation needs to be carefully monitored because too high doses can impair immune function.
- *Vitamin B-12*: B-12 deficiency reduces sperm motility and sperm count and is one of the most frequent vitamin deficiencies so make sure your intake is adequate.
- *Ascorbic Acid (Vitamin C)*: Vitamin C is a water-soluble vitamin and its most important role in male fertility is the prevention of agglutination, when sperm clump together. This often happens when anti-bodies bind to sperm and can be a result of present or past genito-urinary infection. Vitamin C is also a powerful anti-oxidant and present in high levels in seminal fluid. Over heating and smoking easily destroy it.
- *Vitamin E*: Helps to improve the overall health of sperm. This is a fat-soluble vitamin and the main antioxidant in

sperm membranes. It works with selenium in its anti-oxidative capacity.

- *Omega fatty acids*: Omega 3 fatty acids (found in oily fish and flaxseed oils) and omega-6 fatty acids (evening primrose and starflower oils) can help improve the sperm membrane fluidity and male fertility (Tarkovsky, 2006).
- *Selenium*: This antioxidant mineral is vital for healthy sperm formation, particularly motility. It also protects against toxic metal contamination. Consumption of selenium in food is dependant on the amount in the soil where the food is grown, and it is believed that the soil is often highly depleted of this mineral, so supervised supplementation is especially recommended.

In addition, folic acid, the amino acid taurine and the anti-oxidant glutathione are all important for fertility.

Conclusion

Naturopathy is gaining a lot of popularity these days. It is no doubt the safest way to manage diseases and symptoms. Used individually or as a fertility blend, herbs can help to increase fertility significantly and with no side effects. Herbal remedies experiencing fertility problems seem to work best in both men and women with hormonal imbalances. It is very essential to have a proper documentation of medicinal plants and to know their potential for the improvement of health and hygiene through an eco friendly system. Thus importance should be given to the potentiality of ethno medicinal studies as these can provide a very effective strategy for the discovery of useful medicinally active identity. Recently, several important developments have been reported in scientific literature that may help improve male fertility. A detailed and systematic study is required for identification, cataloguing and documentation of herbal medicinal plants for enhancing male fertility which may provide a meaningful way for the promotion of the traditional knowledge of the herbal medicinal plants.

References

Anne, M. Jequier, 1991. *Male Infertility: A Guide for the Children*, p. 1.

Das, Vishnu, 2007. Ayurvedic herbs for male reproductive problems. *Journal of Health.*

Health Science Report. Error! Hyperlink reference not valid.

http://en.wikipedia.org/wiki/Male_infertility

http://upload.wikimedia.org/wikipedia/commons/a/a7/Starr_030612-0067_Tribulus_terrestris.jpg

http://www.bluelotusayurveda.com/male-herbs-art.html

http://www.hunts-osteopaths.co.uk/Resources/Male per cent 20fertility.pdf.

http://www.nativeremedies.com/ailment/natural-male-infertility-treatment.html

Kamal, R., Gupta, R.S. and Lohiya, N.K., 2003. Review Article-Plants for male fertility regulation. *Phytotherapy Research*, 17(6): 579-590.

Keshri Govind, Kumar Sudhir, Kulshreshtha Dinesh Kumar, Rajendran Siron Mani, Singh Man Mohan, 2008. Postcoital interceptive activity of *Wrightia tinctoria* in Sprague–Dawley rats: A preliminary study. *Elsevier-Contraception*. 78: 266–270.

Kidd, S.A., Eskenazi, B. and Wyrobek, A.J., 2001. Effects of male age on semen quality and fertility: A review of the literature. *Fertil. Steril*. 75(2): 237–248. doi:10.1016/S0015-0282(00)01679.

Male Fertility Supplement Proceptin: Male Infertility Supplement Successful in Enhancing Male Fertility and Healthy Sperm Counts. Jul 05, 2009. Global press release.

Ola-Mudathir, F. K., Suru, M. S., Fafunso, A.M., Obioha, E.U. and. Faremi, Y.T., 2008. Protective roles of onion and garlic extracts on cadmium-induced changes in sperm characteristics and testicular oxidative damage in rats. *Food and Chemical Toxicology*, 46(12): 3604-3611.

Patki, P.S., 1998. The role of indigenous drugs in the management of male sexual disorders. *Probe*, 28(1): 25-28.

Sherman, J. Silber, 1991. Effect of age on male fertility. In: *Seminars in Reproductive Endocrinology*.

Tarkovsky, Sacha, 2006. Male Fertility–11 Essential Supplements to Increase Male Fertility. EzineArticles.com.

Tremellen, K., 2008. Oxidative stress and male infertility–a clinical perspective. *Human Reproduction Update*, doi:10.1093/humupd/dmn004.

Zheng, Rong-Liang and Zhang, Hong, 1999. Effects of Ferulic Acid on Fertile and Asthenozoospermic Infertile Human Sperm Motility, Viability, Lipid Peroxidation, and Cyclic Nucleotides. *Elsevier*. doi:10.1016/S0891-5849(96)00272-9.

Chapter 22

Comparative Study on the Induced Spawning of *Clarias batrachus* Using Three Different Hormones Ovatide, Ovaprim and Pituitary Extract

Kavita Sharma, Meenakshi Jindal* and N.K. Yadava

Department of Zoology and Aquaculture,
CCS Haryana Agricultural University,
Hisar – 125 004, Haryana India

ABSTRACT

A comparative study of three hormones (Pituitary gland extract, Ovaprim and Ovatide), with three different doses were tried on the breeding performance of Indian magur, *Clarias batrachus*. In case of Pituitary gland (PG) extract, three different doses were tried at the dose level of 25, 30 and 35 mg/kg body weight of female brood fish, whereas, in case of ovaprim and ovatide the three different doses were tried at the dose level of 0.6, 0.8 and 1.0 ml/kg body weight of female brood fish. When all the three best doses of three hormones were compared, the overall results for spawning, net fecundity, fertilization and hatching have shown that ovatide when used at the dose level of 1.0ml/kg body weight, then, the spawning percentage was 81.97, fecundity was 4919 eggs, total fertilization percentage

* Corresponding author: E-mail: meenjind@gmail.com

was 82.33, hatching percentage was 55.35 and the net survival of fry 98.52 per cent, followed by the ovaprim (at the dose level of 1.0ml/kg body weight), with spawning percentage was 76.91, fecundity was 4711 eggs, total fertilization was 78.37 per cent, hatching percentage was 55.68 and net survival of fry was 97.31 per cent, followed by the PG extract (35mg/kg body weight), the spawning percentage was 67.77, fecundity was 4326 eggs, total fertilization percentage was 40.82, hatching percentage 30.38 and net survival of fry 95.75 per cent. The water quality parameters were also analysed which were found within the optimal range. The survival rate of fry was found to be independent of the types of hormones used and the rate of various doses which concluded that the better survival of fry/seed population was depending on the excellent management practices. Thus, the comparative study recommended the use of ovatide at the dose level of 1 ml/kg body weight followed by ovaprim at the dose level of 1ml/kg body wt. followed by PG extract at the dose level of 35 mg/kg body wt. for better breeding performance of catfish *C. batrachus*.

Keywords: *Breeding, Clarias batrachus, Pituitary gland extract, Ovaprim and Ovatide.*

Introduction

In recent years, culture of catfishes such as singhi (*H. fossilis*), magur (*C. batrachus*) *etc.* has received increased interest, due to their high market price and hardy nature. Among all these catfishes magur got high attention as it is a hardy fish which can thrive where many other fish struggle to survive. In addition to lakes and rivers, they can be found in brackish waters or warm stagnant, often hypoxic water such as muddy pond, canals, ditches, swamps and flooded priories. They can remain dormant through periods of drought and go several months without eating. Due to this reason this fish become an attractive food fish for human being and can easily handled for trade in live condition. It can tolerate a wide range of temperature.

Regarding food and feeding habits, basically, magur is carnivorous, but, occasionally eat plant material. Magur is voracious opportunistic feeder which is mainly active at night. It can consume a wide variety of prey including eggs and larvae of other fishes, small fishes and a number of invertebrates, including, crustacean and insects and sometimes plant material. In densely populated drying ponds, these fish become even more indiscrimmable and quickly consume most other species of fishes present in the pond. It gets easily trained to feed on artificial feeds, such as, trash fish and fish meal mixed with rice bran. Low grade marine trash fish and rice bran, when given as feed bring about profitable conversion with appreciable growth (Thakur, 1991). Males and females are easily distinguished particularly around April. Egg-bearing females are identified by their big, soft and distended belly with swollen and reddish pink vent. Males could easily be identified by their reddish genital opening and oozing of milt, when the abdomen is pressed.

Artificial propagation of fishes is done by induced breeding technique. The natural source provides a negligible amount of fish seed because of higher mortality rate, mixture of cultivable and non cultivable species and shrinkage of spawning ground which impede the extension and expansion of fish culture. After the first attempt of induced spawning in early thirties this technique had been successfully tried in many countries of the world.

Hormones for induced spawning of fish has been in use for almost 60 years. Our biologists have worked for 20 years to develop artificial breeding methods. Hormone in addition to breeding, can be used to produce hybrids, that are different from the parent species, produce sterile polyploidy fish, synchronize reproduction of large numbers of fish for simultaneous spawning, thereby, simplifying production and marketing of the fish, maximize survival of fry under controlled hatchery conditions.

Although, hypophysation is a simple practical technique, but, suffers from the disadvantage that often gonadotropic potency of pituitary glands used, is unknown and difficult to standardize. Because of the above mentioned drawbacks, several fish farmers breed only common carp which does not require pituitary hormone treatment for breeding under tropical conditions.

Dehadrai (1984) reported that only about 15 per cent of the existing carp seed farms use the hypophysation technique for carps breeding. So there was need to develop alternative method to hypophysation technique of induced breeding.

Hence alternative sources *viz.* HCG, human chorionic gonadotropin (Mollah and Tan, 1983; Inyang and Heltiarchchi, 1994)

Leuitinizing releasing hormone (Billard *et al.*, 1984; Dee leeuw *et al.*, 1985 and Ovaprim (Alok *et al.*, 1993; Francis, 1996; Haniffa *et al.*, 1996) have been attempted in air breathing fishes.

The use of synthetic inducing agent for successful ovulation followed by stripping on catfish is of common practice and reported by numerous workers (Banerji, 1974; Dee leeuw *et al.*, 1985; Legendre, 1986; Manickam and Joy, 1989; Tan fermin *et al.*, 1997; Gupta *et al.*, 2002; Sahoo *et al.*, 2003; Sahoo *et al.*, 2004; Sahu *et al.*, 2005). The ever increasing cost of donar pituitary and the cumbersome process, obliged the experts to test alternative hormones, such as, LHRH analogues, ovaprim, ovatide, HCG, wova-fh and ovopel.

The commercially available synthetic inducing hormones in readymade form containing GnRH and dopamine blocker receptor (Ovaprim, Ovopel, Dagin and Aquaspawn) are becoming very popular and found to be efficient in successful spawning of fishes (Peter *et al.*, 1988; Nandeesha, 1990; Brzuska and Adamek, 1999; Cheah and Lee, 2000).

The aim of the present studies is to breed *C. batrachus*, under artificial conditions, by using different hormones *viz.* Pituitary extract (PG), Ovaprim and Ovatide and also to assess their efficiencies, concerns latency period, fecundity, fertilization rate, hatching and survival.

Materials and Methods

The induced breeding was carried out at the Magur hatchery of the Central Institute of freshwater Education (CIFE) at Lahli Centre Rohtak, Haryana, India (Plate 22.1). Brooders were collected from Gazipur fish market, Delhi prior to the breeding season (May-August). During the breeding season both male and female were collected from the brooder's pond and were kept separately in plastic tubs. The fish were fed at 2 per cent body weight daily in the evening hour (17:00h) with supplementary feed containing 40 per cent crude protein. During the breeding season both males and females were collected from the brood stock pond for breeding operation. The males were selected on the basis of pointed and reddish genital papilla, while females by a round and reddish papilla (Plate 22.2).

Three hormones ovaprim, ovatide and PG extract were tried and given in three different doses (Plate 22.3). The treatments were given in following pattern:

Name of the hormone	Various Doses Used per kg of the Female Brood Fish		
PG extract (mg)	25	30	35
Ovaprim (ml)	0.6	0.8	1.0
Ovatide (ml)	0.6	0.8	1.0

Ovaprim and ovatide were synthetic hormones available in the form of prepared solution. Ovaprim is a synthetic drug manufactured by M/s Syndel Laboratories Ltd., Canada, containing 20 µg sGnRH (salmon gonadotropin releasing hormone) and 10 mg domperidone in 1 ml solution. Ovatide is a mixture of a sGnRH-A and domperidone. It came in market in the year 1998-99. This is an outcome of a collaborative research effort of Central Institute of Fisheries Education and M/s Hemmo Pharma, Mumbai.

The males and females were kept separately. Injections were administered intramuscularly, in the dorso-lateral region of the female body of female brood fish (Plate 22.4). This enabled the researchers to find out the optimum dose, required for optimum spawning of the fish. Before injection, individual female body weight was recorded and marked with coloured chips tied to their dorsal fin to study individual breeding performance and egg quality (Table 22.1). The testes were removed from male fish, incised and squeezed to get sperm. The sperms were pooled and diluted with 3 ml of physiological saline to prepare a sperm suspension. Before stripping, individual weight of females was recorded. At the end of the desired latency period of 19h, the females were stripped individually into dry and preweighed petri plates to record the stripped egg weight. Egg were weighed and mixed with 4-5 drops of sperm suspension. After thorough washing with water, they were released into the round plastic tub of 5 l capacity provided with flow-through water system for 2-3 min. (Plate 22.5). After three hours of incubation, the fertilised eggs were counted (Plate 22.6). The translucent eggs containing embryonic eyes were considered fertilised. Unfertilized eggs were removed immediately from the tray to avoid the fouling of water.

Results and Discussion

For pituitary extract, in general, a dose of 15 to 25 mg/kg body weight was found effective for successful breeding. The dose of

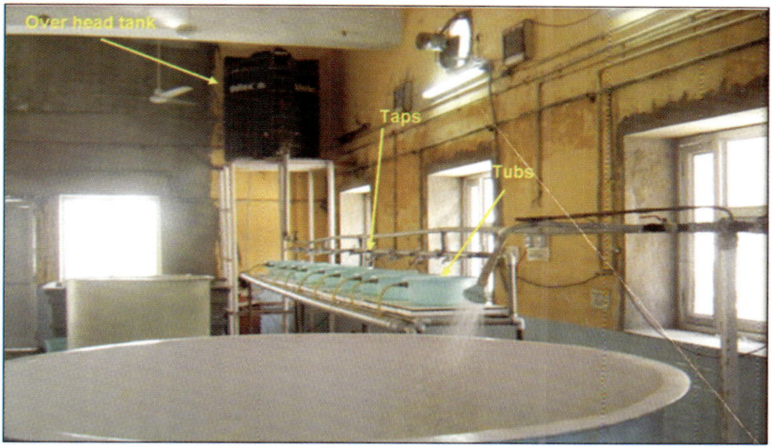

Plate 22.1: Showing a View of Magur Hatchery at (CIFE) Lahli, Rohtak where the Experiments on Induced Breeding of Magur, *Clarias batrachus* were Conducted

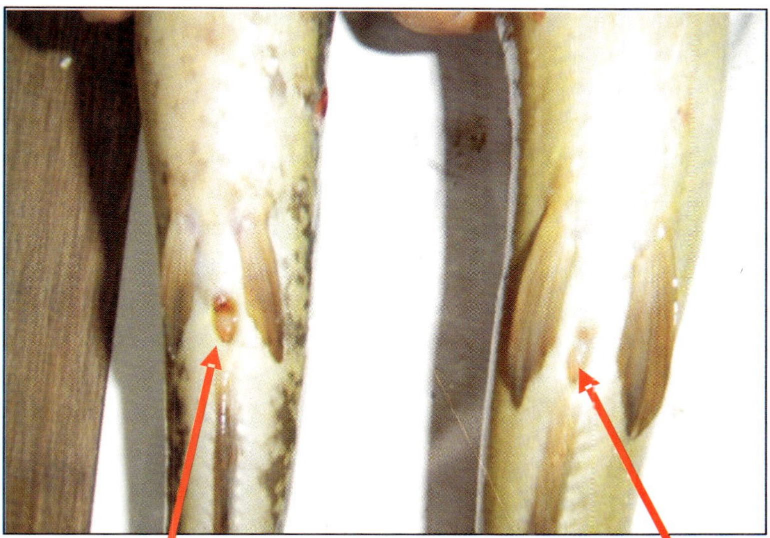

Plate 22.2: Genital papilla of Male and Female Brood fish of *Clarias batrachus*

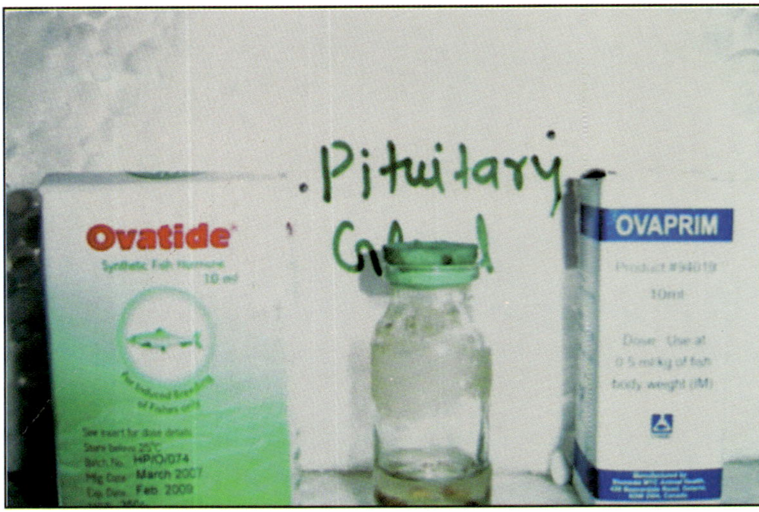

Plate 22.3: Showing Photograph of Various Hormones Used for Induced Breeding of Magur *Clarias batrachus*

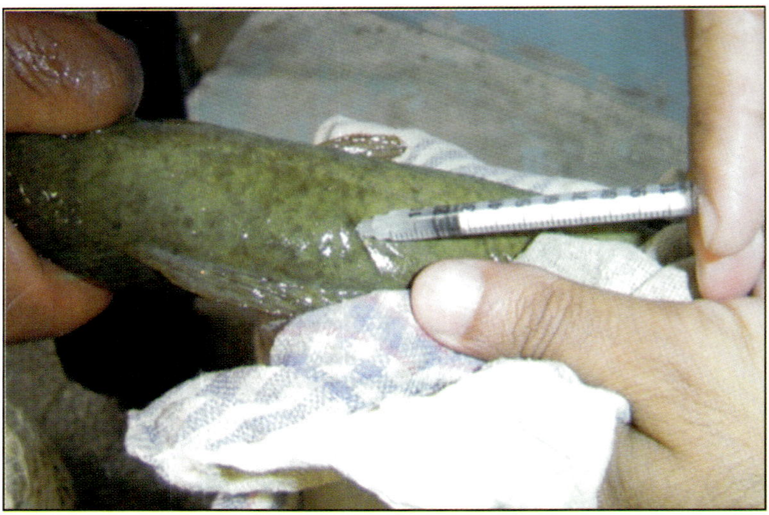

Plate 22.4: Showing Intramuscular Injection Given to Female Brood Fish of Magur *Clarias batrachus* for Induced Breeding

course, is much higher in comparison to major carps which ranges from 2-8 mg/kg body weight and 3-10 mg/kg body weight for the exotic carps. Catfish, in general, requires a higher dose for successful

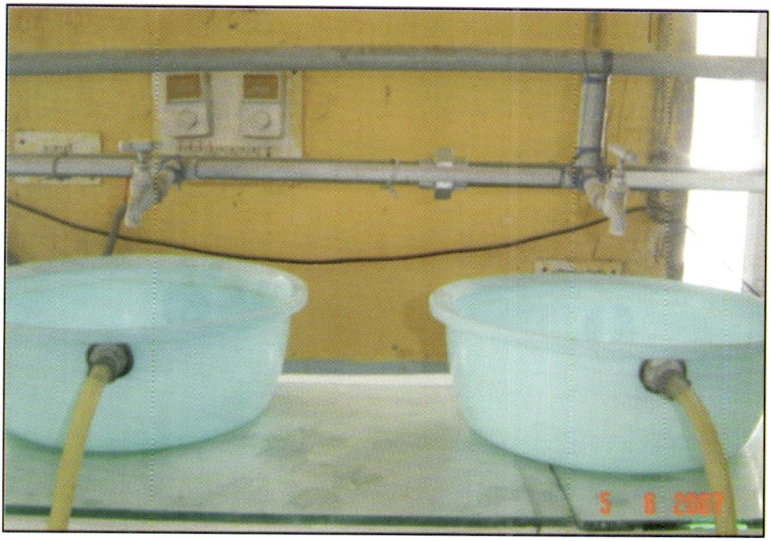

Plate 22.5: Showing Close View of Flow Through System of Magur Hatchery for the Incubation of Fertilized Eggs

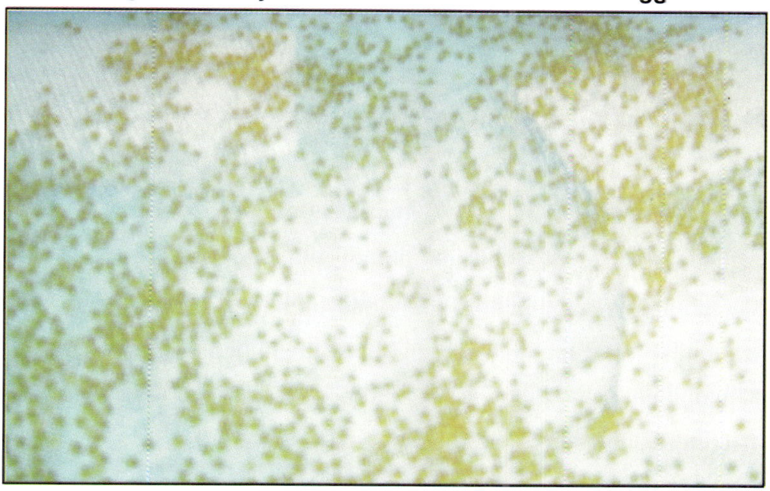

Plate 22.6: Showing Fertilized Eggs of Magur *Clarias batrachus* at Magur Hatchery

breeding. It may be mentioned that carp pituitary extract used for successful breeding of *H. fossilis* is 15-20 mg/kg body weight. Basu *et al.* (2000) reported 5 mg/kg body weight for female and 30 mg/kg

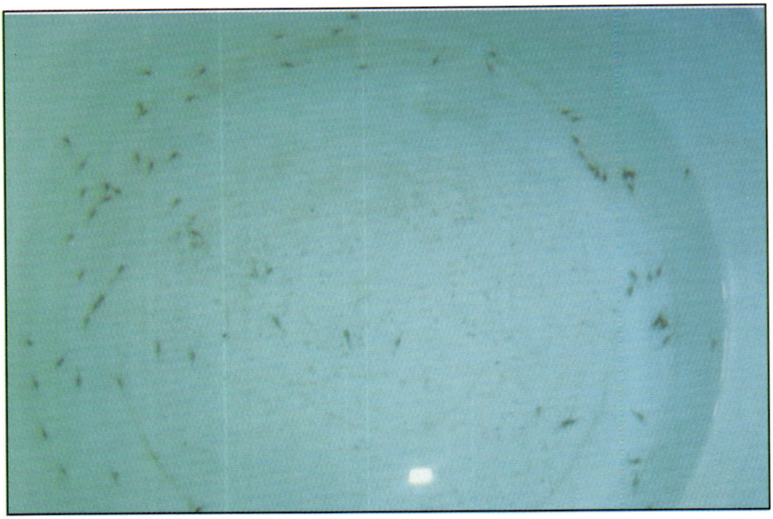

Plate 22.7: Showing Hatchlings (4 days old) of Magur, *Clarias batrachus* at Magur Hatchery

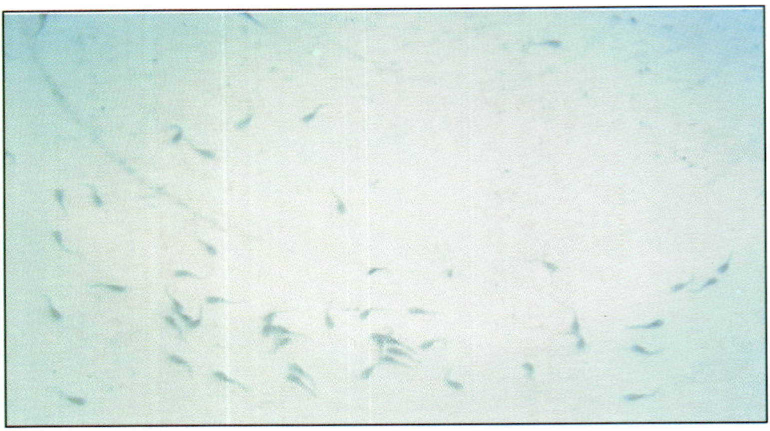

Plate 22.8: Showing Fry (7 days old) of Magur *Clarias batrachus* at Magur Hatchery

body weight for male *Clarias batrachus*. In the present study a dose of 35mg/kg found to be most effective as compared to 25 and 30 mg/kg.

Comparative efficacy of ovaprim and ovatide used for the induced breeding of revealed the *C. batrachus* effectiveness of ovtide over ovaprim. During the study it was observed that highest egg output was found in case of ovatideat the dose level of 1.00ml/kg body weight (17.12g) followed by ovaprim at the dose level of 1.00ml/ kg body weight (15.66g) and PG extract at the dose level of 35mg/kg body weight (12.68g). The observed spawning was also found to highest for the ovatide (81.97 per cent) followed by ovaprim and Pituitary extract (Table 22.1; Figure 22.1).

Haniffa *et al.* (1996) studied the spawning of the *Channa striatus* using Pituitary extract, HCG, LHRHa and Ovaprim. Result shown that in comparison to LHRHa and ovaprim the latency period was long in Pituitary (24 h) and HCG injected (26h) fish. The percentage of fertilization was lowest in the Pituitary injected *Channa striatus* while the duration of hatching was longest followed by HCG, LHRHa and Ovaprim. Overall result of fertilization, hatching and survivality show that the Ovaprim resulted better. Haniffa and Sridhar (2002) studied the induced spawning of spotted murrel, *Channa punctatus* and catfish *H. fossilis* using HCG and ovaprim. Brooder were administered a single intramuscular injection of the hormones at varying dosage. Dhawan and Kaur (2004) studied the comparative efficacy of ovaprim and ovatide used for the induced breeding of Indian major carps. The study revealed the effectiveness of ovaprim over ovatide for the breeding of *Catla catla*. However for *Labeo rohita* and *Cirrihinus mrigala* ovatide resulted better.

As far as latency period, incubation period and survival percentage of the hatchlings concerned, they were found to be independent of the different doses three different hormones applied during the induced breeding of *C. batrachus.*

For all the three hormones, Net fecundity was also found to be highest for ovatide (4919) followed by ovaprim (4,711) and PG extract (4,326) as in Table 22.1 (Figure 22.2). The doses of different hormones were significantly affected the fertilization of eggs in *C. batrachus* (Das,2004; Dhawan and Kaur, 2004; Sahoo *et al.*, 2004). The maximum number of eggs were found to be fertilized with ovatide at the dose level of 1ml/kg of body weight of the female (82.33 per cent) followed by ovaprim at the dose level of 1.00 ml/kg body weight (78.37 per cent) and PG extract at the dose level of 35mg/kg body weight (40.82 per cent) (Table 22.2). During the observations a comparison was made between different doses of different hormones in relation to total fertilized and unfertilized eggs percentage of magur, *C. batrachus* as shown through (Figure 22.3).

Table 22.1: Comparative Influence of Different Doses of Hormones Used for Induced Spawning of *Clarias batrachus*

Name of Hormone	*Doses Used/ kg Body Wt. of Female Brooder*	*Wt. of Female Brood Fish (g)*	*Latency Period (hr.)*	*Net Wt. of Stripped Eggs (g)*	*Observed Spawning (per cent)*	*Net Fecundity (No. of eggs)*
Pituitary	25.00	202.33 ± 8.82	21.00	10.34 ± 0.06	51.06 ± 0.58	3,627 ± 16
extract (mg)	30.00	200.00 ± 1.15	20.50	10.88 ± 0.07	57.87 ± 2.22	3,847 ± 40
	35.00	209.00 ± 2.08	21.00	12.68 ± 0.18	67.77 ± 0.54	4,326 ± 30
Ovaprim (ml)	0.60	198.00 ± 1.73	18.14	13.57 ± 0.33	69.40 ± 0.41	4,318 ± 17
	0.80	199.00 ± 2.08	17.50	14.09 ± 0.41	73.29 ± 0.45	4,565 ± 30
	1.00	198 ± 1.73	18.50	15.66 ± 0.30	76.91 ± 1.15	4,711 ± 5
Ovatide (ml)	0.60	207.66 ± 1.85	20.25	14.78 ± 0.18	76.52 ± 0.35	4,788 ± 40
	0.80	213.00 ± 2.64	19.00	16.81 ± 0.19	79.74 ± 0.43	4,644 ± 71
	1.00	201.00 ± 2.08	19.50	17.12 ± 0.46	81.97 ± 0.19	4,919 ± 50

Each value is a mean value of three replicates ± standard error.

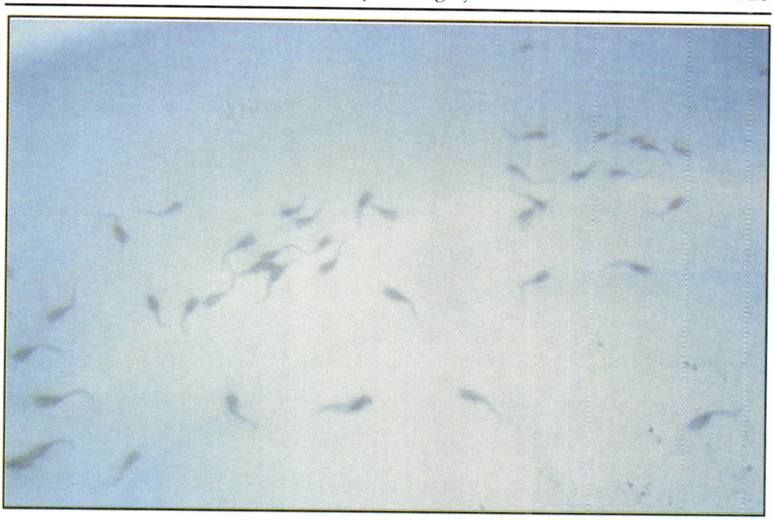

Plate 22.9: Showing Fry (15 days old) of Magur *Clarias batrachus* at Magur Hatchery

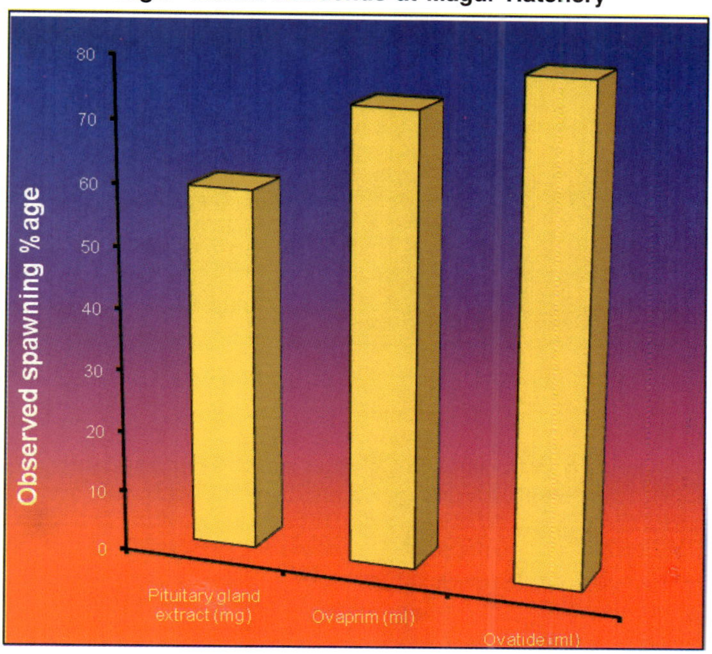

Figure 22.1: Showing a Comparison between Different Hormones in Relation to Observed Spawning in Magur, *Clarias batrachus*

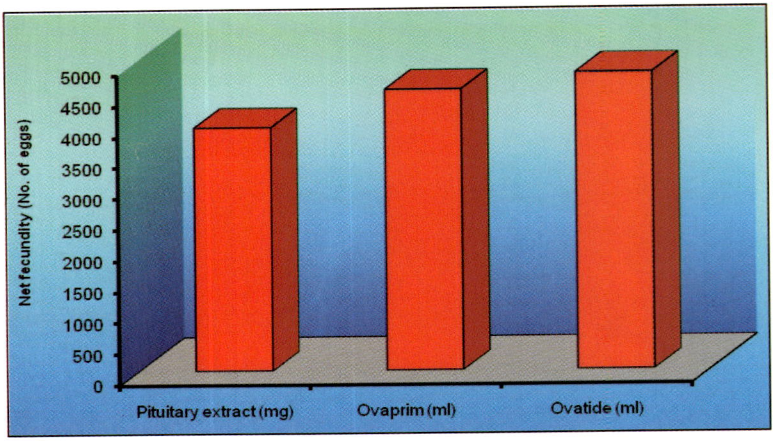

Figure 22.2: Showing a Comparison between Different Hormones in Relation to Net Fecundity of Magur, *Clarias batrachus*

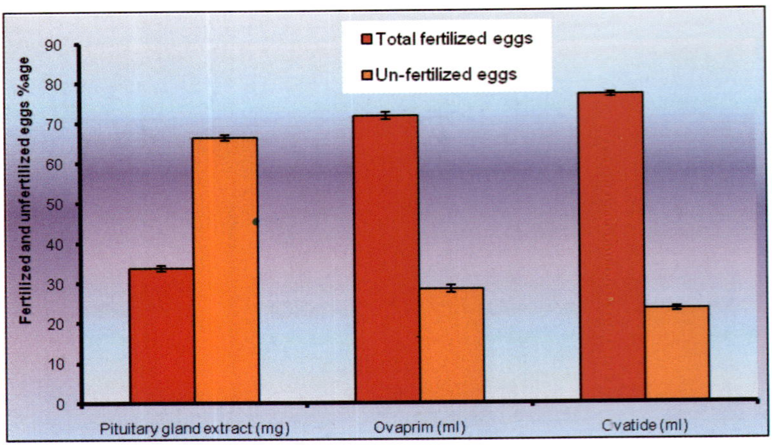

Figure 22.3: Showing a Comparison Between Different Doses of Hormones in Relation to Total Fertilized and Unfertilized Eggs of Magur, *Clarias batrachus*

When all the three doses of three hormones compared the overall results for spawning, egg output, net fecundity fertilization and hatching showed that ovatide at the dose level of 1.C0ml/kg body weight gave best results followed by ovaprim at the dose level of 1.0 ml/kg body weight and PG extract at the dose level of 35mg/kg body weight.

Table 22.2: Comparative Influence of Different Doses of Hormones Used for Induced Spawning of *Clarias batrachus*

Name of Hormone	Doses at the Dose Level of/ kg Body Weight	Wt. of Female Brood Fish (gm)	Total Fertilized Eggs (per cent)	Total Unfertilized Eggs (per cent)	Incubation Period Observed (hr.)	Hatching Success of Fertilized Eggs (per cent)	Survival of Fry upto 15th Day (Adv. Fry stage) (per cent)
Pituitary	25.00	202.33 ± 8.82	26.15 ± 0.55	73.85 ± 0.55	42.00	18.43 ± 0.29	90.31 ± 1.18
extract (mg)	30.00	200.00 ± 1.15	34.20 ± 0.59	65.79 ± 0.59	44.50	25.73 ± 1.66	93.45 ± 0.08
	35.00	209.00 ± 2.08	40.82 ± 0.82	59.17 ± 0.82	45.50	30.38 ± 0.43	95.75 ± 0.29
Ovaprim (ml))	0.60	198.00 ± 1.73	64.79 ± 1.81	35.20 ± 1.81	43.00	45.33 ± 1.06	96.83 ± 0.28
	0.80	199.00 ± 2.08	71.55 ± 057	28.45 ± 0.57	42.75	52.75 ± 0.45	95.87 ± 0.47
	1.00	198 ± 1.73	78.37 ± 0.35	21.63 ± 0.35	40.25	55.68 ± 0.38	97.31 ± 0.36
Ovatide (ml)	0.60	207.66 ± 1.85	67.70 ± 0.51	32.30 ± 0.51	42.50	47.91 ± 0.28	96.00 ± 1.01
	0.80	213.00 ± 2.64	80.22 ± 0.45	19.77 ± 0.45	46.00	52.90 ± 1.28	96.81 ± 0.32
	1.00	201.00 ± 2.08	82.33 ± 0.80	17.67 ± 0.80	44.50	55.35 ± 1.54	98.52 ± 1.46

Each value is a mean value of three replicates ± standard error.

The reasons for better performance of ovatide followed by ovaprim and PG extract was due to the poor quality of pituitary glands supplied by the various firms. In addition to this aspect, the difference in the mode of action between PG extract, ovaprim and ovatide hormones are also appears to be responsible for comparatively better results than pituitary extract. During the present studies it was also concluded that the hormones ovaprim and ovatide are known to act at pituitary level leading to the secretion of endogenous gondotropins while in case of hypophysation technique, exogenous gonadotropins introduced into the body of the female brood fish. The above findings were also supported by Habibi *et al.* (1989).

During the present study 30-36 hours of fertilization, twitching movements in the fertilized eggs were started and after about 40-45 hours, hatching took place (Plate 22.7). The yolk sac in the hatchlings was absorbed after 4 days of hatching. The young fry start feeding before the yolk sac is finally absorbed.

From, 4th day onwards, the hatchlings start feeding, during the present studies, the feeding was carried out with artemia (live zooplankton cultured under laboratory conditions) three times a day (Plates 22.8 and 22.9).

Table 22.3: Physicochemical Parameters of Hatchery Shed Water during the Induced Breeding Period at Lahli, Rohtak (June, 2007)

Sl.No.	Parameters	Range
1.	Temperature(°C)	28-30
2.	Dissolved oxygen (mg/l)	5.53-6.10
3.	pH	7.4-7.6
4.	Alkalinity (mg/l)	227-245
5.	Total hardness (mg/l)	189-195
6.	Free CO_2 (ppm)	1-1.5
7.	Electrical conductivity (m mhos/cm)	0.50

Physicochemical Parameters

Physicochemical parameters of hatchery shed pond water were calculated as water temperature, 28-30°C; pH ranged between 7.4-7.6, Dissolved oxygen(DO)was ranged between 5.53-6.10mg/l, alkalinity ranged between 227-245 mg/l, total hardness ranged between 189-195 mg/l, free carbon dioxide ranged between 1-1.5ppm and Electrical conductivity ranged between 0.50mhos/cm as given in Table 22.3.

Conclusions

The present experiments proved that seed production in *C. batrachus* by adopting induced breeding method can be done successfully provided some preconditions are fulfilled appropriately. In the present work pituitary extract, ovaprim and ovatide have been used for induced breeding of *C. batrachus* and it was found that the ovatide was the best among all the three hormones used for spawning in the above fish. It was also observed during the present studies that PG extract gave best performance at 35mg/kg of body wt. of the female brood fish, where as ovaprim and ovatide indicated best potency for spawning at 1.0ml/kg body wt. of the female brood fish. It is already established that larval rearing is the most critical stage in seed raising. Food selectivity is a major factor here particularly in the artificial environment where they find no option of selecting food, as they can resort to in natural environment. Cases of mortality due to overfeeding and dropsy are much higher at this stage. Mortality rate gradually decreases as the larvae grow. Mortality is almost negligible in the advanced larvae/juvenile stages. So far as inducing agent is concerned, Ovatide has given a better result and more number of eggs could be stripped out easily and fertilization result was also very good. Therefore further work is needed to standardize larval rearing success/farming potentiality.

Acknowledgements

The authors acknowledge Dr. U.K Mahaeshwari, Dr. N.K Chadda and Dr. Ashok Kumar of CIFE centre of Lahli (Rohtak) for their sincere co-operation and help in conducting the breeding experiments of *C. batrachus* and for providing necessary experimental facilities at their centre and also for their valuable guidance whenever required.

References

Alok, D., Krishnan, T., Talwar, G.P. and Garg, L.C., 1993. Induced Spawning of catfish *Heteropneustes fossilis* (Bloch), using D-Lys super (6) salmon gonadotropin releasing hormone analogue. *Aquaculture*, 115: 159-167.

Banerji, S.R., 1974. Hypophysation and life history of *Channa punctatus* (Bloch). *J. Inland Fish. Soc. India*, 6. 62-73.

Basu, D., Rana, G.C., Mondal, B.K., Sengupta, K.K. and Dhar, P.K., 2000. Studies on the comparative efficacy of Ovaprim, HCG and piscine pituitary gland in induced breeding of *Clarias batrachus*,(Linn). *Fishing Chimes*, 19(10–11): 103-104.

Billard, R., Reinaud, P., Hollebecq, M.G. and Breton, B., 1984. Advancement and Synchronization of spawning in *Salmo gairdneri* and *Sital trutta* following administration of LHRHa Combined or not with pimozide. *Aquaculture*, 43: 57-66.

Brzuska, E. and Adamek, J., 1999. Artificial spawning of European catfish, *Silurus glanis*: Stimulation of ovulation using LHRHa, ovaprim and carp pituitary extract. *Aquaculture Research*, 3(1): 59.

Cheah, S.H. and Lee, C.L., 2000. Induced ovulation of the Australian eel-tailed catfish *Neosilurus ater* (Perugia) with Ovaprim. *Asian Fisheries Science*, 13: 87-96.

Das,S.K., 2004. Evaluation of a New spawning agent ovopel in induced breeding of Indian carps. *Asian Fisheries Science*, 17: 313-322.

Dehadrai, P.V., 1984. Carp seed production in India. In: *Summery Report of the Asian Regional Workshop on Carp Hatchery and Nursery Technology*, (Eds.) R.C. May, R.S.V. Pullin and V.G. Jhingran. Asian Development Bank and International Center for Living Aquatic Resources, Manila, Philippines, p. 33.

Deleeuw, R. Goods. H.J.T., Richter, C.J.J. and Edind, E.H., 1985. Pimozide-LHRHa induced breeding in the African Catfish, *Clarias gariepinus* (Burchell). *Aquaculture*, 44: 299-302.

Dhawan, A. and Kaur, K., 2004. Comparative efficacy of ovaprim and ovatide in carp breeding. *Indian Journal of Fisheries*, 51(2): 227-228.

Francis, T., 1996. Studies on the effect of pituitary hormone and feeds on the reproduction of *Heteropneustes fossilis*. *Ph.D. Thesis*. Tamil Nadu Veterinary and Animal Science University, Madras, India.

Gupta, S. D. Mohapatra, B. C. Sahoo, S. K. and Verma, D. K., 2002. Breeding response of rohu, *Labeo rohita* induced with different inducing agents. In: The Sixth Indian Fisheries Forum, Asian Fisheries Society (Indian Branch) and Indian Fisheries Association (CIFE), Mumbai. 17-20 December 2002.

Habibi, H.R., Marchant, T.A., Nahornaik, C.S., Van Der Loo, H., Peter, Haniffa, M.A., Merlin Rose,T., Francis,T., 2000. Induced spawning of the stripped murrel *Channa striatus* using pituitary extracts, human chorionic gonadotropin, LHRHa hormone releasing hormone analogue, and ovaprim. *Acta Icthylogica et pisctoria,* 30 (1): 53-60.

Haniffa M.A., Shaik Mohamed, J., Merlinrose,J., 1996. Induction of ovulation in *Channa striatus* (Bloch) by SGnRH. *Fishing chimes,* 23-24.

Haniffa, M.A. and Sridhar, S., 2002. Induced spawning of sppoted murrel (*Channa punctatus*) and catfish (*Heteropneustes fossilis*) using human chorionic gonadotropin and synthetic hormone (ovaprim). *Veterinarsiki Arhiv.,* 72(1), 51-56.

Inyang, N.M. and Heltiarachchi, M., 1994. Efficacy of human chorionic gonadoropin (HCG) and crude extract of fish and frog in oocyte oraturation and ovulations in African catfish *Clarias gariepinus* Burchell. *Aqua. Fish. Mang.,* 25: 245-258.

Legendre, M., 1986. Seasonal changes in sexual maturity and fecundity and HCG Induced breeding of the catfish *Heterobranchus longifilus* Vd. (Flarriclae) reared in Elorie Lagoon (Ivory Coast). *Aquaculture,* 83: 193-199.

Manickam, P. and Joy, K.P., 1989. Induction of maturation and ovulation by pimozide–LHRH analogue treatment and resulting high quality egg production in the Asian catfish, *Clarias batrachus* (Linn.). *Aquaculture,* 83:193-199.

Mollah, M.F.A. and Tan, E.S.P., 1983. HCG-Induced spawning of the catfish, *Clarias macrocephalus* Gunther. *Aquaculture,* 35(3): 239-247.

Nandeesha, M.C., Rao, K.G., Jayanna, R.N., Parker, N.C., Verghese, T.J., Keshavanath, P. and Shetty, H.P.C., 1990. Induced spawning of Indian major carps through single application of Ovaprim-C. *The Second Asian Fisheries Forum, Tokyo, Japan,* pp. 581-586.

Peter, R. E., Lin, H.R. and Van der Kraak, G., 1988. Induced ovulation and spawning of cultured freshwater fish in China: Advances in application of GnRH analogues and dopamine antagonists. *Aquaculture*, 74:1-10.

Sahoo, S.K., Giri, S.S. and Sahu, A.K., 2004. Induced breeding of *Clarias batrachus* (Linn.): effect of different doses of Ovatide on breeding performance and egg quality. In: *National Seminar on Responsible Fisheries and Aquaculture*, Orissa, India. 12-13 February, pp. 2.

Sahoo, S.K., Giri, S.S., Sahu, A.K. and Ayyappan, S., 2003. Experimental hybridization between catfish *Clarias batrachus* (Linn.) X *Clarias gariepinus* (Bur.) and performance of the offspring in rearing operation. *Asian Fisheries Science*, 16 (In press).

Sahu, A.K., 2005. *Manual on Breeding and Culture of Clarias batrachus (Magur)*. Central Institute of Freshwater Aquaculture. (Indian Council of Agricultural Research) Kausalyaganga, Bhubaneswar, Orissa, India. 33 pp.

Tan-Fermin, J.D., Pagador, R.R. and Chavez, R.C., 1997. LHRHa and pimozide-induced spawning of Asian catfish *Clarias macrocephalus* (Gunther) at different times during an annual reproductive cycle. *Aquaculture*, 148: 323-331.

Thakur, N.K., 1991. Possibilities and problems of catfish culture in India. *J. Inland Fish. Soc. India*, 232: 80-90.

Chapter 23

Reproductive Potential of Freshwater Fish in Fluoride Contaminated Water

*Anand Kumar, Sandeep Bajpai, Nalini Tripathi and Madhu Tripathi**

Aquatic Toxicology Research Laboratory, Department of Zoology, University of Lucknow, Lucknow – 226 007, U.P., India

ABSTRACT

In the present study an attempt was made to assess the impact of fluoride contaminated water on reproduction in freshwater catfish, *Clarias batrachus*. The fishes were exposed to different sub-lethal concentrations (35 mg F/L and 70 mg F/L) of fluoride for a period of 90 days. Various morphometric indices such as average body weight, length, liver weight, gonad weight, hepatosomatic index (HSI), gonadosomatic index (GSI), Condition factor (CF) and Somatic condition factor (SCF) were observed after 90 days of exposure. There was significant decrease in body weight, liver weight, gonad weight, HSI and GSI whereas an insignificant increase in CF and SCF after 90 days of fluoride exposure was also recorded. Insignificant decrease in body length of fish was also observed after exposure to different concentrations. The alterations induced

* Corresponding author: E-mail: drmtripathi@gmail.com

by fluoride were found to be concentration and duration dependent. These findings thus indicate that fluoride is able to induce reproductive toxicity in fishes.

Keywords: Clarias batrachus, Fluoride toxicity, Morphometric indices, Reproductive potential, Walking catfish.

Introduction

Water is the key element in socio-economic development of Nation. It cannot be created through what ever technical advancements we made but at the same time, it is the natural resource which gets polluted easily. Water bodies serve as reservoir for man made pollutions and often contains biological or chemical agents, detrimental to health. Anthropogenic degradation of water quality has created a lot of stress to the aquatic environment and thereby posing a threat to the existence of several species of organisms including fishes (Camargo, 2003). Toxicants initially exert their impact at cellular and sub cellular level, prior to any gross damages in the morphology and behaviour of fish (Masud *et al.*, 2001; Samanta *et al.*, 2005). Fluoride is also one of such toxicant, and it is getting its way into water resources due to both natural as well as anthropogenic activities. Its level is increasing in ground water as well as surface water. It tends to accumulate in the bones and various soft tissues of fishes (Kaur and Singh, 1980; Shashi and Singh, 1987). Fluoride ions act as 'enzymatic poisons' inhibits enzyme activity and ultimately interrupts metabolic processes such as glycolysis and synthesis of proteins. There are reports that fluoride interferes with various biological activities such as growth, reproduction, survival etc (Chinoy, 1991; ATSDR, 2001; Camarago, 2003; Bajpai *et al.*, 2010).

Most of the experimental work regarding fluoride toxicity has been carried out on human beings and other mammalian models such as rats, rabbits, guinea pigs etc, which indicate that fluoride interferes with the reproduction (Arabi *et al.*, 1989; Chinoy and Sequeira, 1992; Chinoy and Patel, 2001; Sharma *et al.*, 2007) but a very few reports are available in fishes regarding the effect of fluoride on reproduction inspite of their great nutritive and economic value. It is well known that presence of xenobiotics in water affects sex differentiation as well as other reproductive stages and activities in fishes (Jalabert *et al.*, 2000).

The present study has been planned to observe the adverse effect of fluoride on reproduction in fishes. This study is useful from the aquaculture point of view because water being used for aquacultural practices is mostly ground water which may be contaminated with fluoride.

Materials and Methods

Sexually mature live and healthy specimens of both male and female catfish, *Clarias batrachus* were collected from nearby areas of Lucknow. Fish weighing 55±2gm and size 15±1.7cm were selected and transported to the laboratory in large plastic containers filled with river water to minimize physical stress. They were acclimatized to the laboratory condition in large glass aquaria for 15 days prior to the experimentation. Before stocking, the fishes as well as aquaria were treated with 0.1 per cent $KMnO_4$ solution to avoid fungal infection. Fishes were not fed initially for 48 hours. The water of the aquaria was changed on alternate days and food was given one hour before the change of water. The physico-chemical properties of holding water during acclimatization of fish in laboratory were determined by methods of APHA (1998) such as, temperature 26±1.5°C, pH 6.9±0.2, dissolved oxygen content 7.8±1.5mg/L, alkalinity as $CaCO_3$ 90-102 mg/L, fluoride 0.1 mg/L and electrical conductivity 269.21±15.65μ ohms/cm.

For the experiment, fishes were divided in three groups, each having six fishes. One group served as control group and the remaining two were exposed to 35mg F/L of water (Low concentration) and 70mgF/L of water (High concentration) respectively. Experiment was conducted for 90 days. After 90 days, weight of all fishes was recorded and they were sacrificed. Their gonads and liver were dissected out to record their weight. Gonado-somatic index (GSI), Hepato-somatic index (HSI), Condition factor (CF) and Somatic condition factor (SCF) were calculated.

Results

There was decrease in the body weight, average length, liver weight and gonad weight of fishes after exposure to fluoride in both concentrations (Tables 23.1 and 23.2). After exposure to fluoride both in male and female fishes, the HSI and GSI decreased as compared to the control values in both the concentrations (Tables 23.3 and 23.4) whereas CF and SCF in both the concentrations were increased in comparison to the control values (Tables 23.3 and 23.4).The decrease in HSI and GSI was concentration dependent. It was observed that the values of CF and SCF in both the exposure groups were increased insignificantly in comparison to control.

Table 23.1: Effect of Fluoride on Body Weight, Length, Liver Weight and Gonad Weight of male *Clarias batrachus* After Exposure for 90 Days

Parameters	*Control Group*	*Experimental Groups*	
		Low Concentration (35mgF/L)	*High Concentration (70mgF/L)*
Body Weight (g)	72.30 ± 0.99	68.80±0.78*	64.80±0.80***
Body length (cm)	19.80±0.34	19.07±0.37^NS	18.04±0.31^NS
Liver Weight (mg)	638.80±13.82	505.20±13.90***	466.00±13.28***
Gonad Weight(mg)	113.00±2.40	79.80±1.87***	59.40±1.08***

Values are Mean ± S.E, n = 6 (observations in each value).

*p<0.05 (in comparison to control), **p<0.01 (in comparison to control);

***p<0.001(in comparison to control).

Table 23.2: Effect of Fluoride on Body Weight, Length, Liver Weight and Gonad Weight of Female *Clarias batrachus* After Exposure for 90 Days

Parameters	*Control Group*	*Experimental Groups*	
		Low Concentration (35mgF/L)	*High Concentration (70mgF/L)*
Body Weight (g)	56.40 ± 1.43	54.46±0.98	51.73±1.05*
Body length (cm)	17.80±0.38	17.61±0.53	16.95±0.88^NS
Liver Weight (mg)	553.80±12.61	500.91±8.58*	482.62±11.83**
Gonad Weight(mg)	3481.73±38.28	1285.67±40.42*	1125.62±33.91**

Values are Mean ± S.E, n = 6 (observations in each value)

*p<0.05 (in comparison to control), **p<0.01 (in comparison to control).

NS: Nonsignificant.

Table 23.3: Effect of Fluoride on HSI, GSI, CF and SCF of Male *Clarias batrachus* after Exposure for 90 Days

Parameters	*Control Group*	*Experimental Groups*	
		Low Concentration (35mgF/L)	*High Concentration (70mgF/L)*
HSI	0.867±0.018	0.606±0.016***	0.587±0.015***
GSI	0.156±0.005	0.105±0.003***	0.086±0.004***
CF	947.07±39.40	999.83±40.91^{NS}	1066.23±36.66^{NS}
SCF	945.83±36.67	990.00±39.05^{NS}	1065.59±36.64^{NS}

Values are Mean ± S.E, n = 6 (observations in each value).

***p<0.001(in comparison to control).

NS: Nonsignificant.

Table 23.4: Effect of Fluoride on HSI, GSI, CF and SCF of Female *Clarias batrachus* After Exposure for 90 Days

Parameters	*Control Group*	*Experimental Groups*	
		Low Concentration (35mgF/L)	*High Concentration (70mgF/L)*
HSI	0.982±0.031	0.791±0.052**	0.665±0.034***
GSI	6.142±0.73	3.354±0.94**	2.887±0.82**
CF	952.08±37.40	987.83±40.20^{NS}	1062.50±39.33^{NS}
SCF	938.31±26.23	978.75±25.81^{NS}	1039.15±30.26^{NS}

Values are Mean ± S.E, n = 6 (observations in each value).

**P<0.01 (in comparison to control, ***P<0.001(in comparison to control).

NS: Nonsignificant.

Discussion

In the present study reduction in body weight of fishes after exposure to fluoride was found. This finding is supported by the observations of other workers (Sarlakumari *et al.*, 1998; Chinoy *et al.*, 1992) who have found reduction in body weight of rat after exposure to NaF. This reduction may be due to decreased feeding frequency and disturbed digestive activities after exposure to fluoride, as it was evident during experimentation. Other possibility may be more utilization of stored materials for carrying out the metabolic activities during exposure period. Similar observations *i.e.* reduction in body weight has been reported by other workers in fishes after exposure to various toxicants such as insecticides, pesticides etc (Gopal and Devi, 1991; Lata *et al.,* 2001; Devi, 2003).

There was reduction in HSI, after exposure to fluoride which indicates reduction in liver weight. It is well known that liver is the first site to be affected by the toxicants. It may be possible that fluoride interferes with the biosynthesizing activities and altering the enzyme activities in liver as has been suggested by Chitra *et al.* (1983). Similarly, Gupta (2003) has reported damage in hepatocytes of *Channa punctatus* after exposure to fluoride. Thus, it seems that degeneration of the hepatocytes and disturbed biosynthesizing activity may be a cause of decrease in HSI and liver weight.

Decrease in the gonadal weight and GSI, in both male and female fish found in the present study indicates toxic effect of fluoride on reproductive activities in fishes. This finding is in accordance with the earlier observations because fluoride has been reported to affect reproduction adversely in other animals (Chinoy, 1991). It affects spermatogenesis (Narayana and Chinoy, 1994) and Oogenesis (Shusheela and Kumar, 1991) in mammals by inhibiting synthesis of steroidal hormones and enzymes which are responsible for maturation and development of reproductive bodies. GSI is considered as a reliable parameters for assessment of gonadal activity in seasonal breeding teleosts and it increases with the advancement of gonadal development and maturation. Decreased GSI after exposure to fluoride indicates that fluoride induces deleterious changes in reproductive process. This is more clear from the dose dependent changes in GSI found in both male and female fishes. Similar findings on reproduction in fishes have been reported after exposure to other toxicants (Ahsan and Ahsan, 1974, Masud *et al.,* 2001 Chandra *et al.,* 2003). They have also suggested that toxicants interfere with normal metabolic relationship between liver and gonad in fishes. It is well known that there is an inverse relationship between HSI and GSI during breeding season.They have reported that gonadal maturation and development of reproductive bodies were affected because energy mobilization from the liver to gonads during gonadal maturation was inhibited. Generally HSI decreases from preparatory phase to spawning phase with increasing GSI. This may be attributed to energy reserve mobilization from liver to gonad during breeding season. Lal *et al.* (1987) have also reported that the liver lipid contributes maximum for the gonadal development and maturation. Thus it is clear that lesser increase in GSI after exposure to fluoride in comparison to control may be due to interference of fluoride at the energy mobilization level. CF and SCF are indicator of good health and nutritional status of fishes (Rijnsdrop, 1990). They are correlated with gonadal activity also. In experimental fishes lesser decrease in CF and SCF in comparison to control may be due to less increase in weight of gonads in comparison to control during breeding season. This observation is supported by the findings of Shanker and Kulkarni (2005) who have reported decreasing trend of CF and SCF from pre spawning phase to post spawning phase in *Notopterus notopterus*. Thus, it is clear that fluoride interferes with the reproductive physiology of fishes and induces deleterious effect on gonadal maturation. On the basis of the study it may be suggested that fluoride affects the fecundity of fishes, inhabiting the areas where fluoride level is higher. At the same time it can be concluded that aquacultural practices will not be economical in places where ground water is having higher fluoride level.

Acknowledgements

The authors are thankful to Prof. Minakshi Shrivastava, Head, Department of Zoology, University of Lucknow for providing necessary laboratory facilities to carry out this work.

References

Ahsan, S.N. and Ahsan, J., 1974. Degenerative changes in the testis of *Clarias batrachus* (Linn) caused by cadmium chloride. *Indian. J. Zool.*, 15: 39-43.

APHA, 1998. *Standard Methods for the Examination of Water and Wastewater*, 20th Edn. American Public Health Association, Washington, DC. 2005-2006.

Araibi, A.A., Yousif, W.H. and Al-Dewachi, O.S., 1989. Effect of high fluoride on the reproductive performance of male rat. *J. Biol. Sci. Res.*, 20: 1-30.

ATSDR, 2001. Draft toxicological profile for fluorine, hydrogen fluoride and fluoride: U.S. Department of health and human services. Agency for Toxic Substances and Disease Registry. Atlanta, Georgia.

Bajpai, S., Tripathi, N., Tewari, S. and Tripathi, M., 2010. Retardation of growth after fluoride exposure in catfish, *Heteropneustes fossilis* (Bloch). In: *Bioresources for Rural Livelihood, Vol. 1*. Narendra Publishing House, pp. 167-173.

Camargo, J.A., 2003. Fluoride toxicity to aquatic organism: A review. *Chemosphere*, 50(3): 251-261.

Chinoy, N.J., 1991. Effects of fluoride on physiology of animals and human beings. *Indian J. Env. Toxicol.*, 1(1): 17-32.

Chinoy, N.J. and Sequeira, E., 1992. Reversible fluoride induced fertility impairment in male mice. *Fluoride*, 25(2): 71-76.

Chinoy, N.J., Pradeep, P.K. and Sequeira, E., 1992. Effect of fluoride ingestion on physiology of reproductive organ of male rat. *J. Environ. Biol.*, 13(1): 55-61.

Chinoy, N.J. and Patel, T.N., 2001. Effects of sodium fluoride and aluminium chloride on ovary and uterus of mice and their reversal by some antidodes. *Fluoride*, 34(1): 9-20.

Chitra, T., Reddy, M.M. and Rao, J.V.R., 1983. Levels of muscle and liver tissue enzymes in *Channa punctatus* (Bloch) exposed to NaF. *Fluoride*, 16: 48-51.

Chandra, S., Ram, R.N. and Singh, I.J., 2003. Testicular recrudescence and recovery responses in common carp, *Cyprinus carpio* after long-term exposure to a carbamate pesticide. *J. Ecophysiol. Occup. Hlth.*, 3: 15-35.

Devi, S., 2003. Behavioural changes in *Oreochromis mossambicus* exposed to endosulfan. *J. Ecobiology.*, 15(6): 425-430.

Gopal, V. and Devi, M., 1991. Biomonitoring of heavy metal and pesticide pollution. *Ind. J. Environ. Hlth.*, 33: 488-491.

Gupta, R., 2003. Pathophysiological consequences to freshwater fish, *Channa punctatus* induced by fluoride. *Ph.D. Thesis*, University of Lucknow, Lucknow.

Jalabert, B., Baroiller, J.F., Breton, B., Fostier, A., Le Gac, F., Guiguen, Y. and Monod, G., 2000. Main neuroendocrine, endocrine and paracrine regulations of fish reproduction and vulnerability to xenobiotics. *Ecotoxicology.*, 9: 25-40.

Kaur, K. and Singh, J., 1980. Histological findings of mice testis following fluoride ingestion. *Fluoride*, 13: 160-162.

Lata, S., Gopal, K. and Singh, N.N., 2001. Toxicological evaluations and morphological studies in cat fish *Clarias batrachus* exposed to carbaryl and carbofuran. *J. Ecophysiol. Occup. Hlth.,* 1: 121-130.

Lal, B., Mohan, R. and Singh, T.P., 1987. Variations in different lipids and their relation to reproduction in the male fish *Clarias batrachus* (Linn). *Indian. J. Exp. Biol.,* 25: 639-640.

Masud, S., Singh, I.J. and Ram, R.N., 2001. Testicular recrudescence and related changes in female *Cyprinus carpio* after longterm exposure to a mercurial compound. *J. Ecophysiol. Occup. Hlth.* 1: 109-120.

Narayana, M.V. and Chinoy, N.J., 1994. Effect of fluoride on rat testicular steroidogenesis. *Fluoride,* 27(1): 7-12.

Rijnsdrop, A.D., 1990. The mechanism of energy allocation over reproduction and somatic growth in female North Sea plaice, *Pleuronectus platessa* (L.). *Netherlands. J. Sea Res.,* 25: 279-290.

Samanta, S., Misra, K., Chandra, K., Saha, K., Bandopadhyay, S. and Ghose, A., 2005. Heavy metals in water of the river Hoogly and Haldia at Haldia and their impact on fish. *J. Environ. Biol.,* 26(3): 517-523.

Shashi, A. and Singh, J.P., 1987. Effect of fluoride administration of organs on gastrointestinal tract. An experimental study on rabbits. Effect on tissue proteins. *Fluoride,* 20(3): 183-188.

Shanker, D.S and Kulkarni, R.S., 2005. Somatic condition of the fish, *Notopterus notopterus* (Pallas) during different phases of the reproductive cycle. *J. Environ. Biol.,* 26(1): 49-53.

Sharma, J.D., Solanki, M. and Solanki, D., 2007. Sodium fluoride toxicity on reproductive organ of female albino rats. *Asian J. Exp. Sci.,* 21(2): 359-364.

Sarlakumari, D., Varadacharyulu, N.Ch. and Ramakrishna Rao, P., 1988. Effect of fluoride toxicity on growth and lipids in liver, kidney and serum in rats. *Arogya. J. Hlth. Sci.,* 14: 24-29.

Susheela, A.K. and Kumar, A., 1991. A study of the effect of high concentration of fluoride on the reproductive organs of male rabbits, using light and scanning electron microscopy. *J. Reprd. Fertil.,* 92: 352-360.

Chapter 24

Sexual Selection and Mating Systems Across the Animal World: A Review

Omkar and Geetanjali Mishra*

Department of Zoology, University of Lucknow, Lucknow – 226 007, U.P., India

ABSTRACT

Most of us have observed the male peacock spread out his tail feathers in the air in beautiful trembling motion to woo the dowdy peahen who passes by. We have heard the shiny black male cuckoo (koel) sing his melodious song to attract the plain unmelodious female. Many of us have also seen the billies (male goats) butt their heads to vanquish competitors for the attention of the female. Other than these common displays, the nature lovers have either seen live or through the wonders of modern day cable television, the wonderfully resounding clashes of the rams for the eves, the fluffing, prancing, and bowing of colourful plumage by male paradise birds for the drab females, the weaving of beautiful gifts by the male spiders for the hungry and murderous females, the rolling of bigger dung balls by male dung beetles for attracting their females, the dance of the snakes to appease the females and many more such wonders of the animal world.

* Corresponding author: E-mail: omkaar55@hotmail.com

The common aim of all these displays is to impress a potential mate with their prowess or appease to enable the procurement of an able mate. The bigger, the more beautiful, the more capable or the fitter the animal within a species, the more suitable is he or she deemed as a mate. It is this selection of the best possible mate through competition or choice that has resulted in the evolution of numerous displayable morphological and behavioural manifestations of individual capabilities. These mechanisms help in the search of better mate and have thus been perfected with the passage of time.

Though initially considered as merely natural selection, this entire process was later deemed separate and termed and studied as sexual selection. The study of sexual selection can be termed in layman's language as the study of the various means of mate procurement displayed in the animals, their role in evolution and the reasons involved thereof. Further relevant extension of this entire exercise of sexual selection is to study the myriad mating systems displayed after selection and the reasons thereof. Here in this chapter it is aimed to discuss in detail the various aspects of sexual selection and the numerous mating systems present in the animals.

Keywords: *Sexual selection, Polyandry, Polygynandry, Mating systems.*

I. Sexual Selection

(A) What is Sexual Selection?

Generations of naturalists have observed a distinctive preference during mate search for certain conspecific individuals of opposite sex bearing certain traits. This prominent preference has led to the favourable evolution of these particular traits even though they probably compromise survival while enhancing reproduction. This process was earlier considered akin to natural selection. Later, the great naturalist Charles Darwin concretely studied, defined and differentiated it as sexual selection by his following statement in the book, *The Descent of Man and Selection in Relation to Sex*:

" Sexual selection depends on the success of certain individuals over others of the same sex in relation to the propagation of the species; while natural selection depends on the success of both sexes, at all ages, in relation to the general conditions of life"

Darwin's assumption was that natural selection is the selection for the evolution of survival increasing traits which also promoted the reproductive success of individuals. Sexual selection theory was however proposed by him to explain the evolution of traits that decreased fitness but nevertheless enhanced reproductive success.

More simple definition of sexual selection is:

"A form of natural selection that occurs when individuals differ in their ability to compete with others for mates or to attract members of the opposite sex" – Alcock, 2001

Sexual selection is the process in which competition for mates between individuals of the same sex (typically males) or selection by females drives the evolution of certain traits. Within a species, one sex is relatively rare or more choosy and thus acts as a limiting resource for the other. It is to obtain access to this limiting resource or sex that competition occurs and the mechanism of this process is known as sexual selection. It is distinct from ecological or natural selection which is the competition for limiting resources, other than the mates, such as food, within the ecological niche of the species. Though Darwin's theory of sexual selection is now widely accepted, it had to face numerous ups and downs from its proposal to its present state of acceptance; a brief history of which is discussed below.

(B) Origin of the Concept of Sexual Selection

Darwin in his commendable and extensive works in 1859 and 1871 on evolution and the process of natural selection realized that there were numerous ornamentations in animals that reduced the fitness and survival of individuals. Their presence could not be explained by the theory of natural selection which advocates gradual elimination or reduction of such characters. The examples were the extravagant tails of the male peacock and the antlers of the male deer which decrease survival ability. Darwin through his studies realized that these traits helped in competing for and acquiring sexual partners. He thus through numerous such observations concluded that any inheritable trait in a sexually reproducing species that helps in competing for and obtaining mates will tend to spread through the species, even if it somewhat compromises the survival.

Darwin termed this process favouring evolution of (*i*) better sensory, visual and motor abilities for finding mates, (*ii*) development of gifts and ornaments to attract, (*iii*) weapons to repel and compete with same-sex competitors, and (*iv*) genitals and gametes that maximize fertilization rates, as *sexual selection*. In this process, Darwin distinguished between male competition for female mates (which typically gives rise to weapons), and female choice of male mates (which typically gives rise to gifts and ornaments). Darwin however could not lend a proper explanation as to why it was the males that compete and the females that do the choosing in most animal species (Darwin, 1871).

Though at present, the concept of sexual selection is widely accepted, it was met with great resistance and was confined to the dungeons of history soon after its presentation. The resistance to this concept was owing to its radical nature. The 18th and 19th century thinkers, such as Lamarck, Cuvier, Malthus (Richards, 1987) and Wallace (1870, 1889) had at that time come around to the idea of natural selection after considerable debate and thought. The concept of evolution being a resultant of differential reproduction and not differential survival was absolutely against every scientific conviction held at that time.

Further in the male dominated society of the 19th century, Darwin's theory put females into a powerful evolutionary role. He proposed that mate choice by the females shaped the future of a species. He considered this not radically different from that consciously done by the animal breeders and expressed his opinion in the following words:

"All animals present individual differences, and as man can modify his domesticated birds by selecting the individuals which appear to him the most beautiful, so the habitual or even occasional preference by the female of the more attractive males would almost certainly lead to their modification; and such modification might in the course of time be augmented to almost any extent, compatible with the existence of the species." (Darwin, 1871, p. 750-751).

Thus, though his views on male competition were widely accepted by the peers as important, necessary, and a general evolutionary process, his ideas on the possibility of female choice driving evolution was almost universally mocked and dismissed (Cronin, 1991). Wallace (1889, p. 293) was highly skeptical about the role of females in shaping male ornaments and described these as mere "surplus of strength, vitality, and growth-power which is able to expend itself in this way without injury". Huxley (1938) and Cott (1940) deemed male ornaments to be mere objects of intimidation or 'species recognition markers'. Such a cold reception of the theory of sexual selection led to it being almost forgotten (Cronin, 1991). However, there were still a few evolutionary biologists; chief amongst them was R.A Fisher who took this concept seriously. In his seminal work (Fisher, 1915, 1930), he viewed mate preferences as legitimate biological traits subject to inheritable variation, and this insight led him to postulate a process he called *runaway sexual selection* (details later in the chapter). However, it was not until the 1970's that the concept of sexual selection began to come into its own after a century of condemnation.

Campbell (1972) brought some attention to this erstwhile neglected idea, while Trivers (1972) could finally explain the possible reasons for choosy females and competing males (details later in chapter). Zahavi (1975) further added to the revival of interest by describing ornaments as reliable guaranteed displays of genetic quality as they are handicaps to the general way of life in terms of the costs involved in their production. The mathematical feasibility of Fisher's runaway sexual selection process was also proved (O'Donald, 1980; Lande, 1981; Kirkpatrick, 1982). New behavioural experiments on animals showed that females of many species do exhibit strong preferences for certain male traits (*e.g.* Andersson, 1982; Moller, 1988; Ryan, 1985) and that the preference of female for certain kinds of genital stimulation had led to the diverse array of complex male genitalia (Eberhard, 1985). Books on sexual selection in insects (Blum and Blum, 1979) and humans (Betzig *et al.*, 1988) have added to the information and interest on sexual selection. The role of sexual selection in primate social systems (De Waal, 1982; Dunbar, 1988; Smuts, 1985; Byrne and Whiten, 1988) has now been accepted, and this whole process has percolated down to the successful application of sexual selection theory to the humans beginning with Symons (1979). The circle of proposition, rejection, neglect, revival and almost complete universal acceptance for this theory is now complete (see Cronin, 1991; Andersson, 1994).

(C) Classification of Sexual Selection

Sexual selection can be broadly classified into intrasexual and intersexual selection. The differences between these two and the various means through which they are displayed are mentioned below.

(*i*) Intrasexual Selection

To quote Darwin (1871) once again, intrasexual selection is *"between the individuals of the same sex, generally the males in order to drive away or kill their rivals, the females remaining passive"*. That is intrasexual selection involves the competition between males for the attention and favours of the conspecific females. This is sometimes reversed and in certain cases, like that of the empid files and pipe fishes, it is the females that compete for the attention of males. The reasons behind this differential role of mates are given in the section dealing with role of paternal investment. Intrasexual selection can occur both prior to or post copulation of the animal.

When this selection occurs prior to copulation, it involves competition between conspecific adults of the same sex for procuring the attention of opposite sex. In such a scenario of vigourous competition, the winner male gets an opportunity to mate with a female. Winning males are usually either larger in size, more dextrous in their motor abilities, or have larger and/or more effective weapons. The battles amongst the members of the goat family (Figure 24.1), the contests between the lions, tigers, the massive elephant seals, *etc.* for mating with the females are examples of the pre-copulatory intrasexual selection.

The event of intrasexual selection post copulation mainly involves the competition amongst sperm of the males within the

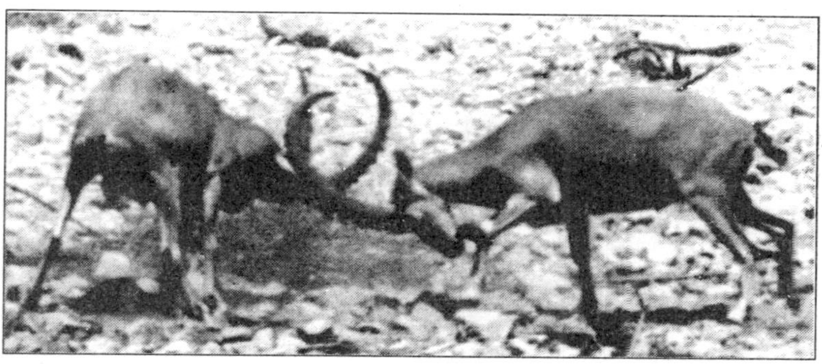

Figure 24.1: Males of the Mountain Goats (The ibex) Locking their Antlers in Competition for Procuring a Mating with a Female

female genital tract. The result depends primarily on the motility of the sperm, the amount of ejaculate and the number of sperm in each ejaculate. While these aspects are indicative of the physiological condition of the males that have mated, there are numerous other tricks that the males resort to in order to ensure that their sperm fertilizes the eggs of the female. These tricks involve, release of chemicals in female genital tract to kill or incapacitate the sperm of the previously mated male and also the use of their uniquely shaped male copulatory organ to clean the female tract of sperm from previous mating. In extreme conditions, males are known to resort to damaging the female genital tract with their copulatory organ and also to plug the female genital tract to prevent further mating, hence ensuring success of their sperm in fertilizing the ova. These aspects of sperm competition are described exclusively in a later section.

(*ii*) Intersexual Selection

Intersexual competition is defined as, "*the struggle is likewise between the individuals of the same sex, in order to excite or charm those of the opposite sex generally the females, which no longer remain passive, but select the more agreeable partners* (Darwin, 1871)"

Under this kind of sexual selection, the more beautiful, the more ornamented the potential mates, the more are the chances of being selected as a mate. Most instances under this selection are of the highly ornamented males (*e.g.* peacocks), of the males that create extensive dwellings (*e.g.* bowerbirds) or provide food packets (*e.g.* spiders) and of those that sing (*e.g.* cuckoo, crickets), dance (*e.g.* paradise birds) or behave in peculiar manners to impress the females. Details are given in the section on sexual selection in the animal world.

(D) Theories of Sexual Selection

Theories accepting competition or intrasexual selection as a means of sexual selection are well documented as the scientists are almost unanimous in the reasoning that the mating with the winner of the competition ensures increased fecundity and healthier offspring.

However, study of sexual selection also involves paying attention to various aspects of mate choice and the criteria involved. The term 'choice' is considered inclusive of processes that are conscious as well as unconscious, and also both psychological and physiological. Numerous theories attempting to explain the basis and the benefits of mate choice have been propounded. Broadly speaking, there are two schools of thought on mate choice criteria. Selection of *genetic indicators* or the so called *good genes, healthy offspring* or *healthy mate* have been discussed in the *theory of handicaps* or the *handicap principle* propounded earliest by Zahavi (1975). The description about *good genes* proposes that the displays and ornaments provide information to the females about the viability promoting genes in the courting males. These genes might advance the chances of offspring survival by conferring hereditary resistance to parasitic infection or disease or by promoting adaptive foraging skills or the ability to avoid predators. The *healthy mate theory* states that male courtship displays and ornaments inform females of a potential sexual partner's health. For example the dominant jungle fowl roosters have larger and redder combs along with stronger immune systems than their subordinate ones (Zuk and Johnson, 1999). Combining both the theories, Zahavi's handicap principle propounded that displays and ornaments used in intersexual competition as means for aiding mate choice worked as handicaps owing to their high maintenance costs and could thus be borne only by those who had good health and good genes.

In the other major theory on sexual selection through mate choice, *runaway sexual selection* (Figure 24.2), Fisher (1930) discussed selection for certain aesthetic displays and ornaments with the intention of producing 'sexy sons'. As per theory, females preferably procure sperm containing genes whose primary effect is to make their daughters select attractive mates and to endow their sons with traits that make them attractive to other conspecific females. This theory states that if a slight majority of females in an ancestral population preferably mated with males possessing certain traits that perhaps initially conferred with some survival advantage; females that mated with such males would give rise to daughter that selected more such trait bearing males and sons which would bear attractive character(s). Such sons would enjoy higher fitness levels due to increased chances of mating, while the females would respond positively only to certain traits as determined by their genes. The coinheritance of mate preference genes in females and attractive genes in males would create a runaway process in which increasingly more extreme female preferences and male traits would

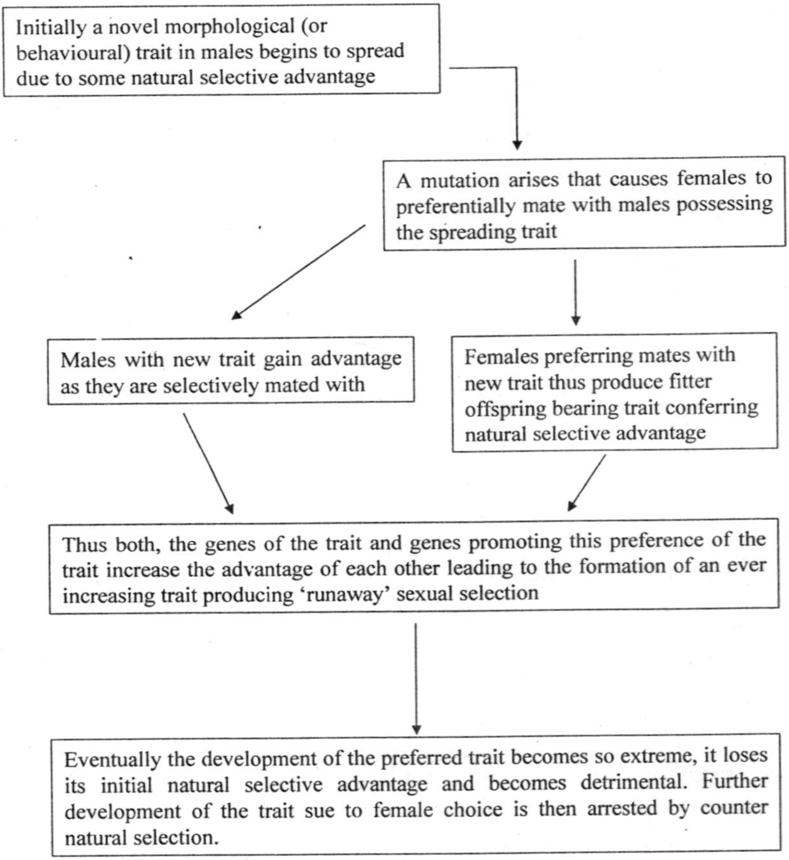

Figure 24.2: Fisher's Runaway Sexual Selection Theory or "Sexy Sons" Hypothesis of Evolution of Sexual Selection Through Female Choice

spread together as new mutations occur. This spread would only stop when natural selection against risky or costly displays will balance sexual selection in favour of traits that are appealing to females. To use as an example, peahens initially preferred males with long tails indicating foraging prowess but now owing to the runaway sexual selection this preference for a long tail has persisted and has been imbibed into the subconscious selection regardless of any other ability, such as food gathering or defense against predators. A theory on food as a mate criterion states that the number of eyes in the tail of a peacock indicate the blueberries, and increased food search ability and is thus attractive to peahens.

These two models of *handicap* and *runaway* sexual selection are considered competitors for explaining the process of sexual selection, but recent work has established sufficient evidence for each (Andersson, 1994). They often act as complementary selective forces. Mate choice favours many other important qualities, including parental ability and resources (Clutton-Brock, 1991; Hoelzer, 1989; Price *et al.*, 1993), fertility through sperm quality in males or fecundity in females (Baker and Bellis, 1995; Singh, 1993), avoidance of inbreeding (Thornhill, 1991, 1993), and similarity in appearance, behaviour, and personality (Rushton, 1989).

(E) Mechanisms of Sexual Selection

(*i*) Competition for Mates

This mechanism of sexual selection involves competition between individuals of one sex for sexual favours from the opposite sex. The winner of this competition is usually the one with larger or more robust size and athletic ability. Mating with the winner ensures benefit of protection to the mate and also healthier offspring. The competitors are usually the sex that is less in number, *i.e.* the operative sex ratio (ratio of sexually receptive males to sexually receptive females) is biased either in favour of the females or the males. In the animals, this ratio is usually biased in favour of the males, making females the scarce source, leading to competition for mating favours. This ratio is not merely based on the number of individuals present in a population but is intricately weaved with the parental investment involved; an aspect described later in this chapter.

(*ii*) Selection for Indicators

Mate preference, which involves selection for indicators of viability (likelihood of survival) and fertility (likelihood of reproduction), is the most fundamental form of operating sexual selection. Any bodily or behavioural trait revealing age, health, nutritional status, size, strength, aggressive dominance, social status, resistance to diseases or overall vigour can work as a reliable indicator of (1) inheritable genetic traits that are likely to be passed on to offspring (the good genes hypothesis), and (2) increased chances of mate survival so as to provide provisioning, protection, and support to offspring (selection for 'good parents').

Avoidance of mating with dead, injured or sick animals is not surprising as it leads to deterioration of fitness parameters. Such decisions ought to be based on easily observable cues of fitness. Evolution of such observable cues of health and innate fitness ought to have thus evolved to exaggerated limits after ages of mate choice. Weak, ambiguous cues would indicate dead or sick individuals while prominent and clearly visible similar cues would indicate vigourous and healthy adults. For example, females of rhesus macaques are known to prefer males with red faces over those with pale faces (Waitt *et al.*, 2003). The colour of the face is considered an indicator of testosterone levels, hence activity and also general state of fitness of the males. Similarly, in peacocks, tail quality reflects some underlying physiological activity as it has been observed that poor tail quality is an indication of sickness which increases the chances of falling prey to predatory attempts (Petri, 1992).

Such qualities as indicated by morphological characteristics are likely to be inheritable by the offspring and the bearers of such displays are thus probably preferred by the females, as seen in the active preference for long tailed males in peacocks (Petrie *et al.*, 1991). Bird plumage (Hamilton and Zuk, 1982; Moller, 1988), loudness and complexity of songs in both birds (Catchpole, 1987) and insects (Omkar and James, 2001; Omkar and Mishra, 2003), body symmetry and body size (Ryan, 1985) are also classical indicators of animal viability. However, other than these, any body part that is expensive to produce and requires much energy or resources from the animal can be used as an indicator.

High costs should be involved in producing an indicator, as this prevents their easy imitation and this theory was mentioned in detail in the *handicap principle* (Zahavi, 1975, 1991). Mathematical models and computer simulations show that good parenting indicators can evolve to display even non-heritable resources, such as good territories (Grafen, 1990; Heywood, 1989; Hoelzer, 1989; Price *et al.*, 1993). Thus, not all indicators are necessarily advertising genetic quality; they could simply be advertising resources and health relevant to raising offspring.

The co-occurrence of runaway sexual selection with the handicap development leads to better evolution of relevant indicators (Andersson, 1986; Heywood, 1989; Pomiankowski, 1988; Tomlinson, 1988) as has been discussed above. However, even the absence of runaway selection, other processes can be sufficient for the evolution of extravagant male ornaments and extreme female preferences (Grafen, 1990).

The idea of morphological characteristics working as indicators of genetic health is not fully acceptable owing to the 'behaviour of the *lek*' or what is also known as the '*lek* paradox' (*e.g.* Williams, 1975; Kirkpatrick, 1987; Pomiankowski, 1987, 1995; Reynolds and Gross, 1990). *Leks* are aggregations of animals, in which females select their mates from among dozens receiving nothing but sperm from them. In such situations, an attractive male might mate up to 30 times (in the sage grouse), while the average male might not receive a single mating (Boyce, 1990). Such high preference would lead to the slow but steady selection of the attractive trait thereby leading to its prevalence and dominance in the genetic pool. This would lead to the slow elimination of genes responsible for unwanted or less desirable traits (Fisher, 1930). Once the attractive genes permeate completely or is fixed (100 per cent) in the gene pool, indicators would become irrelevant. The entire population would become genetically homogenous for a particular preferred trait ending mate choice.

The persistence of mate choice and maintenance of inheritable fitness variation in the animal kingdom and even in animals displaying the *lek* model could be attributed to the temporal and spatial variation in selection, and the mutation pressure (Andersson, 1994). Temporally varying selection can result from co-evolution between ecological competitors, between predators and prey, or perhaps most importantly, between hosts and parasites (Hamilton and Zuk, 1982; Hamilton *et al.*, 1990; Low, 1990; Miller, 1998). Different processes of selection in geographical areas along with the process of migration can maintain inheritable variation in a population, which will be spatial in nature. Occurrence of mutations resulting in individuals with a low fitness levels can also maintain inheritable variation in a population (Lande, 1981; Charlesworth, 1987; Kondrashov, 1988; Rice, 1988), thus continuing and maintaining the process of mate choice.

Biased mutations lead to better evolution of indicators (Iwasa *et al.*, 1991). There are some suggestions that sexually-selected traits have much higher heritabilities and genetic variances than naturally-selected traits (Moller and Pomiankowski, 1993; Pomiankowski,

1995; Wilcockson *et al.*, 1995). The importance of inheritable variation is indicated by studies, which show that females allowed to choose their mates have offspring with higher phenotypic as well as genetic qualities than those not allowed to choose (*e.g.* Reynolds and Gross, 1992; Omkar and Mishra, 2006). Through female choice, males have been forced to clearly display the quality of their genes. In this sense, females shape males to function as a kind of genetic sieve for the species (Atmar, 1991; Michod and Levin, 1988) separating the bad genes from the good like chaff from the crop.

(*iii*) Selection for Aesthetic Displays

Aesthetic displays are designed to attract attention, to excite, to provoke and to increase the desire of the opposite sex to mate. These displays play on the perception of the receiver. Such biases in perception can occur in either of two complementary ways: (1) these may exist already as subconscious perceptions or adaptations to particular environments and side effects of basic evolutionary processes, and/or (2) they may be a result of co-evolution with preferred courtship traits, through Fisher's runaway process.

Recent work reveals that certain ornaments that have not evolved in a species are also preferred when provided as experimental additions to normal morphological outline of the animal. In zebra finches, males bearing red or black plastic bands are preferred over those having blue or green bands (Burley, 1988). In an experiment, plastic swords were attached to a few male platyfish and the female allowed to choose between such males and normal males (without swords). The females exhibited choice for males that bore plastic swords. This was despite the fact that this species does not bear any such ornamentation. This preference is perhaps a subconscious response to the time previous to their divergent evolution from their close relatives' swordtails (Basolo, 1990). Artificially lowered frequencies of calling songs are preferred by females as it indicates extra-large size of frogs (Ryan 1985, 1990). This preference for non-existent traits supports the first mechanism, *viz.* that aesthetic displays may exist as subconscious perceptions or adaptations to particular environments and side effects of basic evolutionary processes

The more prominent the aesthetic displays are in terms of their loudness, size, colours, frequency and novelty the more easily they are perceived and preferred during mate choice (Miller, 1993). These perceptions may also vary considerably across species owing to the niche specialization, *i.e.* birds eating blue berries would probably evolve eyes perceptive to the blue colour, thereby showing an innate preference to blue while another closely related species that eats red berries might prefer the red colour. Such specializations in perception may help explain the rapid divergence of sexually-selected traits across closely-related species (Endler, 1993).

The difference between indicators and aesthetic displays is that the latter evolve to manipulate the receiver to promote the interest of the signaller and not to always communicate truthful information for the benefit of both.

(*iv*) Selection for Provisioning, Territories, and Protection

Females can gain nongenetic benefits from mate choice by favouring males that offer material gifts (Searcy, 1982). Such examples of provisioning come from male insects giving nuptial gifts, such as spermatophores or caught prey (Thornhill and Alcock, 1983) and male birds provisioning offspring and building nests in certain bird species (see Clutton-Brock, 1991). Such provisioning by males eases the burden on the females for producing eggs and providing for the young ones. This feature of providing for offspring is most common in monogamous birds (Clutton-Brock, 1991) and rare elsewhere, though feeding and caring during courtship is quite common in the insects.

The above mentioned selection is quite different from that for good territories defended by males. It has been long recognized by the socioecologists that female animals tend to distribute themselves around their habitat to exploit the available food resources and protect themselves against the local predators, and the males distribute themselves to exploit the available females as reproductive resources (Dunbar, 1988). In such cases, males fight to hold prime territories, and the females prefer to mate with the owners of these territories. This entire behaviour can be assessed as female choice in favour of sexy, healthy, high-status, territory-holding males. In some cases females prefer males that act as protectors. This is prevalent in species where females and/or infants are subject to strong predation risk or strong risk of infanticide by rival males (Hausfater and Hardy, 1984).

(*v*) Sperm Competition

Though initially it was thought that the process of sexual selection was limited to the pre-copulatory phase, researches have shown this to be not the case. The process of sexual selection is a more intricate process and continues even once copulation is secured by the female. Of the myriad processes of sexual selection that take place post copulation, sperm competition is a major one. It is a means of intrasexual competition.

As the term suggests, this process of sexual selection involves the competition between sperm of different males for the fertilization with of ova (Parker, 1990). It thus understandably occurs in polyandrous females, *i.e.* those that mate with multiple males. To ensure the fertilization of ova with their own sperm, the males compete through larger testicle size, ejaculate volume, sperm morphology, sperm concentration, sperm motility and directional movement, sperm longevity, the chemical composition of semen, devices to remove previous competitors' sperm from the female reproductive tract, and various plugs to keep future competitors' sperm excluded entirely (Smith, 1984; Parker, 1984).

The competition for testicle size can result in dramatic developments. A case in point is the 2000-pound testicles of the male North Atlantic right whale. In primates too, the increase in sperm competition across species results in increased testicle size (Harcourt and Harvey, 1984). Rats, which are highly promiscuous, are known to have large sized testicles to ensure larger ejaculate volume and thus probable success in sperm competition. In gorillas, the testicle size is a mere one ounce in relation to their 400 pound or more body size, owing to their largely monogamous nature. However, in the highly promiscuous chimpanzees, the testicle size is about 4 ounces while they are only about 100 pounds in weight (Harcourt and Harvey, 1984; Kenagy and Trombulak, 1986). Thus, testicle size is considered a reliable indicator of mating systems of the species concerned. Human males have medium sized testicles indicating neither monogamous nor highly promiscuous behaviour. The production of about 400 million sperm per ejaculate in humans, suggests that ancestral females had multiple sex partners fairly often (Baker and Bellis, 1995).

In chimpanzees, the large ejaculate involves yet another means of sperm competition. In chimpanzees, only a very small percentage of sperm, possibly as little as 1 per cent, are capable of fertilization. The other 99 per cent work as blockers or are known as kamikaze sperm. These are of two types: Type A block the passage of sperm that enter the female tract after copulation and Type B attack sperm delivered prior to them (Baker and Bellis, 1988).

Sperm length determines speed, because a longer flagellum renders a stronger propulsive force (Gomendio and Roldan, 1991). The increase in sperm size with intensity in sperm competition was predicted by Stockley *et al.* (1997) but his analysis on the same in fishes showed it not to be true. However, the assumption of Stockley *et al.* (1997) found support in butterflies (Gage, 1994), frogs (Bryne *et al.*, 2003), rodents and primates (Gomendio and Roldan, 1991). Sperm longevity in lieu of sperm motility and sperm length are selected for in certain fishes since external fertilization basically requires long lived sperm owing to the distance to be covered to reach eggs and thus the increased amount of time taken.

Studies reveal that a male's chances of fathering a female's offspring may be increased if he delays or prevents her from re-mating (*e.g.* Birkhead and Moller, 1998). This may be achieved by mate-guarding, prolonged copulation, or physical removal of the female from the mating arena (*e.g.* Parker, 1970; Andersson, 1994; Birkhead and Moller, 1998) or by effectively occluding the female's reproductive tract after copulation (*i.e.* by producing a 'chastity belt' or putting a 'mating plug'), so that she is physically incapable of additional copulation at least for some time.

The mating plug is an effective means of sperm competition. Such structures have evolved independently in many groups of animals like nematodes (Barker, 1994), crustaceans (Diesel, 1990), bumblebees (Duvoisin *et al.*, 1999; Baer *et al.*, 2000), ants (Bourke and Franks, 1995), spiders (Masumoto, 1993), snakes (Shine *et al.*, 2000) and several mammals, such as squirrels, bats and primates (Koprowski, 1992; Tidemann, 1993; Dixson and Mundy, 1994). These plugs may be either mechanical as in case of damselfly where a part of the penis is left behind in the female tract after mating (Shine *et al.*, 2000) or through a cocktail of chemicals (Duvoisin *et al.*, 1999; Baer *et al.*, 2000).

The male genitalia of Argentine lake duck has a brush-like tip, which they probably use to scrub the sperm of previous mates from the female's oviduct (McCracken *et al.*, 2001). Similarly, the male damselfly scrubs the female genital tract to clean of sperm of previous males prior to ejaculation with the help of its genitalia that bears spines for the purpose (Waage, 1979). Such behaviour ensures that the higher number of progeny are sired by the last male to mate and is also known as the last male sperm precedence theory. Release of a cocktail of chemicals to ensure death of sperm of prior males is also a means to ensure higher fertilization rate of sperm of last male.

(*vi*) Cryptic Female Choice

The myriad processes of sperm competition discussed in the section above seem to indicate almost passive role of the female once the competing males have managed to mate and release their sperm. However, this is not the case. Females in quite a number of animals are known to possess the ability to choose which from amongst the sperm of a number of males present in her genital tract will fertilize her eggs. This is known as *cryptic female choice* and the term was coined by Randy Thornhill of University of Mexico in 1983.

Eberhard (1996) studied and reviewed the process in much detail. He argues that the females have greater post-copulatory potential to influence paternity than males and listed the ways by which females influence success of a particular copulation (Table 24.1). Pizzari and Birkhead (2000) have found that wild female chickens eject the sperm of subdominant males, while in mallard ducks the females alter the resources to be put into eggs depending on the mating drake (Cunnigham and Russell, 2000). In cricket, *Gryllus bimaculatus*, females are known to consume spermatophores of males attached to their body quickly while letting spermatophores of some males attached for longer, thereby increasing the chances of their sperm to fuse with the eggs.

(F) Examples of Sexual Selection across the Animal World

The animal world is full of numerous examples of sexual selection occurring through various mechanisms discussed above. Here a few vivid, eye catching and interesting examples of sexual selection in different groups of animals are being given in brief.

(*i*) Insects

Size is an important determinant of mating success and is well recorded in the insects, especially the dipterans. In the dance fly,

Table 24.1: List of Female Behaviour for Showing Cryptic Female Choice Adapted from Eberhard (1996)

Mechanism for which cases are known	*Potential Mechanisms for which examples are yet not known*
Premature interruption of copulation	Lack of sperm activation
Denial of deeper penetration of the male genitalia to internal sites where the males will have a better chance of being used	Lack of sperm nourishment
Lack of sperm transport to storage and/or fertilization sites within the female	Failure to seize and open spermatophores in the females bursa copulatrix
Discharge or digestion of the male's sperm	Changes in sperm leakage
Lack of ovulation	Changes in the efficiency of sperm usage
Lack of preparation of the uterus for implantation of embryos	
Abortion	
Lack of oviposition	
Rejection or removal of mating plugs	
Prevention of removal of mating plugs by subsequent males	
Removal of spermatophores before transferring contents	
Selective use of stored sperm	
Failure to trigger sperm-injecting mechanisms of spermatophores	
Failure to modify insemination ducts making remating more difficult	
Selective fusion with sperm that have reached the egg	
Failure to fully resource a particular male's offspring	
Lack of rejection of subsequent advances by other males	

Empis borealis, the mated females were larger than the refused females and also had lower wing wear indices, indicating the role of female size in the mate selection process (Svensson and Peterson, 1989). Gravid females of the yellow dung fly show clear preference for large males as they move towards the larger males on the dung pad and also towards the prime oviposition sites near the centre, where large males are already present. Large males of the dung fly are usually found on the pad whereas the smaller ones are usually found in the surrounding grass probably after their ouster by the large males (Borgia, 1982). In the fruit fly, *Drosophila melanogaster*, larger males have mating advantages over the smaller ones owing to both a longevity advantage and higher mating success for a given age (Partridge and Farquhar, 1983).

The size of the males is assessed by the form and intensity of the calling song of the Caribbean fruitfly, *Anaestrepha suspense*. The larger and sexually more successful males were found to have a higher calling propensity. They won more fights, and were observed repeating pulses of the calling song more quickly than rejected males (Burk and Webb, 1983). The sound pressure level of the approach of the male papaya fruit fly, *Toxotrypana curvicauda*, plays a crucial role in selection of the mate with the noisier larger males being preferred for mating (Silvinski and Webb, 1985).

Males of Japanese scorpionfly, *Panorpa japonica*, compete for sexual favours. First the male captures a nuptial gift preferably a caterpillar for the female and then releases a pheromone to attract the female which in turn also brings more competing males along. A fight ensues for the possession of the caterpillar which is usually lost to the more aggressive male who in turn presents it to the female, thereby winning copulation with her. Females are known to prefer aggressive males possessing nearly symmetrical forewings while rejecting those with higher fluctuating asymmetries (Thornhill, 1993).

The male white-tailed skimmer dragonfly, *Plathemis lydia*, displays the white upper surface of the abdomen toward other males competing for reproductive resources. Artificial blackening of the white surface diminishes territorial success of the males. This experimental elimination of the white colour pattern results in greater expenditure of energy on the part of the blackened males (Moller, 1992).

The strongest creatures on earth, the rhinoceros beetles, which can lift up to 850 times their own weight, fight with their long horns (about 2–3½ inches) for prime feeding site. The victorious males are then able to attract the hornless females. The stag beetle, so named for his enormous jaws that resemble the antlers of the stag, uses them to strut around the females in an attempt to impress her. However, if two males become interested for the same mate, they will fight each other using their jaws like the antler of the stage. The fight is over, once the stronger one of the two turns the other over on the back.

In ant *Cardiocondyla*, the males use their mandibles to pierce or crush the soft cuticle of young males, to sever their antennae or legs, to decapitate them or to cut their bodies into two (Heinze *et al.*, 1998). These ants have evolved powerful mandibles to end competition posed by young adults for the few virgin females present.

Female ladybirds are known to reject males attempting to mate by moving fast, kicking his genitalia, rolling around, dropping from height, *etc*. Two theories, *viz.* the rape and test hypotheses have been proposed to explain this behaviour. Rape hypothesis suggests that the female rejection behaviour is a means of preventing unwanted matings with male. While the test hypothesis regards these rejection attempts as the females plan to assess the ability of the male. The male able to overcome the rejection attempts is likely to bear good genes and it would be advantageous to the female to mate with him (Majerus, 1994).

Insects also possess some amazing examples of sperm competition. The pulse beetle, *Callasobruchus maculatus*, removes about 90-100 per cent of any competing sperm prior to releasing his own sperm in the female tract. The damselfly male too removes sperm with help of his brush tipped male genitalia structure prior to ejaculating his own sperm. After mating, the male tiger swallowtail butterfly deposits a small "mating plug" inside the female genital tract to prevent her from mating again (Russell, 2003). The Apollo butterfly goes one step further; after mating he secretes and glues a rigid structure called a "sphragis" over the abdomen of female mates. Unlike the mating plug, which is eventually dislodged, the heavy and awkward sphragis is meant to last a lifetime. The male zebra longwing stoops even lower, keeping watch over female pupae metamorphosing on the passion vines and, after puncturing the pupal skin, inserts his genitalia and rapes the female just before she emerges. Occasionally, she is injured during the rape and dies

(Russell, 2003). In the 2-spot ladybird, *Adalia bipunctata*, females were found to exert choice and preferred melanic males over non-melanic ones (Majerus, 1994). This has also been seen in C. *septempunctata* (Srivastava and Omkar, 2005) and *P. dissecta* (Mishra and Omkar, unpubl. data).

(*ii*) Vertebrates Other than Mammals

Fishes

Fishes present a few examples of the various types of competitions between males and the mate choice displays. The males of the beautiful mandarin fish, famed for its beauty and elusiveness are known to display their spiked dorsal fin on encountering another male competing for the female's attention. If this display does not lead to the backing of any one of the two, both the males then fight out till the death of any one (Norvich, 2001). Other than this apparent competition, larger males are known to be preferred by the females because it is likely that in the fight the larger one will win. However, the smaller males use alternative tactics; they swim near the mating pair and release their sperm hoping for a random fertilization to take place (Norvich, 2001).

The male Pacific blue eye, another fish, was found to spend more time courting larger females than the smaller ones (Wong and Jennions, 2003) perhaps owing to their higher fecundity (Wong and Jennions, 2003) and/or preference for males that actively court (Wong, 2004; Wong *et al.*, 2004). The guppies show a preference for bright orange coloured males over those that are less orange. In two-spotted gobies, males selected their mates based on the orange belly colouration in the females. When provided with differently coloured females, the males court the brightly coloured females more (Amundsen and Forsgren, 2001). This preference for bright colours is also reported in the stickle backs (Bakker and Mundwiller, 1994).

Amphibians

In the anurans, vocalizations usually play a role in sex recognition and mate choice (Halliday and Tejedo, 1995; Stebbins and Cohen, 1995). However, this chorusing behaviour is lacking in species that indulge in scramble (struggle or contend frantically) competition in high density populations (Hoglund and Robertson, 1988). The males of white-lipped tree frog are usually found perched

on creepers which entwine bamboo fencing or on tall grass near a water source. The first male call is influenced by the weather and may be anytime between 04:30 to 6:00 pm Indian time. This is followed by the call of the second male. The female responds by climbing from the leaf litter to about 10 cm from the male and utters a weak reciprocal call which then results in amplexus (Roy, 1997). The first male is at the highest position and thus his call is likely to be less attenuated and he is also the largest and heaviest and thus owing to both the reasons, attracts the maximum number of females.

In the gray tree frog, the females were found to prefer males' evocating calls with long duration. Females of this species do not derive any direct benefits from mate choice because males do not provide resources, protection or care and there is no difference in fertilization success between matings with males delivering short or long calls (Doty and Welch, 2001). However, it was demonstrated that offspring sired by males with calls of longer duration showed greater larval survival and growth, and greater juvenile growth (Doty and Welch, 2001). These offspring also metamorphosed earlier or at a larger size than those sired by males with short call durations. Therefore, call duration in male frogs appears to advertise genetic qual[illegible]fect female mate choice (Doty and Welch, 2001). In the mi[illegible], the selection is for the male who can provide better ca[illegible].

Reptiles

In the reptilians, mate choice has been studied most widely in lizards with that of snakes and crocodiles being largely ignored owing to the dangers involved. Among the lizards, the green anole lizard presents a bright and colourful example of competition for mate. Display for territory or winning in combat causes males to turn bright green. They also use their dewlaps and crest to impress the females (Tokarz, 1995).

Birds

The birds have some of the most interesting examples of mate choice. Other than the peacock, dealt with earlier in this chapter, there are numerous other examples of mate preference displays. The male satin bowerbird bearing blue plumage and blue irises decorates and displays his bower with lots of blue objects, usually blue fruits and flowers and also paints his bower blue with regurgitated food.

The male on preparing his bower, prances and preens in front to attract the female to his bower (Figure 24.3). The female enters and inspects the bower and then leaves to see the bower of another male. The bluer the bower, the more likely is the male to be selected for mating. While a chain of thought thinks of bower building as a means to display the male prowess, yet another interprets it as proof of food gathering ability as evinced through the decorations and the blueness of the walls, since their prime food is blueberries. The regent bowerbird, *Sericulus chrysocephalis,* with yellow patches on his plumage and yellow eye irises, uses yellow fruits in a similar manner as the satin bowerbird and thus probably supports the theory of decorations indicating food gathering and provisioning abilities. The males of the Laysan Albatross that are breeding for the first time indulge in elaborate courtship display involving twenty five different postures to impress the females. This bird is monogamous and pair bonds remain intact until death or disappearance of the partner. Figure 24.4 shows the "Sky Call" posture of the courtship dance.

The male paradise bird with his bright plumage dances and fluffs his feathers in front of the female to impress her with his colours and win a mating with her. The brighter and better displayed the plumage, the more are the chances to be selected by the female (Jacobs, 1999). Frith and Beehler (1998) in their book on birds of paradise have elaborated on their vivid courtship rituals. In some species, the males of these birds perform courtship displays on special branches or on carefully prepared courts on the forest floor. The male of the magnificent bird of paradise, spends most of his time, trimming the twigs, leaves and branches of trees to enable a bright shaft light to penetrate and illuminate his display patch like a spotlight on the stage. He then under the arc lights and with the female as his audience performs his displays with his beautiful, iridescent plumage shimmering with dazzling highlights. If the female is impressed she consents to mate and after the copulation flies away to lay eggs, while the male switches on his charms for yet another female. The brilliant orange plumes of the male raggianas, or Count Raggi's birds of paradise, are seen at their best during the birds' spectacular courtship dances. Males gather in groups at traditional courting sites on trees, each defending its own perch. When the brown females arrive, the males begin a frenzied bout of songs and dance, hopping about, flapping their wings and shaking their orange tail feathers. They then freeze in a head-down posture that shows off their tail

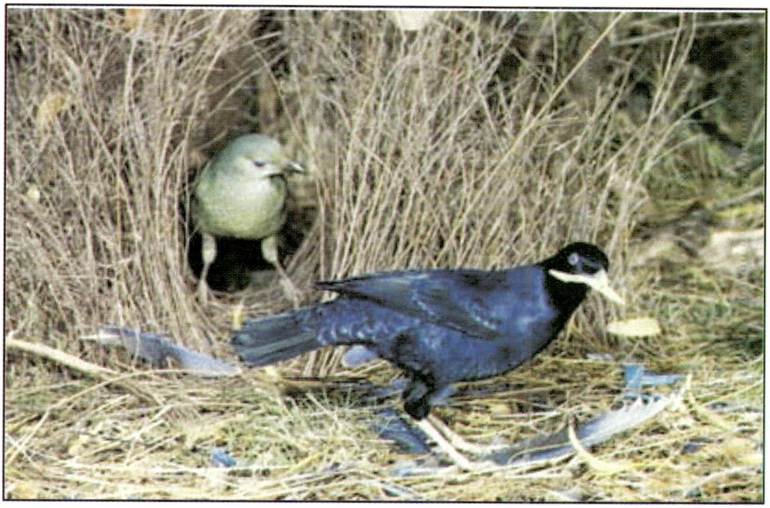

Figure 24.3: The Iridescently Blue Male of the Blue Satin Bowerbird Waits Eagerly Outside his Decorated Bower as the Plain Green Female Inspects it

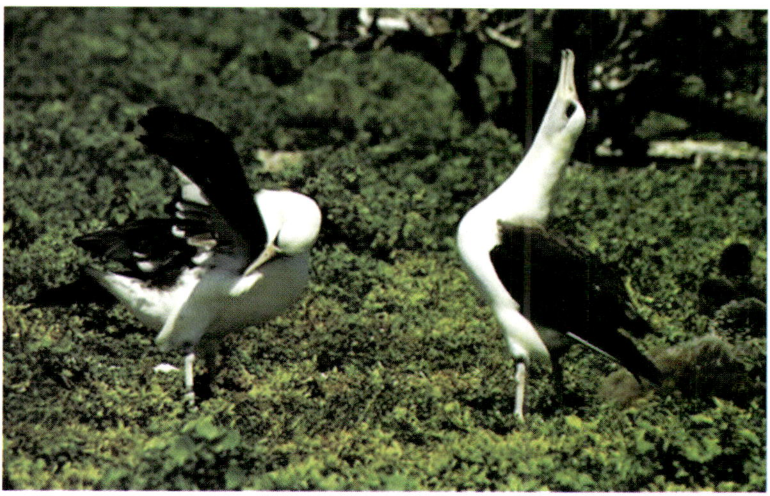

Figure 24.4: The Male of the Laysan Albatross (The one to the right) Shows the Sky-Call Posture of Courtship in an Attempt to Impress the Female who is Preening her Feathers

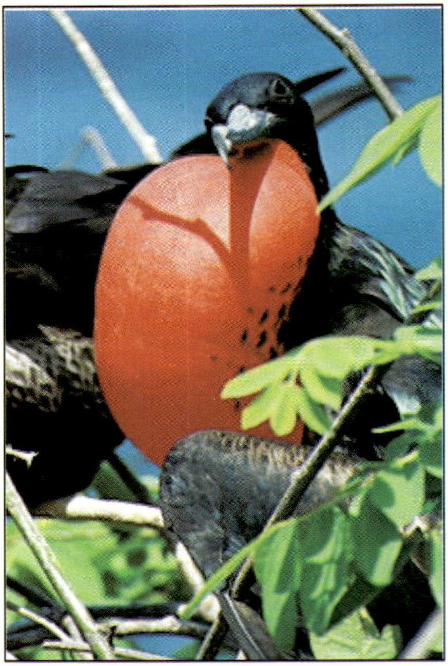

Figure 24.5: The Male of the Frigatebird can be seen Inflating his Bright Red Throat Pouch like a Balloon to Court the Females

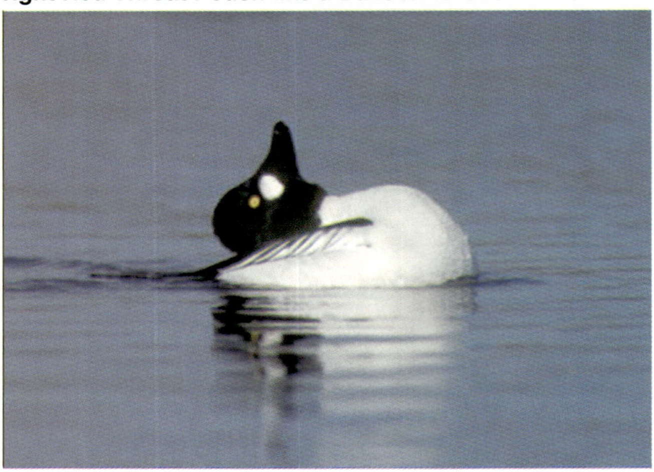

Figure 24.6: The Male of the Common Goldeneye Drake can be seen Dramatically Throwing their Head Backwards as part of their Courtship Display

feathers and allows female visitors to inspect them. If the female is unimpressed, she flies away to another site or else sits besides the male. The chosen mate then performs a brief pre-mating dance in an almost inverted position and by throwing his feathers over his head and into her face, while she plucks at his feathers. The males of the blue bird of paradise hang upside down and display beautiful performance by spreading out his iridescent blue tail plumes in a shimmering mass above the velvety black head and breast and his two-extra long black tail straps rise skywards in graceful curves. He then in this position proceeds to swing to and fro making strange grating calls.

Male frigatebirds seen along the coast of Ecuador and the Galapagos are known to inflate their red throat pouches during courtship to attract females (Figure 24.5). The courtship displays of waterfowl are prominently displayed. Drake Ruddy Ducks inflate tracheal air sacs in their necks, rapidly drum them with their bills, and then utter a low "squeak". Common Golden eye drakes dramatically throw their heads forward and back to their rumps, kick up a spray of water and give calls of "beep-beep" (Figure 24.6). Male Northern Pintails are known to gracefully arch their long necks, fluff up their scapulars, and point their tails skyward as they whistle low trills. Male drakes court the female through dramatic aerial displays with as many as ten drakes chasing a hen, with spectacular aerobatic performances at incredible speeds.

Møller (1992) found that experimental lengthening of the tail of barn swallow males led to earlier mating and therefore an increase in offspring. The elongated tail is probably used as a status symbol in competition for foraging territories (100-500m from the nesting sites). It acts as display of the male swallow's capabilities and avoids the usage of energy in activities such as physical fighting and competitive racing that would have to be undertaken to impress the females into mating in the absence of the morphological manifestations.

(*iii*) Mammals Other Than Humans

Male elephant seals collide violently with each other in a display of power and intense competition to find favour of mating with watching female. The dominant male is usually involved in a number of such fights ranging from 14 to 157 and has been successful in these. The number of matings received by the male elephant seals was found to be directly related to their status based on the number of fights won (Dewsbury, 1982; Hoelzel *et al.*, 1999).

In hamadryas baboon, colobus monkeys, langurs and gorillas, there is strong sexual selection for aggressiveness, including male size, strength, and weaponry (*e.g.* large canine teeth), resulting in high degrees of sexual dimorphism in body size and behaviour. The male is also allowed to mate with the female based on his ability to protect them and their offspring against predators (Dunbar, 1988) and infanticide by strange males (Hrdy, 1979).

In primate groups, where females move in groups of more than 10 or so, some males usually form coalitions to exclude other potential male mates. In such a system, males compete at several levels for mating and fertilization success such as sperm competition owing to female promiscuity, status competition since females prefer dominant males, development of individual aggressiveness as well as offspring and females protection and grooming qualities since females also prefer nice males (Smuts, 1987; De Waal, 1989).

An interesting display of sexual selection and female mate choice is seen in the baboons. The females do not differentiate between males within the social hierarchy in terms of the number of couplings (Hausfater, 1975). Almost all males in the baboon society receive an equal number of matings. From the outside, it seems that the females do not differentiate between statuses of males, then why has a hierarchical society evolved in male baboons? In depth research reveals that though the females do not seem to differentiate between males in terms of the number of matings, they do differentiate in the time of mating. Dominant males receive matings on the days when the female fertility is at highest (Hausfater, 1975). This was also found to be true for chimpanzees (Matsumoto-Odo, 1999). But weaker males can also trick the females into mating with him on her days of high fertility by demonstrating his willingness to provide protection to the female as well as her infants (Strum, 1987).

Thus, in the multi-male, multi-female groups of most primates, females exercise choice by joining groups that contain favoured males, initiating sex with them during estrus, supporting them during conflicts, and developing long-term social relationships with them. Females are also known to reject certain males by refusing to cooperate during copulation attempts, driving males away, or leaving the group themselves.

The displayed preference for parental care is not true since this display is to mate with a female since such a displayer is usually not the father of the infant and is attempting only to impress the female (Seyfarth, 1978; Smuts, 1985). Female primates may choose to mate promiscuously to maximize sperm competition and to confuse paternity, thereby inducing several males to protect the offspring and to guard against infanticide (Hrdy, 1979; Small, 1993). Despite Darwin's (1871) view of sexual selection for the various beards, tufts, and colourful hair styles that adorn male primates, female choice for aesthetic displays and indicators has rarely been investigated in primates.

In primates, examples of female competition and male mate choice are also present. In monogamous marmosets and tamarins, female compete to form pairs with quality males and drive off competing females. In unimale polygynous systems, the dominant male's sperm becomes a limiting resource, and high-ranking females prevent low-ranking females from mating through aggression and harassment (Small, 1988). This is also reported in the spotted hyenas and African wild dogs, where the females at alpha position in the pack mate almost exclusively with the male members of the pack and do not let the subordinate females procure matings (Creel *et al.*, 1997).

(*iv*) Human Beings

The process of sexual selection, which has usually been subconscious and innate in the animals has been refined and taken to realms of consciousness by the human beings.

The subconscious realm of sexual selection that has evolved in the humans dictates the innate selection for certain physical characteristics. Men are known to value physical characteristics, such as smooth skin, a small waist-to-hip ratio, and a youthful appearance in women (Buss, 1995), probably because these signal fertility and general health. On the other hand women prefer in men physical traits, such as height, muscularity, and broad shoulders (Buss, 1994; Barber, 1995) and personality traits, such as power, ascendance, and dominance (Botwin *et al.*, 1997) as they perhaps indicate their ability to provide resources. The desire for these traits is however malleable with reports suggesting that hungry women prefer taller men more than satiated women (Nelson and Morrison, 2002; Cate *et al.*, 2003). This is probably owing to some subconscious evolutionary correlation of height with the male's protective and food hunting abilities. The psychologists have shown that women are attracted to more masculine-looking men at the most fertile time of their menstrual cycle. During the less fertile times, they choose men with more feminine-looking faces. These are seen as kinder and more co-operative, but less strong and healthy genetically.

The lesser hair on bodies, more on heads, whiter eyes, longer noses, larger ear lobes, more everted lips, smaller and safer teeth, more expressive faces and more dextrous hands (Margulis and Sagan, 1991; Miller, 1993; Morris, 1985; Napier, 1993; Stoddart, 1990) have evolved to a persistent mate choice for such feature. The boom in studies on facial aesthetics (Alley and Cunningham, 1991; Brown and Perrett, 1993; Langlois and Roggman, 1990; Perrett, May, and Yoshikawa, 1994) reveals that average faces are attractive, but that females with more child-like faces, including large eyes, small noses, and full lips, are more attractive (Thornhill and Gangestad, 1993). On the other hand males bearing testosterone-enlarged features, such as high cheekbones, strong jaws, strong chins, and large noses, are preferred over others (Thornhill and Gangestad, 1993).

Evolutionary biologists believe that the process of male mate choice has shaped female breasts, buttocks, and orgasms, while mate choice by females has shaped male body size, beards, and penises. Mutual mate choice has probably influenced human hair, skin, eyes, lips, ears, face shape, hands, and pheromones (see Cate *et al.*, 2003). The preference for intelligence (Chance, 1962), leadership (Fox, 1972) better organizational and vocational capabilities (Caspari, 1972) in mates has played a role in the evolution of larger brains (Cate *et al.*, 2003).

The conscious process to select the best for the offspring is displayed by the institution of arranged marriage, where based on the fitness of the individual, in terms of family background, social and monetary status, looks, and physique, the potential bride or groom is selected. The wills of the humans to procure the best for the offspring and its conscious commercialization is best displayed by the latest trend to hit the masses, the concept of designer babies.

(G) Sexual Selection, Parental Investment and Mate Choice

It is quite apparent from the above account that the displayed choice by one sex for certain traits in the opposite sex during search for mate has shaped the morphology, physiology and behaviour of most animals on earth. What most of the above examples of intra- as well as inter-sexual selection reveal is that it is the males that generally compete and the females that usually choose and thus shape the future of the species. Why have these two sexes evolved such radically different roles? Why has the onus of selecting the mate been placed on the female's shoulders and not the males? Why do the males have to compete for females attention? These are the many questions that are yet to be answered. In this section it is aimed to present accounts to provide answers to these myriad questions.

To understand differences in the roles of the two sexes, it is necessary to go down to one of the most basic differences in the sexes, "the males produce sperm and the females produce eggs". Sperm are the smaller gametes that are produced to the count of millions and are more simply put just a set of genes placed in a package with just enough energy to reach its ultimate destination, the egg. The energy expenditure per sperm during production is thus not very high. The egg on the other hand utilizes a major amount of resources of the female. It is produced in exceedingly small quantities. Also, the role of this gamete is to ensure the development of the zygote, through the embryonic stages, till birth and thus, is loaded with enough energy to easily complete this process. An egg may constitute up to 15-20 per cent of the female body weight and sometimes even as high as 30 per cent (Lack, 1968). The fairy wren, a common bird in Australia, lays only about six eggs per nesting attempt while the male stores about 8 billion sperm at any given time in his testis (Tuttle *et al.*, 1996). In the case of humans, while a woman ovulates not more than 500 eggs in a lifetime, 5 million sperm are present in a single drop of the ejaculate of a normal man (http://www.sirinet.net/~jgjohnso/reproduction.html). The male of the ladybird *Adalia bipunctata* is capable of producing 42,415 offspring while the female's capability is a mere 2,341 (Majerus, 2003). Another example of this discriminating ability to produce offspring is evident in the elephant seals; the males are known to produce 100 offspring while the female is limited to just 8 (Krebs and Davies, 1987).

The point to make through these examples is that sperm is relatively easier and cheaper to produce and thus easier to dispense away with. The egg being a costly as well as scarce resource needs to be used with much caution. Thus in view of the immense reproductive resources available to the male, it seems quite obvious that their reproductive success will be governed by the increased number of offspring they sire. The higher the rate of fertilization, the greater is their fitness levels. On the other hand the female's success is limited by the number of eggs produced by them and the survival of these costly products. Moreover, the females often spend additional amount of time to raise their offspring and thus expend further more resources. Thus, in view of the large amount of expended energy by the females, they need to be more careful about whom they mate with and hence are choosy.

Due to the female occupation with nest building or caring for offspring, in most species, the number of females who are free to mate is significantly lower than the males who do not have any such responsibility and only need to mate to increase their fitness. This leads to a highly male biased operative sex ratio (*i.e.* number of sexually receptive males to sexually receptive females), indicating that either the males need to compete to gain access to the females or vow her with their vivid courtship endeavours.

All expenditures of time, energy and risks by a parent to increase the survival chance of their offspring while decreasing the chance of having more offspring is known as parental investment (Trivers, 1972). While increased parental investment increases the probability of existing offspring to reach its reproductive stage, it reduces their own chances of producing more offspring. The examples above indicate that it is usually the female that makes the larger parental investment.

The accepted pattern of scientific thought suggests that the two different types of sexual selection, *i.e.* intra- and inter-sexual selection, arise as a result of the differential parental investment. Further, females are choosy as they are the large investors, and males compete to make a space for themselves or attempt to impress owing to their larger number of gametes and subsequently lower parental investment. A flow chart depicting the evolutionary theory of differences between the sexes in sexual behaviour is given below (Figure 24.7).

The theories explaining male competition and female choice based on parental investment stand reversed when faced with examples in the animals of larger parental investment by the males and also lower reproductive potential. This can be witnessed in the empid flies, where the males are usually away from the swarm searching for food to bring to the females. When a food laden male re-enters the swarm, females advertise themselves in front of him to gain both food and mating (Funk and Tallamy, 2000). In the pipe fish and the sea horse where the male carries the young ones, and his reproductive potential is lower as it can carry only one brood at a given time, it is the females who compete and attract the males for their offspring caring resource. In ladybird species such as

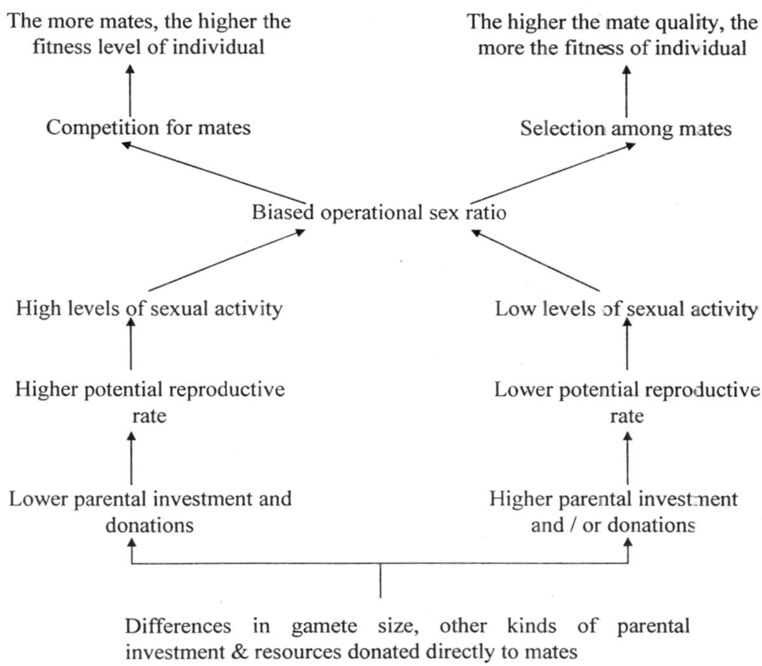

Figure 24.7: Flow Chart Depicting the Evolution of Differences Between Sexes as a Result of Differences in Parental Investment (Modified from Alcock, 2001)

Adalia bipunctata, which shows prominent female biased sex ratios (owing to infection with male killing bacteria); reversal of sex roles is likely to be seen (Majerus, 2006). Thus males will then be the limiting sex and would be likely to indulge in increased levels of mate choice while the females show varying levels of competition. This has been seen in the ladybird *Harmonia axyridis.* The levels of mating preference shown by the female members were found to vary with the prevailing sex ratios in the population (Osawa and Nishida, 1992).

(H) The Concept of Sexual Conflict

Till now, it is dealt with as to how the selection patterns of the more choosy sex shape the evolution of morphology and behavioural characteristics of species. The more popular conceived mechanism regarding the evolution of outstanding characteristics in animals indicating good health and genes was that of cooperation between the two sexes. However, recent studies now suggest the role of antagonism in shaping of ornamentations and energy draining displays.

The advocates of the latter theory believe that there is a basic conflict between the two sexes with regards to the attainment of their highest fitness levels; males attain high fitness by siring as many offspring as possible by indiscriminate matings, females on the contrary are expected to reach fitness peaks by allowing only a few matings with the best mates. This basic difference in the approach of the two sexes is known as *sexual conflict.*

The shaping of species specific highly exaggerated morphological and behavioural traits *via* sexual conflict has been explained by the chase-selection theory propounded by Holland and Rice (1998). As per this theory, at some point of time in the history of the species, a mutation probably led to the formation of a novel display trait which signals favourably to some pre-existing sensory preference of the female. Owing to this tapping into the subconscious preference, such a male would be preferred over other males even though he might provide only sensory satisfaction and not any material or genetic benefits. The population of such males would increase over the time owing to their success in procuring matings. Also under the influence of their sensory biases, the females would continue to select such males which are not of any benefit to the females. This prominent preference would lead to the evolution of exaggerated male traits which do not provide any benefit but rather fool the female into mating with the male; thereby increasing male fitness while decreasing that of the female. Hence, the occurrence of sexual conflict.

(II) Mating Systems

A study of the animals reveals myriad mating systems. In sociobiology and behavioural ecology the term mating system is used to describe the ways in which animal societies are structured in relation to sexual behaviour. The mating system specifies the number of males mating with the number of females under specific or different circumstances. There are cases where a male and female pair and live together until death and cases where the male remains faithful to the female who mates with other males. The reverse scenario of the female being faithful while the male mates with other females and a system where both males and females mate multiply with multiple males is also known in the animals. It is a matter of wonder why such myriad systems occur and why a single system does not meet the requirement of all animals. This section discusses the different types of mating systems, their examples in the animals and the reasons for their evolution.

(A) Classification of Mating Systems

A number of mating systems are recognized amongst animals and the below listed classification encompassess most widely accepted examples. The terminologies used to describe animal mating systems have been borrowed from a social anthropolgical approach where they are used to describe human mating systems realtive to marriage.

1. *Monogamy or Pair bonding*: This system deals with an exclusive sexual relationship between one male and one female. The word monogamy is of Greek etymology, with monos meaning single or only and gamos meaning mating.
2. *Polygamy*: Here one or more males have an exclusive sexual relationship with one or more females. This is divided into three sub classes:
   (*a*) *Polygyny*: This is one of the most common mating systems found in the vertebrates. In this a single male has a sexual relationship with two or more females.

(*b*) *Polyandry*: This is the reverse of polygyny and a single female maintains sexual relationship with two or more males

(*c*) *Polygynandry*: In this system as apparent by the terminology, two or more males have a sexual relationship with two or more females; the numbers of males and females need not be equal, and in vertebrate species studied so far, the number of males is usually less.

3. *Promiscuity*: This system is one step ahead of the polygamy setup and in this there are no exclusive sexual relationships, with any male within a social group mating freely with any female.

All the above mating relationships may or may not be social in nature, *i.e.* the sexual partners may or may not stay together as parenting partners. In case the mating partners stay together as parenting partners too, the mating sytsem would be known as *social* or else it is *genetic*. This is usually found in the monogamous pairs thus monogamy can be either social or genetic. However, this is not only restricted to the mongamous sytems. In many polyandrous systems, the male and females stay together to rear the young. In polygynous systems, where a number of females pair with a single male, the male usually transfers his attention and parenting skills to rearing the offspring of one female, while the other females rear them on their own. In the system of polygynandry, each of the males may assist one female. If all adults get together to rear the young then it is known as *communal breeding*. Any type of parental care is rare or completely absent in highly polygynous or promiscuous systems.

Before moving further, it is essential to understand that the study of such social relationships is easier than studying mating systems because the truth of the mating systems lies at the genetic level. DNA fingerprinting of offspring to verify paternity and thus the mating systems show that even in cases of monogamous systems, some offspring show different paternity. In certain species, these mating systems are liable to change with geographical location or food availability.

(B) Monogamy in Animals

Monogamy in the words of an absolute lay man would mean having only one sexual partner in a lifetime. It is already described earlier that male fitness in most animals is dependent on the number of matings they secure and the number of offspring they sire. In such a scenario, it would be more feasible for the males to procure and mate with as many females as possible because it is easier to mate with numerous females. Then the question arises, why are cases of monogamy evident in the animals, with a staggering 90 per cent of the bird species, 9 per cent of the mammals, 18 per cent of the primates, and 20 per cent of humans (in traditional societies) showing such a mating system.

Various explanations have been proffered to understand why males stop hunting for more mates after having found a sexual partner. The preferred and widely accepted explanations are (*i*) Mate-guarding, (*ii*) mate-assistance, and (*iii*) female-enforced monogamy.

The line of reasoning proposed by *Mate-guarding* hypothesis argues that monogamous behaviour would be adaptive in cases where females are sexually receptive even after a recent mating and thus it would be advantageous for the male to guard his mate against unwanted mating attempts from other males. A mating with another male leads to a possible sperm competition thus reducing the possible percentage of sired offspring from the first male (Emlen and Oring, 1977). In cases, where the females are difficult to locate and widely scattered, this hypothesis is likely to hold true. In the clown shrimp, the females are receptive for only a short duration every 3 weeks and are also widely scattered; thus, it is feasible for the male to pair off with a female rather than search for another. His behaviour is likely to result in 100 per cent siring of all eggs by the monogamous male, thereby increasing fitness (Wicker and Seibt, 1981).

The *mate-assistance* hypothesis promulgates that increased reproductive success of both mating partners as a result of parental care by male and his assistance of female would be enough to compensate for the opportunities lost by staying monogamous. This hypothesis is usually found relevant in explaining monogamous mating systems in birds. In the cave dwelling oil birds, the temperature of the nesting sites within the cave is always low necessitating the continuous presence of the female in order to keep her eggs warm and hence viable. Here, the male pairs for life, and increases his fitness levels by searching for food and feeding the female through the gestation of their clutches. This also results in the female's continuous presence over her eggs, thereby increasing their hatching success.

Another example of altricial birds (having relatively immobile young ones, with closed eyes and lacking hair), constant parental care is required to feed and protect the young ones. Pair-bonding or monogamy increases the reproductive success as one partner cares for the young ones while the other searches for food and provides protection. A single parent may not be able to collect enough food for a large brood and so would have to raise fewer young and hence be less reproductively successful. This is also reported in the penguins and herring gulls, where the female needs male to incubate and guard eggs while she feeds.

The hypothesis, female-enforced monogamy proposes as suggested by the name itself that the female per force stops the male from exploiting his polygynist tendencies. This hypothesis lends explanation to the behaviour shown by females of two absolutely different groups of animals: the insects and the birds. The females of the burying beetles and the razorbills attack the males with which they have mated if they show interest in other females. Here though it may be adaptive for the males to be polygynous, the females prevent this from happening.

Having discussed the probable reasons behind the occurrence of monogamy, a few more interesting examples of monogamy are being described. Unlike birds, the event of monogamy, social or otherwise, is very rare in mammals. This is probably because in most cases very little parental care is required of the males as the newly born young ones are precocial and the females have a steady supply of food (milk) available. Thus the males owing to their extremely low parental investment tend towards polygyny. There however are some outstanding examples of parental care and monogamy, chief amongst which is that of the male Djungarian hamster, which mate for life and also helps deliver their children. Without help of the male, it is not possible for the female to give birth as the male helps in the birthing process by pulling out the young ones out of the birth canal.

Certain examples of genetic monogamy have now been proved to be merely social involving only commitment to provide exclusive caring for offspring but none for exclusive mating. This differentiation between social and genetic monogamy has been tested through the process of DNA fingerprinting of the offspring of a monogamous pair. DNA fingerprinting of offspring of many species that were erstwhile considered as showing exclusive or genetic monogamy has revealed that they have been sired by more than one male through what are known as extra-pair copulations (EPC's). Such EPC's indicate the risk that a male may be spending his energy by caring for eggs and offspring that have been fertilized by the sperm of another male. However, there are still some examples of social as well as genetic monogamy, such as the common loons and the Florida scrub jays in which almost all the young ones were genetic offspring of the pair that cared for them (Piper *et al.*, 1997; Quinn *et al.*, 1999).

The occurrence of extra pair copulations from the female perspective carries more benefits than costs. The females by avoiding genetic monogamy gain both genetically and materially. The genetic benefits of extra-pair copulations are that through these females are able to (*i*) ensure fertility of their eggs in case their social partner is a partially or completely infertile male, (*ii*) increase the chance of their offspring bearing good genes, in the possibility of the social partner bearing poorer genes, and (*iii*) increase the chances of increased genetic compatibility between her eggs and sperm. The material benefits of extra pair copulations are that the females are able to (*i*) procure more resources or parental care, (*ii*) protection from sexual harassment, and (*iii*) reduce the likelihood of infanticide by creating confusion amongst males regarding the paternity of offspring.

(C) Polygamy in Animals

The term polygamy can also trace its roots to the Greeks with *polos* meaning multiple and *gamos* meaning mating. This is a more common mating system in the animals and can be subdivided into three mating systems, *viz.* polygyny, polyandry and polygynandry.

(*i*) Polygyny

Polygyny is a form of mating system in which males can monopolize sexual access to several females. This may be of four types, *viz.* female defense polygyny, resource defense polygyny, scramble competition polygyny and lek polygyny.

In *female defense polygyny*, receptive females live in defensible clusters for access to which the males compete. The winning male then has sexual access to almost all females of the clusters, thereby siring all offspring. This system can be found in the big horn sheep, gorillas (Harcourt *et al.*, 1981; Hogg, 1984), tropical bats (McCracken and Bradbury, 1981) and black birds (Webster, 1994). Dominant male in the tropical black bird tries to gain access to groups of nesting females in a tree and once successful is able to secure up to 80 per cent of the matings. These males do not defend a resource or a nesting site but rather shift from one nest trèe to another (Webster, 1994). In the impalas, during the rainy season, the females come into their estrous cycle probably owing to the presence of lush territories, which males defend vigorously. This is evolutionarily adaptive because females then receive an opportunity to build up energy reserves to help sustain her through her pregnancy and lactation (Macdonald 1984; van Rooyen 1996; Dunham and Murray, 1982). Female herds move through territories eating the food on them, and territory owner receives exclusive mating rights for these females (Estes 1999; Nowak 1991), thus exhibiting female-defense polygyny. The famous black faced Hanuman langurs of India also exhibit female defense polygyny.

In *resource defense polygyny*, females do not live in permanent groups but are spatially concentrated at food, nesting sites or other resources which are under the control of males. But how can it be advantageous for a female to share resources with a male that already has one or more sexual partners? Studies reveal that females of polygynous species benefit by sharing resources of a rich male rather than monopolizing those of a poor one. This was found to be true in the great reed warbler, where the offspring from predatory attacks of females sharing attractive nesting sites of a particular male were found to be safer than in the nesting sites of the less preferred males (Hansson *et al.*, 2000). In view of the safety of eggs, it is thus more advantageous to be polygynous. In the female African cichilid fish, *Lamprologus callipterus*, the females deposit eggs in empty gastropod shells which are searched and scavenged by males. The larger and more protected the collection of shells, the greater reproductive success is enjoyed by the males, thereby putting up an interesting example of resource defense polygyny (Alcock, 1998).

The *scramble competition polygyny* is found in the fireflies, ladybirds, thirteen-lined ground squirrels, etc. As suggested by the name, it involves an ungainly scramble for the females. This mating system occurs when females may be scattered or clustered. Males race to contact as many receptive females as possible without engaging in territorial defense. This is also reported in water striders where males run and compete for the attention of the females so as to grab a mating opportunity. The males of the thirteen lined ground squirrels also run and scramble for the female, and display overt conflict, sperm competition and competitive mate searching (Schwagmeyer, 1994).

In the *lek polygyny* mating system, males compete for high dominance ranking within a group, usually in a traditional display arena and the winner is selected by many females. This can be exemplified in hammer headed bats, white bearded manakins and a number of other bird species. It is the females who come to watch the males display their wares and abilities and the dominant one or the winner is then selected and mates with many females. The manakin males do beautiful leapfrog dances in front of the females hoping to catch attention. The possible reasons for formation of lek are (i) reduced chances of predation while displaying, (ii) requirement by males of specific habitat qualities that are patchily distributed, (iii) clumping in areas of females passage, (iv) preference of females for male clumps as it reduces predatory attempts, and (v) preference of females for clumped males as it facilitates mate choice since it reduces time and energy expenditure and also the risk of predation (Bradbury and Gibson, 1983).

(*ii*) Polyandry

In polyandry, the individual females may mate with more than one male per breeding season. Polyandry takes up a number of forms and can be broadly categorized into: (i) Polyandry without sex role reversal, and (ii) Polyandry with sex role reversal (Alcock, 1988).

In polyandry that does not involve sex role reversal; the females can be a part of this system for the purpose of sperm replenishment or for what is known as prostitution polyandry (Alcock, 1988). In *sperm replenishment* polyandry, the females mate with more than one male to secure additional sperm with which to fertilize a new clutch of eggs and is known in fruit flies and anoles. In *prostitution polyandry*, the females do this to gain access to the resources that the males control and offer only to females as in the case of humming birds, sources of nectar act as the resources.

In polyandry that occurs with reversal in sex role, the females indulge in this behaviour either owing to what is known as resource defense polyandry or male defense polyandry (Alcock, 1988). In *resource defense polyandry*, females control resources that are attractive to more than one male; males thus provide more parental care per offspring to gain access to resources. This behaviour is quite often seen in fishes. On the other hand in *male defense polyandry*, males provide neither resources nor greater parental investment but rather compete to monopolize mates in female aggregations as most evident in phalaropes and sandpipers. In phalaropes and the wattled jacanas, the females are larger and brighter than the males and they fight for males to whom they provide a clutch of eggs of mixed paternity to incubate. If the males fail to accept these mixed clutches, they are likely not to leave any sired offspring of their own; this behaviour thus being suicidal (Crews and Moore, 1986; Dale *et al.*, 1999). In some new world monkeys, such as callimicos, the dominant female suppresses ovulation in other subordinate females and monopolizes almost all males in the group for caring for the young ones, whether they are the fathers or not. The cooperative males are selected as mates.

(*iii*) Polygynandry

In this system, the animals of both the sexes have multiple sexual partners and would almost be similar to promiscuity, except for the fact that all the partners belong to a social group. For example, in the lions, promiscuity is prevented by the complex pride unit, *i.e.* the lions of both sexes mate randomly and have multiple partners but only within the pride. Since the pride limits the number of females and males available for mating, lions are termed as being polygynandrous (Bertram, 1975). Mating within a pride is first come first served. Since there is no dominance hierarchy amongst males or females, no mate selection is found to occur (Viljoen 2003).

(D) Promiscuity in Animals

In this system as explained earlier there is no limit on where you obtain your partner from or how many individuals you mate with. In the wildebeest mating systems, males gather in a ground with each male defending a patch of ground and competing for dominance (McFarland, 1985). These patches do not contain any resources but are rather display grounds. In the breeding season when the females pass through such an area, the males increase their territorial behaviour to such an extent that they begin to foam at the mouth, make pelvic thrusts, and spontaneously ejaculate (Moss, 1975). By doing so they attempt to impress females and break them into smaller groups that has only one estrus female and the rest are protectors. The male then mates with the estrus female (Moss, 1975). If the female cooperates with the male's intentions, the bull may mount her several times within the next few minutes. The female may then continue to move through other territories and mate with other bulls (Moss, 1975), while the male waits for another herd of females.

(E) Evolution of Mating Systems

Study of the myriad mating systems in the world leads us to question the possible factors responsible for their evolution. One of the major factors responsible for these vividly different mating systems is the process of sexual selection. This process specially plays a major role when understood in terms of parental investment. The degree of parental care and investment shown by the males determines which mating system is likely to be present in the species concerned. Species with more parental care and investment evolve to be monogamous, while those in which females put in more parental effort and males more mating effort usually evolve to be polygynous. In polygyny there is stronger or more intense sexual selection, but in monogamy it's not so intense.

Ecological factors also determine the evolution of mating systems. To explain this a term Environmental Potential for Polygyny (EPP) has been formulated. This term is an indicator of the distribution of the limiting resources of each sex, *i.e.* food for female and female for the male, within the species. Males are under constant pressure to monopolize multiple females. However, this tendency to monopolize will be dependent on the whether they will be able to gain sexual access to the females, which in turn is space and time dependent. Even distribution of females is likely to favour monogamy as it is harder to hold on to multiple females. But if the distribution of females is dependent on patchy food distribution they are likely to be found in clumps, which encourage the evolution of polygyny. The female distribution in time in terms of their sexual receptivity is also likely to evolve mating systems. If females of a species tend to become sexually receptive within a similar time period, it will be difficult for the males to be polygynous.

Thus to conclude with monogamy per se has evolved in conditions where either sex has the ability to monopolize multiple members of the opposite sex but do neither because of the impositions of ecological factors or parental care. That is monogamous behaviour evolves in animals in which parental care is indispensable to female reproduction and where females are spatially spirited or have synchronous sexual receptivity.

Polygyny on the other hand can evolve only if it the benefits of defending females outweigh the costs in males. Also, the males must be able to capitalize on their potential for polygyny, *i.e.* in scenarios where despite high potential for polygyny, if offspring are not likely to survive without the care of the male, the species is likely to display and evolve monogamy and not polygyny.

On the other hand, the evolution of polyandry is probably dependent on the outweighing of benefits to the female. Multiple matings with multiple males are deleterious to the females as they carry with them numerous costs, such as time and energy consumption (Thornhill and Alcock, 1983; Omkar and Mishra, 2005), increased risk of predation (Arnqvist, 1989) and disease transmission (Hurst *et al.*, 1995). It is only when these costs are outweighed by benefits like: (i) multiple nuptial gifts or resources from the males, (2) multiple males to help brood, (iii) reduced cost of sexual harassment, (iv) reduced cost of sexual competition between mates, (v) to hedge against possible infertility of a mate, (vi) acquisition of sufficient sperm to fertilize large number of eggs, (vii) guard against deterioration of too long storage of sperm, (viii) more genetically diverse offspring, (ix) promote sperm competition, and (x) possible female expression of a trait selected for in males, that polyandry is likely to evolve.

Through the descriptive account of myriad modes of sexual selection and also the different mating systems of animals contained in this chapter, it is hoped to ignite in the readers an appreciation for the beautiful workings of the animal world and also a scientific appreciation of the reasons for their occurrence and evolution.

References

Alcock, J., 1998. *Animal Behaviour: An Evolutionary Approach*. Sinauer Associates, Inc., Massachusetts.

Alcock, J., 2001. *Animal Behaviour*. Sinauer, Sunderland, MA, p. 543.

Alley, T.R. and Cunningham, M.R., 1991. Average faces are attractive, but very attractive faces are not average. *Psychological Science*, 2(2): 123-125.

Amundsen, T. and Forsgren, E., 2001. Male mate choice selects for female coloration in a fish. *PNAS*, 98 (23): 13155–13160

Andersson, M., 1982. Sexual selection, natural selection, and quality advertisements. *Biological Journal of the Linnean Society*, 17: 375-393.

Andersson, M., 1986. Evolution of condition-dependent sex ornaments and mating preferences: Sexual selection based on viability differences. *Evolution*, 40: 804-820.

Andersson, M., 1994. *Sexual Selection*. Princeton University Press, Princeton, New Jersey.

Atmar, W., 1991. On the role of males. *Animal Behaviour*, 41: 195-205.

Baer, B., Maile, R., Schmid-Hempel, P., Morgan, E.D. and Jones, G.R., 2000. Chemistry of a mating plug in bumblebees. *Journal of Chemical Ecology*, 26: 1869–1875.

Baker, R. R., and Bellis, M. A., 1995. *Human Sperm Competition*. Chapman and Hall, London.

Baker, R.R. and Bellis, M.A., 1988. "Kamikaze" sperm in mammals? *Animal Behaviour*, 36: 936-939.

Bakker, T.C.M. and Mundwiler, B., 1994. Female mate choice and male red coloration in a natural three-spined stickleback (*Gasterosteus aculeatus*) population. *Behavioural Ecology*, 5: 74-80.

Barber, N., 1995. The evolutionary psychology of physical attractiveness: Sexual selection and human morphology. *Ethology and Sociobiology*, 16: 395-424.

Barker, D.M., 1994. Copulatory plugs and paternity assurance in the nematode *Caenorhabditis elegans*. *Animal Behaviour* 48: 147–156.

Basolo, A.L., 1990. Female preference predates the evolution of the sword in swordfish. *Science,* 250: 808-810.

Bertram, B., 1975. Social factors influencing reproduction in wild lions. *Journal of Zoology,* 177: 463-482.

Betzig, L., Borgerhoff Mulder, M., and Turke, P., 1988. *Human Reproductive Behaviour: A Darwinian Perspective*. Cambridge University Press.

Birkhead, T.R., and Møller, A.P., 1998. *Sperm Competition and Sexual Selection*. Academic Press, San Diego, CA.

Blum, M.S., and Blum, N.A., 1979. *Sexual Selection and Reproductive Competition in Insects*. Academic Press, New York.

Borgia, G., 1982. Experimental changes in resource structure and male density: size related differences in mating success among male *Scatophaga stercoraria*. *Evolution,* 36: 307-315.

Botwin, M. D., Buss, D. M., and Shackelford, T. K., 1997. Personality and mate preference: Five factors in mate selection and marital satisfaction. *Journal of Personality,* 65: 107-136.

Bourke, A.F.G. and Franks, N.R., 1995. *Social Evolution in Ants*. Princeton University Press, Princeton, New Jersey, 529 pp.

Boyce, M. S., 1990. The Red Queen visits sage grouse leks. *American Zoologist,* 30: 263-270.

Bradbury, J.W. and Gibson, R., 1983. Leks and mate choice. In: *Mate Choice,* (Ed.) P. Bateson. Cambridge University Press, Cambridge, p. 109-139.

Brown, E., and Perrett, D.I., 1993. What gives a face its gender? *Perception,* 22: 829-840.

Burk, T., and Webb, J.C., 1983. Effect of male size on calling propensity, song parameters, and mating success in Caribbean fruit flies, *Anastrepha suspensa* (Loew) (Diptera: Tephritidae). *Annals of the Entomological Society of America,* 76: 678-681.

Burley, N., 1988. Wild zebra finches have band-color preferences. *Animal Behaviour,* 36: 1235-1237.

Buss, D.M., 1994. *The Evolution of Desire: Strategies of Human Mating*. Basic Books, New York.

Buss, D.M., 1995. Evolutionary desire: A new paradigm for psychological science. *Psychological Inventory*, 6: 1-30.

Byrne, P.G., Simmons, L.W. and Roberts, J.D., 2003. Sperm competition and the evolution of gamete morphology in frogs. *Proceedings of Biological Sciences*, 270: 2079-2086.

Byrne, R., and Whiten, A., 1988. *Machiavellian Intelligence: Social Expertise and the Evolution of Intellect in Monkeys, Apes and Humans*. Oxford University Press.

Campbell, B., 1972. *Sexual Selection and the Descent of Man, 1871-1971*. Aldine Atherton, Chicago.

Caspari, E., 1972. Sexual selection in human evolution. In: *Sexual Selection and the Descent of Man*, (Ed.) B. Campbell. Aldine, Chicago, pp. 87-104.

Catchpole, C.K., 1987. Bird song, sexual selection and female choice. *Trends in Evolution and Ecology*, 2: 94-97.

Cate, K.L., Bassett, J.F. and Dabbs, J.M. Jr., 2003. Fear Primes may not affect women's implicit and explicit mate preferences. *JASNH*, 1(4): 49-56.

Chance, M.R.A., 1962. Social behaviour and primate evolution. In: *Culture and the Evolution of Man*, (Ed.) M.F.A. Montagu. Oxford University Press, pp. 84-130.

Charlesworth, B., 1987. The heritability of fitness. In: *Sexual Selection: Testing the Alternatives*, (Eds.) J.W. Bradbury and M.B. Andersson. John Wiley, New York, pp. 21-40.

Clutton-Brock, T.H., 1991. *The Evolution of Parental Care*. Princeton University Press.

Cott, H.B., 1940. *Adaptive Coloration in Animals*. Methuen, London.

Creel, S., Creel, N.M., Mills, M.G.L. and Monfort, S.L., 1997. Rank and reproduction in cooperatively breeding African wild dogs: Behavioural and endocrine correlates. *Behavioural Ecology*, 8: 298-306.

Crews, D. and Moore, M.C., 1986. Evolution of mechanisms controlling mating behaviour. *Science*, 231: 121-125.

Cronin, H., 1991. *The Ant and the Peacock: Altruism and Sexual Selection from Darwin to Today*. Cambridge University Press.

Cunnigham, E.J.A., and Russell, A.F., 2000. Egg investment is influenced by male attractiveness in the mallard. *Nature,* 404: 74-77.

Dale, J., Montogomerie, R., Michaud, D and Boag, P., 1999. Frequency and timing of extrapair fertilization in the polyandrous red phalarope (*Phalaropus fucilarius*). *Behavioural Ecology and Sociobiology,* 46: 50-56.

Darwin, C.A., 1859. *On the Origin of Species*. Murray, London.

Darwin, C.A., 1871. *The Descent of Man and Selection in Relation to Sex*. John Murray, London; A.L. Burt Publ., 2nd Ed., 1874, New York.

De Waal, F., 1982. *Chimpanzee Politics*. Harper and Row, New York.

De Waal, F., 1989. *Peacemaking Among Primates*. Harvard University Press, Cambridge, MA.

Dewsbury, D.A., 1982. Dominance rank, copulatory behaviour, and differential reproduction. *Quarterly Review of Biology,* 57: 135-158.

Diesel, R., 1990. Sperm competition and reproductive success in the decapod *Inachus phalangium* (*Majidae*): A male ghost spider crab that seals off rivals' sperm. *Journal of Zoology,* 220: 213–224.

Dixson, A.F. and Mundy, N.I., 1994. Sexual behaviour, sexual swelling, and penile evolution in chimpanzees (*Pan troglodytes*). *Archives of Sexual Behaviour,* 23: 267–280.

Doty, G.V. and Welch, A.M. 2001. Advertisement call duration indicates good genes for offspring feeding rate in gray tree frogs (*Hyla versicolor*). *Behavioural Ecology and Sociobiology,* 49: 150-156.

Dunbar, 1988. *Primate Social Systems*. Chapman Hall and Yale University Press.

Dunham, K.M. and Murray, M.G., 1982. The fat reserves of impala, *Aepyceros melampus*. *African Journal of Ecology,* 20(2): 81-88.

Duvoisin, N., Baer, B., and Schmid-Hempel, P., 1999. Sperm transfer and male competition in the bumblebee *Bombus terrestris*. *Animal Behaviour,* 58: 743–749.

Eberhard, W.G., 1985. *Sexual Selection and Animal Genitalia*. Harvard University Press, Cambridge.

Eberhard, W.G., 1996. *Female Control: Sexual Selection by Cryptic Female Choice*. Princeton University Press, Princeton, New Jersey.

Emlen, S.T. and Oring, W.L., 1977. Ecology, sexual selection and the evolution of mating systems. *Science*, 197: 215-223.

Endler, J.A., 1993. Some general comments on the evolution and design of animal communication systems. *Philosophical Transaction of the Royal Society, London, B*. 340: 215-225.

Estes, R.D., 1999. *The Safari Companion*. Rev. Ed. Chelsea Green Publishing Company: White River Junction, pp. 459.

Fisher, R.A., 1915. The evolution of sexual preference. *Eugenics Review*, 7: 184-192.

Fisher, R.A., 1930. *The Genetical Theory of Natural Selection*. Clarendon Press.

Fox, R., 1972. Alliance and constraint: Sexual selection in the evolution of human kinship systems. In: *Sexual Selection and the Descent of Man, 1871-1971*, (Ed.) B. Campbell. Aldine Atherton, Chicago, pp. 282-311.

Frith, C.B. and Beehler, B.M., 1998. *The Birds of Paradise*. Oxford University Press, Oxford.

Funk, D.H. and Tallamy, D.W., 2000. Courtship role reversal and deceptive signals in the long-tailed dance fly, *Rhamphomyia longicauda*. *Animal Behaviour*, 59: 411-421.

Gage, M.J.G., 1994. Associations between body size, sperm competition, testis size and sperm sizes across butterflies. *Proc. R. Soc. London Ser. B*, 258: 247-254.

Gomendio, M. and Roldan, E.M.S., 1991. Sperm competition influences sperm size in mammals. *Proc. R. Soc. London Ser. B*, 243: 181-185.

Grafen, A., 1990. Biological signals as handicaps. *Journal of Theoretical Biology*, 144: 517-546.

Halliday, T.R. and Tejedo, M. 1995. Intrasexual selection and alternative mating behaviour. In: *Amphibian Biology, Vol. 2: Social Behaviour*, (Eds.) H. Heatwole and B.K. Sullivan. Chipping Norton: Surrey Beatty, pp. 419–468.

Hamilton, W.D., Axelrod, R., and Tanese, R., 1990. Sexual reproduction as an adaptation to resist parasites: A review.

Proceedings of the National Academy of Sciences, USA, 87: 3566-3573.

Hamilton, W.D. and Zuk, M., 1982. Heritable true fitness and bright birds: A role for parasites? *Science,* 218: 384-387.

Hansson, B., Bensch, S. and Hasselquist, D., 2000. Patterns of nest predation contribute to polygyny in the great reed warbler. *Ecology,* 81: 319-328.

Harcourt, A. H., and Harvey, P. H., 1984. Sperm competition, testes size, and breeding systems in primates. In: *Sperm Competition and the Evolution of Animal Mating Systems,* (Ed.) R. Smith. Academic Press, New York.

Harcourt, A.H., Harvey, P.H., Larson, S.G. and Short, R.V., 1981. Testis weight, body weight and breeding system in primates. *Nature,* 293: 55-57.

Hausfater, G., 1975. Dominance and reproduction in baboons (*Papio cynocephalus*): A quantitative analysis. *Contributions in Primatology,* 7: 1-150.

Hausfater, G., and Hrdy, S.B., 1984. *Infanticide: Comparative and Evolutionary Perspectives.* Aldine, New York.

Heinze, J., Holldobler, B. and Yamuchi, K., 1998. Male competition in *Cardiocondyla* ants. *Behavioural Ecology and Sociobiology,* 29: 9-12.

Heywood, J.S., 1989. Sexual selection by the handicap mechanism. *Evolution,* 43: 1387-1397.

Hoelzel, A.R., Le Boeuf, B.J., Reiter, J. and Campagna, C., 1999. Alpha-male paternity in elephant seals. *Behavioural Ecology and Sociobiology,* 46: 298-306.

Hoelzer, G.A., 1989. The good parent process of sexual selection. *Animal Behaviour,* 38(6): 1067-1078.

Hogg, J.T., 1984. Mating in bighorn sheep: Multiple creative male strategies. *Science,* 225: 526-529.

Hoglund, J. and Robertson, G.M., 1988. Chorusing behaviour, a density-dependent alternative mating strategy in male common toads (*Bufo bufo*). *Ethology,* 79: 324–332.

Holland, B., and Rice, W.R., 1998. Chase-away sexual selection; antagonistic seduction versus resistance. *Evolution,* 52: 1-7.

Hrdy, S. B., 1979. Infanticide among animals: A review, classification, and examination of the implications for the reproductive strategies of females. *Ethology and Sociobiology*, 1: 13-40.

Huxley, J.S., 1938. Darwin's theory of sexual selection and the data subsumed by it in the light of recent research. *American Naturalist* 72: 416-433

Iwasa, Y., Pomiankowski, A., and Nee, S., 1991. The evolution of costly mate preferences. II. The 'handicap' principle. *Evolution*, 45(6): 1431-1442.

Jacobs, M.E., 1999. Mr. Darwin misread Miss Peacock's mind: a new look at mate selection in light of lessons from nature. Nature Books.

Kenagy, G.J. and Trombulak, S.C., 1986. Size and function of mammalian testes in relation to body size. *Journal of Mammalogy*, 67: 1-22

Kirkpatrick, M., 1982. Sexual selection and the evolution of female choice. *Evolution*, 36: 1-12.

Kirkpatrick, M., 1987. The evolutionary forces acting on female preferences in polygynous animals. In: *Sexual Selection: Testing the Alternatives*, (Eds.) J.W. Bradbury and M.B. Andersson. John Wiley, New York, pp. 67-82.

Kondrashov, A., 1988. Deleterious mutations as an evolutionary factor III. Mating preference and some general remarks. *Journal of Theoretical Biology*, 131: 487-496.

Koprowski, J.L., 1992. Removal of copulatory plugs by female tree squirrels. *Journal of Mammalogy*, 73: 572–576.

Krebs, J.R. and Davies, N.B., 1987. *An Introduction to Behavioural Ecology*. Blackwell Scientific Publications, Oxford.

Lack, D., 1968. *Ecological Adaptations for Breeding in Birds*. Methuen, London.

Lande, R., 1981. Models of speciation by sexual selection on polygenic characters. *Proc. Nat. Acad. Sciences USA*, 78: 3721-3725.

Langlois, J. H., and Roggman, L. A., 1990. Attractive faces are only average. *Psychological Science*, 1(2): 115-121.

Low, B., 1990. Marriage systems and pathogen stress in human societies. *American Zoologist*, 30: 325-339.

Macdonald, D., 1984. *The Encyclopedia of Mammals*. Facts on File, Inc., New York.

Majerus, M.E.N., 1994. *Ladybirds*. Harper Collins, UK, p. 359.

Majerus, M.E.N., 2003. *Sex Wars: Genes, Bacteria, and Biased Sex Ratios*. Princeton University Press, Princeton and Oxford, pp. 250.

Majerus, M.E.N., 2006. The impact of male-killing bacteria on the evolution of aphidophagous coccinellids. *European Journal of Entomology*, 103: 1-7.

Margulis, L., and Sagan, D., 1991. *Mystery Dance: On the Evolution of Human Sexuality*. Summit Books, New York.

Masumoto, T., 1993. The effect of the copulatory plug in the funnel-web spider, *Agelena limbata* (Araneae: Agelenidae). *Journal of Arachanology*, 21: 55–59.

Matsumoto-Oda, A., 1999. Female choice in the opportunistic mating of wild chimpanzees (*Pan troglodytes schweinfurthii*) at Mahale. *Behavioural Ecology and Sociobiology*, 46: 258-266.

McCracken, G.F. and Bradbury, J.W., 1981. Social organization and kinship in the polygynous bat *Phyllostomus hastatus*. *Behavioural Ecology and Sociobiology*, 8: 11-34.

McCracken, K.G., Wilson, R. E., McCracken, P.J. and Johnson, K.P., 2001. Are ducks impressed by drakes' display. *Nature*, 413: 128.

McFarland, D., 1985. *Animal Behaviour*. Benjamin Cummings.

Michod, R.E. and Levin, B.R., 1988. *The Evolution of Sex: An Examination of Current Ideas*. Sinauer.

Miller, G.F., 1993. Evolution of the human brain through runaway sexual selection: The mind as a protean courtship device. *Ph.D. Thesis*, Stanford Psych Dept, Stanford University, USA.

Miller, G.F., 1998. How mate choice shaped human nature: A review of sexual selection and human evolution. In: *Handbook of Evolutionary Psychology: Ideas, Issues and Applications*, (Eds.) C. Crawford and D. Krebs . Lawrence Erlbaum, pp. 87-130.

Moller, A.P., 1988. Female choice selects for male sexual tail ornaments in the monogamous swallow. *Nature*, 332(6165): 640-642.

Moller, A.P., 1992. Female swallow preference for symmetrical male sexual ornaments. *Nature*, 357: 238-240.

Moller, A.P. and Pomiankowski, A., 1993. Fluctuating asymmetry and sexual selection. *Genetics*, 89: 267-279

Morris, D., 1985. *Bodywatching: A Field Guide to the Human Species*. Crown Books, New York.

Moss, C., 1975. *Portraits in the Wild Boston*. Houghton Mifflin Company.

Napier, J., 1993. *Hands*. Princeton University Press.

Nelson, L.D. and Morrison, E.L., 2005. The symptoms of resource scarcity: judgments of food and finances impact preferences for potential partners. *Psychological Science*, 16: 167-173.

Norvich, S.N., 2001. *The Magical Mandarins*. http://underwaterphotos.com/article3.htm

Nowak, R. M., 1991. *Walker's Mammals of the World*. John's Hopkins University Press, Baltimore.

O'Donald, P., 1980. *Genetic Models of Sexual Selection*. Cambridge University Press.

Omkar and Mishra, G., 2003. Chrysopids: An effective pest management tool. In: *Biopesticides and Bioagents in Integrated Pest Management of Agricultural Crops*, (Ed.) R.P. Srivastava. International Book Distributing Co., Lucknow, p. 671-719.

Omkar and Mishra, G., 2005. Evolutionary significance of promiscuity in an aphidophagous ladybird, *Propylea dissecta* (Coleoptera: Coccinellidae). *Bulletin of Entomological Research*, 95(6): 527-533.

Omkar and Mishra, G., 2005. Mating in aphidophagous ladybirds: costs and benefits. *Journal of Applied Entomology*, 129(8): 32-436.

Parker, G.A., 1984. Sperm competition. In: *Sperm Competition and Animal Mating Systems*, (Ed.) R.L. Smith. Academic Press, New York.

Parker, G.A., 1990. Sperm competition games: raffles and roles. *Proceedings of the Royal Society of London, Series B*, 242:120-126.

Parker, G.A. 1970. Sperm competition and its evolutionary consequences in insects. *Biological Reviews*, 45: 525-567.

Patridge, L., and Farquhar, M., 1983. Lifetime mating success of male fruitflies (*Drosiphila melanogaster*) is relared to their size. *Animal Behaviour*, 31: 871-877.

Perrett, D.I., May, K.A., and Yoshikawa, S., 1994. Facial shape and judgments of female attractiveness. *Nature*, 368: 239-242.

Petrie, M., 1992. Peacocks with low mating success are more likely to suffer predation. *Animal Behaviour*, 44: 585-586.

Petrie, M., Halliday, T. and Sanders, C. 1991. Peahens prefer peacocks with elaborate trains. *Animal Behaviour*, 41: 323-331.

Piper, W.H., Evers, D.C., Meyer, M.W., Tischler, K.B., Kaplan, J.D. and Feischler, R.C., 1997. Genetic monogamy in the common loon (*Gavia immer*). *Behavioural Ecology and Sociobiology*, 41: 25-32.

Pizzari, T. and Birkhead, T.R., 2000. Female feral fowl eject sperm of sub-dominant males. *Nature*, 405: 787-789.

Pomiankowski, A., 1987. The costs of choice in sexual selection. *Journal of Theoretical Biology*, 128: 195-218

Pomiankowski, A., 1988. The evolution of female mate preferences for male genetic quality. *Oxford Surveys in Evolutionary Biology*, 5: 136-184.

Pomiankowski, A., 1995. A resolution of the lek paradox. *Proceedings of the Royal Society London Series B*, 260 (1357), 21-29.

Price, T. D., Schluter, D., and Heckman, N. E., 1993. Sexual selection when the female directly benefits. *Biological Journal of the Linnean Society*, 48: 187-211.

Quinn, J.S., Woolfenden, G.E., Fitzpatrick, J.W. and White, B.N., 1999. Multi-locus DNA fingerprinting supports genetic monogamy in Florida scrub-jays. *Behavioural Ecology and Sociobiology*, 45:1-10.

Reynolds, J.D. and Gross, M.R., 1992. Female mate preference enhances offspring growth and reproduction in a fish, *Poecilia reticulata*. *Proceedings of the Royal Society London Series B*, 250: 57-62.

Reynolds, J.D. and Gross, M.R., 1990. Costs and benefits of female choice: Is there a lek paradox? *American Naturalist*, 136: 230-243.

Rice, W.R., 1988. Heritable variation in fitness as a prerequisite for adaptive female choice: The effect of mutation-selection balance. *Evolution*, 42: 817-820.

Richards, R. J., 1987. *Darwin and the Emergence of Evolutionary Theory of Mind and Behaviour*. University of Chicago Press.

Roy, D., 1997. Communication signals and sexual selection in amphibians. *Current Science*, 72: 923-927.

Rushton, J.P., 1989. Genetic similarity, human altruism, and group selection. *Behavioural and Brain Sciences*, 12: 503-559.

Russell, S.A., 2003. *An Obsession with Butterflies*. William Heinemann.

Ryan, M.J., 1985. *The Tungara Frog: A Study in Sexual Selection and Communication*. University of Chicago Press.

Ryan, M.J., 1990. Sexual selection, sensory systems, and sensory exploitation. *Oxford Surveys of Evolutionary Biology*, 7: 156-195.

Schwagmeyer, P.L., 1994. Competitive mate searching in the 13-lined ground squirrel: potential role of spatial memory? *Ethology*, 98: 265-276.

Searcy, W.A., 1982. The evolutionary effects of mate selection. *Annual Reviews of Ecology and Systematics*, 13: 57-85.

Seyfarth, R. M., 1978. Social relationships among adult male and female baboons, 1: Behaviour during sexual courtship. *Behaviour*, 64: 204-226.

Shine, R., Olsson, M.M. and Mason, R.T., 2000. Chastity belts in gartersnakes: the functional significance of mating plugs *Biological Journal of the Linnean Society*, 70: 377–390

Silvinski, J., and Webb, J.C., 1985. The form and function of acoustic courtships signals of the papaya fruit fly *Toxotrypana curricauda* (Tephritidae) *Florida Entomoogical Society*, 68: 634-641.

Singh, D., 1993. Waist-to-hip ratio (WHR): A defining morphological feature of health and female attractiveness. *Journal of Personality and Social Psychology*, 65(2): 293-307.

Small, M., 1988. Female primate sexual behaviour and conception: Are there really sperm to spare? *Current Anthropology*, 29(1): 81-100.

Small, M., 1993. *Female Choices: Sexual Behaviour of Female Primates*. Cornell University Press.

Smith, R., 1984. Human sperm competition. In: *Sperm Competition and the Evolution of Animal Mating Systems*, (Ed.) R. Smith. Academic Press, New York.

Smuts, B.B., 1985. *Sex and Friendship in Baboons*. Aldine, New York.

Smuts, B.B., 1987. Sexual competition and mate choice. In: *Primate Societies*, (Eds.) B.B. Smuts, D.L. Cheney, R.M. Seyfarth, R.W. Wrangham, and T.T. Struthsaker. University of Chicago Press, pp. 385-399.

Srivastava, S. and Omkar, 2005. Short and long term benefits of promiscuity in a seven-spotted ladybird, *Coccinella septempunctata*. *International Journal of Tropical Insect Science*, 25(3): 176-181.

Stebbins, R.C. and Cohen, N.W. 1995. *A Natural History of Amphibians*. Princeton University Press, Princeton, New Jersey.

Stockley, P.M., Gage, J.G., Parker, G.A. and Møller, A.P., 1997. Sperm competition in fishes: the evolution of testis size and ejaculate characteristics. *American Naturalist*, 149: 933-954.

Stoddart, D. M., 1990. *The Scented Ape: The Biology and Culture of Human Odour*. Cambridge University Press.

Strum, S.C., 1987. *Almost Human*. W.W. Norton, New York.

Svensson, B.G. and Petersson, E., 1987. Sex-role reversed courtship behaviour, sexual dimorphism and nuptial gifts in the dance fly, *Empis borealis* (L.). *Annales Zoologica Fennica*, 24: 323-334.

Symons, D., 1979. *The Evolution of Human Sexuality*. Oxford University Press.

Thornhill, N.W., 1991. An evolutionary analysis of rules regulating human inbreeding and marriage. *Behavioural and Brain Sciences*, 14: 247-293.

Thornhill, N.W., 1993. *The Natural History of Inbreeding and Outbreeding*. Chicago University Press.

Thornhill, R. and Gangestad, S.W., 1993. Human facial beauty: Averageness, symmetry, and parasite resistance. *Human Nature*, 4(3): 237-269.

Thornhill, R., and Alcock, J., 1983. *The Evolution of Insect Mating Systems*. Harvard University Press, Cambridge, Massachusetts.

Tidemann, C.R., 1993. Reproduction in the bats *Vespadelus vulturnus*, *Vespadelus regulus* and *Vespadelus darlingtoni* (Microchiroptera: Vespertilionidae) in coastal south-eastern Australia. *Australian Journal of Zoology*, 41: 21–35.

Tokarz, R.R., 1995. Mate choice in lizards: A review. *Herpetological Monographs*, 9: 17-40.

Tomlinson, I.P.M., 1988. Diploid models of the handicap principle. *Heredity*, 60: 283-293.

Trivers, R., 1972. Parental investment and sexual selection. In: *Sexual Selection and the Descent of Man 1871-1971*, (Ed.) B. Campbell. Aldine, Chicago, pp. 136-179.

Tuttle, E.M., Pruett-Jones, S. and Webster, M.S., 1996. Cloacal protuberances and extreme sperm production in Australian fairy-wrens. *Proceedings of the Royal Society London, B*, 263: 1359-1364.

van Rooyen, A.F., 1996. Simulated protein requirements and seasonal breeding in Impala Aepyceros Melampus. *South African Journal of Wildlife Research*, 26(3): 77-81.

Viljoen, P., 2003. African Lion Working Group: Dedicated to African Lion Conservation. 2003, African Lion Working Group. http://www.african-lion.org/lions_e.htm.

Waage, J.K., 1979. Dual function of the damselfly penis: Sperm removal and transfer. *Science*, 203: 916–918.

Waitt, C., Little, A.C., Wolfensohn, S. Honess, P., Brown, A.P., Buchanan-Smith, H.M. and Perrett, D.I., 2003. Evidence from rhesus macaques suggests male colouration plays a role in female primate mate choice. *Proceedings of the Royal Society: Biology Letters*, 270: 144-146.

Wallace, A.R., 1870. *Contributions to the Theory of Natural Selection*. Macmillan, London.

Wallace, A.R., 1889. *Darwinism*, 3rd edn. Macmillan, London.

Webster, M.S., 1994. Female-defence polygyny in a neotropical bird, the *Montezuma oropendula*. *Animal Behaviour*, 48: 779-794.

Wickler, W. and Seibt, U., 1981. Monogamy in crustacea and man. *Zeitschrift fur Tierpsychologie*, 57: 215-234.

Wilcockson, R.W., Crean, C.S. and Day, T.H., 1995. Heritability of a sexually selected character in both sexes. *Nature*, 374(6518): 158-159.

Williams, G.C., 1975. *Sex and Evolution*. Princeton University Press.

Wong, B.B.M., 2004. Superior fighters make mediocre fathers in the Pacific blue-eye fish. *Animal Behaviour*, 67: 583–590.

Wong, B.B.M. and Jennions, M.D., 2003. Costs influence male mate choice in a freshwater fish. In: *Proceedings of the Royal Society of London Series* B [Suppl] 270: s36–s38 (DOI 10.1098/rsbl.2003.0003)

Wong, B.B.M., Jennions, M.D. and Keogh, J.S., 2004. Sequential male mate choice in a fish, the Pacific blue-eye *Pseudomugil signifier*. *Behavioural Ecology and Sociobiology*, 56: 253–256.

Zahavi, A., 1975. Mate selection: A selection of handicap. *Journal of Theoretical Biology*, 53: 205-214.

Zahavi, A., 1991. On the definition of sexual selection, Fisher's model, and the evolution of waste and of signals in general. *Animal Behaviour*, 42(3): 501-503.

Zuk, M. and Johnson, T.S., 1999. Social environment and immunity in male red jungle fowl. *Behavioural Ecology*, 11: 146-153.

Previous Volumes

— Volume 1 —

2002, xiii+308p., figs., tabls., ind., 23 cm Rs. 650

ISBN 81-7035-272-X

Section I: Animal Ecology

Section II: Animal Reproduction

— Volume 2 —

2004, xi+387p., figs., tabls., ind., 23 cm Rs. 850

ISBN 81-7035-322-X

Section I: Animal Ecology

Section II: Animal Reproduction

— Volume 3 —

2006, xvii+443p., figs., tabls., ind., 23 cm **Rs. 1150**

ISBN 81-7035-424-2

Section I: Animal Ecology

Section II: Animal Reproduction

— Volume 4 —

2007, xiv+550p., figs., tabls., ind., 23 cm Rs. 1400

ISBN 81-7035-459-5

Section I: Animal Ecology

— Volume 5 —

2008, xiv+476p., col. plts., figs., tabls., ind., 23 cm Rs. 1600

ISBN 81-7035-563-X; 978-81-7035-563-2

Section I: Animal Ecology

Section II: Animal Reproduction

— Volume 6 —

2010, xiv+497p., col. plts., figs., tabls., ind., 23 cm Rs. 1500

ISBN 81-7035-635-0; 978-81-7035-635-6

Section I: Animal Ecology

Section II: Animal Reproduction

— Volume 7 —

2011, xiv+494p., col. plts., figs., tabls., ind., 23 cm **Rs. 1700**

ISBN 81-7035-746-2; 978-81-7035-746-9

Section I: Animal Ecology

Section II: Animal Reproduction

Index

B

C

D

Q

R

S

T